NUTRITION AND CHEMICAL TOXICITY

Current Toxicology Series

Series Editors

Diana Anderson	**Michael D Waters**	**Timothy C Marrs**
BIBRA Toxicology	Consultant	Department of Health
International	Chapel Hill	London, UK
Surrey, UK	NC, USA	

Toxicology is now considered to be a topic worthy of study and research in its own right, having originally arisen as a subsection of pharmacology. This rapid growth in the significance of toxicology necessitates specialised yet comprehensive information that is easily accessible both to professionals and to the increasing number of students with an interest in the subject area.

Comprising professional and reference books, primarily aimed at an academic/industrial/professional audience, the *Current Toxicology Series* will cover a wide variety of 'core' toxicology topics, thus building into a comprehensive range of books suitable for use both as an updating tool and as a reference source.

Forthcoming titles

Toxicology of Contact Dermatitis: Allergy, Irritancy and Urticaria
D Basketter, F Gerberick, I Kimber and C Willis (0 471 97201 0)

Food Borne Carcinogens: Heterocyclic Amines
Edited by M Nagao and T Sugimura (0 471 98399 3)

NUTRITION AND CHEMICAL TOXICITY

Edited by

Costas Ioannides
University of Surrey, Guildford, UK

JOHN WILEY & SONS
Chichester • New York • Weinheim • Brisbane • Singapore • Toronto

Other Wiley Editorial Offices

John Wiley & Sons, Inc., 605 Third Avenue,
New York, NY 10158-0012, USA

WILEY-VCH Verlag GmbH, Pappelallee 3,
D-69469 Weinheim, Germany

Jacaranda Wiley Ltd, 33 Park Road, Milton,
Queensland 4064, Australia

John Wiley & Sons (Asia) Pte Ltd, 2 Clementi Loop #02-01,
Jin Xing Distripark, Singapore 129809

John Wiley & Sons (Canada) Ltd, 22 Worcester Road,
Rexdale, Ontario M9W 1L1, Canada

Library of Congress Cataloging-in-Publication Data

Nutrition and chemical toxicity / edited by Costas Ioannides.
      p.   cm. — (Current toxicology series)
   Includes bibliographical references and index.
   ISBN 0-471-97453-6 (hc. : alk. paper)
   1. Food—Toxicology.   2. Nutrition.   I. Ioannides. Costas.
II. Series.
RA1258.N865   1998
613.2—dc21   98-24067
                                                  CIP

British Library Cataloguing in Publication Data
A catalogue record for this book is available from the British Library

ISBN 0 471 97453 6
Typeset in 10/12 pt Optima by Keyword Publishing.
Printed and bound in Great Britain by Biddles Ltd, Guildford and King's Lynn.
This book is printed on acid-free paper responsibly manufactured from sustainable forestry,
in which at least two trees are planted for each one used for paper production.

Contents

Contributors

Nihal Ahmad, Department of Dermatology, University Hospitals of Cleveland, Case Western Reserve University, 2074 Abington Road, Cleveland, OH 44106, USA

William T Allaben, Associate Director for Scientific Coordination, National Center for Toxicological Research, Food and Drug Administration, 3900 NCTR Road, Jefferson, AR 72079, USA

Tammy M Bray, Department of Human Nutrition, The Ohio State University, 347 Campbell Hall, 1787 Neil Avenue, Columbus, OH 43210-1295, USA

Emmanuel Farber, Department of Pathology, Anatomy and Cell Biology, Jefferson Medical College, Thomas Jefferson University, 1020 Locus Street, Philadelphia, PA 19107-6799, USA

Amiya K Ghoshal, Department of Pathology, University of Toronto, Toronto, Ontario, Canada M5S 1A8

John D Groopman, Department of Environmental Health Sciences, School of Hygiene and Public Health, Johns Hopkins University, Baltimore, MD 21205, USA

Ronald W Hart, Office of the Director, National Center for Toxicological Research, Food and Drug Administration, 3800 NCTR Road, Jefferson, AR 72079, USA

John N Hathcock, Nutritional and Regulatory Science, Council for Responsible Nutrition, 1300 19th Street NW, Suite 310, Washington DC 20036-1609, USA

Iwao Hirono, Fujita-Gakuen Health University School of Medicine, Toyoake, Aichi 470-11, Japan

Emily Ho, Department of Human Nutrition,The Ohio State University, 347 Campbell Hall, 1787 Neil Avenue, Columbus, OH 43210-1295, USA

Costas Ioannides, Molecular Toxicology Group, School of Biological Sciences, University of Surrey, Guildford, Surrey GU2 5XH, UK

Margaretha Jägerstad, Department of Food Science, Swedish University of Agricultural Sciences, PO Box 7051, SE-750 07 Uppsala, Sweden

Santosh K Katiyar, Department of Dermatology, University Hospitals of Cleveland, Case Western Reserve University, 2074 Abington Road, Cleveland, OH 44106, USA

Thomas W Kensler, Department of Environmental Health Sciences, School of Hygiene and Public Health, Johns Hopkins University, Baltimore, MD 21205, USA

Joseph J Knapka, National Center for Research Services, National Institutes of Health, Bethesda, MD 20892, USA

Julian E Leakey, Division of Microbiology and Chemistry, National Center for Toxicological Research, Food and Drug Administration, 3900 NCTR Road, Jefferson, AR 72079, USA

Samuel B Lehrer, Department of Medicine, Section of Allergy and Clinical Immunology, Tulane University School of Medicine, 1700 Perdido Street, New Orleans, LA 70112-1293, USA

Mark A Levy, Department of Human Nutrition, The Ohio State University, 347 Campbell Hall, 1787 Neil Avenue, Columbus, OH 43210-1295, USA

Hideki Mori, Department of Pathology, Gifu University School of Medicine, 40 Tsukasa-machi, Gifu 500-8705, Japan

Hasan Mukhtar, Department of Dermatology, University Hospitals of Cleveland, Case Western Reserve University, 1100 Euclid Avenue, Cleveland, OH 44106, USA

Akiyoshi Nishikawa, Division of Pathology, National Institute of Public Health Sciences, 1-18-1 Kamiyoga, Setagaya-ku, Tokyo 158-0098, Japan

Ghanta N Rao, National Institute of Environmental Health Sciences, MD B3-08, National Institutes of Health, PO Box 12233, Research Triangle Park, NC 27709, USA

Gerald Reese, Department of Medicine, Section of Allergy and Chemical Immunology, Tulane University School of Medicine, 1700 Perdido Street, New Orleans, LA 70112, USA

Kerstin I Skog, Department of Applied Nutrition and Food Chemistry, Centre for Chemistry and Chemical Engineering, PO Box 124, SE-221 00 Lund, Sweden

W Wayne Stargel, Monsanto Company, 5200 Old Orchard Road, Skokie, IL 60077, USA

Takuji Tanaka, Department of Pathology, Kanazawa Medical University, Uchinada, Ishikawa 920-0293, Japan

John A Thomas, Department of Pharmacology, University of Texas Health Science Center, 7703 Floyd Curl Drive, San Antonio, TX 78284-7722, USA

Christian Tschanz, Monsanto Company, 5200 Old Orchard Road, Skokie, IL 60077, USA

Angelo Turturro, Division of Biometry and Risk Assessment, National Center for Toxicological Research, Food and Drug Administration, 3900 NCTR Road, Jefferson, AR 72079, USA

Jia-Sheng Wang, Department of Environmental Health Sciences, School of Hygiene and Public Health, Johns Hopkins University, Baltimore, MD 21205, USA

Gary Williamson, Biochemistry Department, Institute of Food Research, Norwich Research Park, Colney, Norwich NR4 7UA, UK

Foreword

The past 40 years have been exciting in providing key information in the field of nutrition and health as well as regards the mechanisms of toxicity. In the first area, important knowledge accrued through geographic pathology, namely to investigate the rationale for the great international differences in disease incidence as a function of area residence. For example, people in the countries of the Orient such as Japan and China suffer from high blood pressure and stroke. These conditions occur also in Western countries, but to a much lower extent than in the Orient. On the other hand, in the Western world, atherosclerosis and coronary heart disease display a high incidence. In parts of Africa and Asia, chronic liver disease and liver cancer are observed frequently.

These basic data have been the subject of detailed research on the underlying causes, and extended through investigations in animal models or *in vitro* approaches. In most instances, these causative elements were complex. Nutritional habits play a controlling role in defining causes of disease and toxicity. There were not only causative factors that were the primary reason for the occurrence of a given disease, but there were also modulating factors lowering the risk, as a function of area of residence. In fact, while genetic parameters could be postulated to play a role in the diverse occurrence of a given disease, it was clear from pioneering studies in migrants from a region of high risk to one of lower risk or vice versa, that genetics played a minor role. For example, migrants from China or Japan displayed much lower risk of hypertension and stroke or of stomach cancer in the second generation of migration to places such as the USA or Europe. Migrants from Scotland or Ireland with a high risk for colon cancer eventually had a lower incidence upon migration to Australia. With the development of techniques in molecular biology, it will be possible to sort out the question of the role of genetic constitution in a given individual and that of environmental elements.

In many parts of the world, the public and political bodies speak of the environment as an important element in the occurrence of chronic diseases. Diverse types of cancer were attributed to a person's constitution and environmental contamination, especially by chemicals. We need to consider the important role of quantitation. A high-level exposure to a causative agent represents a high-risk situation, but there may be lower levels of environmental contamination that may not represent a significant risk. In any case, there are excellent laboratory procedures that can be carried out efficiently and rapidly to determine whether a given environmental chemical might represent a human cancer risk. If there is a suspicion of risk due to an environmental agent, one can clearly protect humans from exposure. It is important to classify a chemical as to genotoxic or not, since the dose–response and the existence of a clear threshold dose depends on this attribute.

A major human cancer in the Western world is lung cancer. Through epidemiological studies, Wynder in the USA and shortly thereafter, Doll in the UK, made the important discovery that most lung cancers in men in the USA and in the UK were observed in addicted smokers of cigarettes. Wynder reproduced with tobacco tar the famous experiments of the British School of Kennaway that demonstrated that coal tar applied to mouse skin elicited cancer. Tobacco tar had the same effect and mouse skin was the tool that permitted Wynder and his chemist colleague, Hoffmann, to identify the major risk factors in tobacco tar, polycyclic aromatic hydrocarbons; in addition they observed powerful promoting chemicals in the so-called acidic fraction, that contained phenolic compounds. Here was a disease involving carcinogens and promoting factors. This is important, for basic cancer research has revealed that the dose–response curves for genotoxic carcinogens were quite different from those applying to promoters. Moreover, the effect of promoters is totally or partially reversible, a factor explaining why smoking cessation, especially after limited years of smoking, leads to a progressive decreased risk. In turn, these findings provide the basis for an important means of disease control by encouraging individuals to stop smoking.

Lung cancer is not the only disease caused by smoking. It was found that the incidence of cancer of the pancreas, kidney, urinary bladder, cervix was also higher in smokers compared with non-smokers. Furthermore, in people on a Western high saturated fat diet with a demonstrated higher risk of atherosclerosis and heart disease, a much higher incidence of these cancers was observed in smokers. Of current interest is the fact that more Japanese males are smokers but the lung cancer rate in Japan is lower than in the Western countries. One explanation is that the traditional Japanese diet is lower in fat and, in fact, the fat consumed includes ω-3-polyunsaturated oils from fish that in other situations have displayed a lower risk for many types of cancer and heart disease. Also, the Japanese are prodigious consumers of green tea, that in animal models has shown a protective effect.

In the Orient, stomach cancer has been a high-incidence disease, and in addition, in parts of China there is a high incidence of cancer of the oesophagus. Joossens in Belgium has proposed that there is an association between the incidence of stroke and that of gastric cancer, and suggested that a high intake of salt and pickled foods was the causative element. This has been fully documented and we have identified a totally new chemical, 2-chloro-4-methylthiobutanoic acid in a salted, pickled Japanese fish consumed in a high-risk region of Japan. Sugimura convinced the then Prime Minister, Nakasone, in 1982 to institute a plan to decrease salt intake in Japan. This scheme is in its second decade and appears to be successful since both stroke and gastric cancer are declining in Japan. This is a situation that deserves to be imitated anywhere in the world. Salt in excess can exert toxic effects, including promoting gastric cancer in humans, and the recommended daily intake is 3 g, or less, per day per adult.

In the Western world, heart disease continues to be a major killer, albeit with the lower rate of cigarette smoking, it has a declining trend. Many types of cancer such as those in the colon, breast, pancreas, prostate, ovary and endometrium are not yet decreasing. Geographic pathology provides the clues on the underlying causative elements. These diseases have a low incidence in Japan, and migrants acquired the risk. These neoplastic diseases are clearly not related to the environment as such, but the personal environment of individuals on certain dietary traditions. In fact, with the progressive Westernisation of dietary customs in Japan, these cancers are increasing, providing solid evidence on the role of nutrition in cancer and in toxicology. Westerners consume fried or broiled meat. The surface of fried meat contains powerful mutagens, a discovery originally made by Sugimura and associates in Tokyo. These mutagens belong to a new class of chemicals, the heterocyclic amines, formed by reaction of creatinine with Maillard-type products. In animal models, these chemicals induce many of the cancers discussed in this paragraph. There is epidemiological evidence that individuals consuming well-done meat have a higher risk of colon and breast cancer. The formation of heterocyclic amines during cooking can be partially inhibited by either removing creatinine from the food (brief microwave heating), or through the addition of antioxidants.

Western nutrition also is a source of fat, saturated fat from meats and dairy products, ω-6 polyunsaturated fats from edible oils, and monounsaturated fats from sources such as olive oil. The intake of fat in the Western world is 37–45% of calories that exert a powerful promoting effect in the cancers mentioned. These findings have been the basis for health recommendations to lower the total fat intake to 20% of calories. Also, in the Mediterranean region such as Southern Italy or Greece, these diseases have a lower incidence, in part accounted for by the regular use of olive oil, a monounsaturated oil. In animal models for colon or breast cancer, olive oil does not display a promoting effect, unlike the ω-6 polyunsaturated oils that are powerful promoters. An additional element is the regular intake of fruits and vegetables, including tomatoes which have been shown to be protective in the nutritionally linked cancers. Another interesting finding is the high heart disease risk in Finland, but a low colon cancer rate, and a lower breast cancer rate than in the Western world. This was accounted for by the traditional intake of a high-bran fibre bread, yielding a larger stool bulk and thus, elimination of carcinogens, and of bile acids, acting as promoters. Incidentally, the higher heart attack rate in Finland may be due to their traditional high intake of milk. It has been suggested that lactose in milk may be atherogenic. The lower rate of heart disease in France or Italy, despite their rich diet, may be due to the fact that adult French or Italian people rarely consume milk. Red wine with the antioxidant resveratrol has also been cited as protective in heart disease. Research with tea suggests that antioxidant tea polyphenols are, likewise, protective.

In the context of nutrition and toxicity it is clear that regular consumption of vegetables is beneficial. This element does not depend only on the content in essential or non-essential vitamins or minerals, but rather to other powerful antioxidants such as quercetin, isothiocyanates, lycopene in tomatoes, or the tea polyphenols. These chemicals act as radical traps. They also can induce selectively Phase I enzymes of the cytochrome P450 systems, or Phase II enzymes such as glucuronyl transferase, GSH transferase and the like. These systems can detoxify endogenous or exogenous harmful chemicals.

In this volume, most of these topics are reviewed in detail and provide an excellent overview on the influence of overall nutrition or specific nutrients in lowering the effect of toxicants and provide an understanding of the relevant mechanisms. We can always benefit by more research in the general area of lifestyle-related medicine. However, the time has come to apply to human populations worldwide what has been learned over the past 40 years. The goal of medical and toxicologic research is to extend the lifespan of humans under conditions of minimal disease, especially the chronic diseases that were so rampant decades ago. We also need to look to the future to provide better data on the occurrene of mental diseases and the diseases of ageing such as Alzheimer's disease, so as to be in a position to prevent these afflictions. This book is designed to provide background information ready to be applied to disease prevention.

John H Weisburger, PhD, MD(hc)
American Health Foundation
Valhalla, NY 10595, USA

1 Toxicants in Food: Naturally Occurring

Hideki Mori[1], Takuji Tanaka[2] and Iwao Hirono[3]

[1]*Department of Pathology, Gifu University School of Medicine, 40 Tsukasa-machi, Gifu 500–8705, Japan*
[2]*Department of Pathology, Kanazawa Medical University, Uchinada, Ishikawa 920-0293, Japan*
[3]*Fujita-Gakuen Health University School of Medicine, Toyoake, Aichi 470-11, Japan*

Introduction

There are a number of naturally occurring toxicants in food. Most of these are toxins in plants and plant products, but some marine toxins such as those present in fish could be also considered naturally occurring toxicants in food. Many toxicants in food have been known since ancient times, and discovery of some toxins and multidisciplinary information on their behaviour have provided a great benefit to modern sciences. Enormous progress in the toxicology, pathology and biochemistry of these agents has contributed to the understanding of human diseases, although the ecology of each toxin is poorly understood.

The human diet contains nutrients (macro- and micro-) and a variable amount of non-nutrients. The latter is largely composed of inert, non-absorbable compounds of plant origin. The extreme complexity of the food situation provides almost endless opportunities for problems, including malnutrition, overnutrition, toxicity and carcinogenicity. Food may contain harmful substances either of natural or human origin. It may be contaminated with harmful microorganisms or their metabolic products, or it may have acquired other unrecognised environmental contaminants. Even if all such difficulties are avoided, serious ill health can, and apparently does, result from unwise use of some of the very food chemicals that are normally desirable or even essential for life. Some potent toxic metabolites of animals and plants used as food are

Nutrition and Chemical Toxicity. Edited by Costas Ioannides. © John Wiley & Sons Ltd. ISBN 0 471 97453 6

formed during their normal course of metabolism and growth, while others may be acquired under conditions including microbial infection, mechanical and chemical injury, and insect parasitism. There is little doubt, that the major classes of toxic substances present in the diet of early humans were similar to those that may be found in today's foods. We have adapted means of dealing with this problem through the application of scientific knowledge and new technologies. In fact, modern food-processing techniques have greatly reduced the possibility of illness from food-borne microorganisms, while improved agricultural marketing practices have increased the availability of wholesome and nutritious food. The main consideration of the Committee on Food Protection, National Research Council (1973) (Committee on Food Protection, 1973), when reviewing natural toxicants in food was 'the hope that it may contribute to a more informed, realistic, and sensible attitude on the part of the public toward the food supply'. Today, as was the case earlier, natural toxic components in foods have received little attention (Committee on Food Protection, 1966). Most people routinely accept that plants eaten in their 'pristine' state are not only absolutely safe for one's health, but are better than plants 'manipulated' by man. This review aims to place some perspective on certain aspects of the problem relative to our current level of toxicological understanding of naturally occurring toxic factors found in food.

Food-derived naturally occurring carcinogens

CYCASIN

Cycads are widely distributed throughout tropical and subtropical regions, and the species indigenous to Amami and Okinawa, the southwestern islands of Japan, is *Cycas revoluta* Thunb. In these islands, the seeds and trunks of cycad were invaluable food when other food supplies were destroyed by typhoons before and during World War II. The cycad seeds are still used in some parts of the islands as a source of starch and as a constituent of the bean paste miso. The inhabitants of Guam also use nuts of the cycad as a source of food starch (Hirono, 1987a). Discovery of the carcinogenicity of cycasin, a toxic glucoside occurring in the seeds, trunks and leaves of cycads, originated from the finding of an unusually high incidence of amiotrophic lateral sclerosis on the island of Guam (Kurland and Mulder, 1954) where *Cycas circinalis* had long been used as a source of food starch, in an exploratory study at the National Institutes of Health on the possible existence of neurotoxins in cycads, Laquer *et al.* (1963) found that rats fed crude cycad meal developed hepatocellular, kidney and intestinal tumours, whereas neurological disorder was not confirmed. The responsible carcinogen in cycads was later found to be cycasin which had been identified by Nishida *et al.* (1955). Cycasin was toxic only when given orally (Nishida *et al.*, 1956), suggesting that a metabolite of cycasin was the toxic compound. Studies on the excretion of cycasin suggested that intestinal microorganisms contained the enzyme which hydrolyses cycasin *in vivo* (Spatz *et al.*, 1967). Later, methylazoxymethanol (MAM), the aglycone of cycasin, was shown to be the proximate carcinogen appearing after passage through the gastrointestinal tract. Subsequently, it was proved that MAM acetate was formed by the oxidation of 1,2-dimethylhydrazine to azoxymethane (Hirono 1987a). It is noteworthy that the tumorigenic effects of cycasin are not limited to rats, but have also been demonstrated in mice (Hirono *et al.*, 1969), hamsters (Hirono *et al.*, 1971), guinea pigs (Spatz, 1964), rabbits (Watanabe *et al.*, 1975), fish (Stanton, 1966) and monkeys (Sieber *et al.*, 1980). Even upon single exposure, cycasin and MAM acetate induce tumours in the kidney and large intestine of rats, tumours in the liver and lung of mice, and intrahepatic bile duct tumours in hamsters (Hirono, 1972).

Zedeck *et al.* (1970) reported that a single non-lethal dose of MAM acetate inhibited thymidine incorporation into DNA of liver, small intestine and kidney of rats. Thus, it was suggested that cycasin and dimethylnitrosamine are metabolized to the same biochemically active compound, perhaps diazomethane (Miller, 1964) and methyldiazonium hydroxide (Druckrey, 1970). Matsumoto and Higa (1966) and Nagata and Matsumoto (1969) who studied the methylation of nucleic acids by MAM *in vitro* and in foetal rat brain, respectively found that MAM reacted with nucleic acids and foetal proteins in rats when the compound was given on the 14th day of gestation. Guanine methylated in the 7-position was found in both DNA and RNA (Matsumoto and Higa, 1966; Nagata and Matsumoto, 1969). It was then suggested that the conversion of the primary alcohol group of cycasin to a carboxylic acid group changed the organotropy of the compound from a predominantly kidney tumour inducer to an intestinal tumour inducer (Matsumoto, 1979). It is known that MAM is mutagenic to *Salmonella typhimurium* (Smith, 1966). Teas and Dyson (1967) reported a marked rise in sex-linked recessive lethal mutations in *Drosophila melanogaster* after addition of MAM or MAM acetate to the nutrient medium. Genotoxicity of cycasin in mammalian hepatocytes was demonstrated by Williams *et al.* (1981) with supplementation of β-glucosidase in the test medium.

BRACKEN FERN

Bracken fern, *Pteridium aquilinum*, is widely distributed in many parts of the world and used as human food in Japan and other countries. The toxic syndrome induced by ingestion of sufficient quantities of bracken fern differs in horses, cattle and sheep (Radeleff, 1970; Evans *et al.*, 1982). Ingestion of bracken fern by horses leads to a thiamine deficiency since the ferns contain the enzyme thiaminase that can cleave the thiamine molecules. Chronic enzootic haematuria in cattle is well established (Rosenberger, 1971) and is characterized by haemorrhages in the urinary bladder mucosa. Thrombocytopenia and leukopenia are present in advanced cases. Evans *et al.* (1961) reported that bracken rhizomes caused bovine bracken poisoning and that the toxic factor was present in the rhizomes in much larger quantities than in the fronds. Initial evidence for the carcinogenicity of bracken fern was reported by Rosenberger and Heeschen (1960) who described changes of a polypous-tumorous nature in the urinary bladder mucosa accompanied by haematuria in cattle given bracken fern for long periods. The carcinogenicity of bracken fern was clearly shown by the studies of Evans and Mason (1965), where rats fed diets containing bracken fern developed intestinal carcinomas. Subsequently, induction of urinary bladder tumours by bracken in cows and rats was also confirmed (Pamukcu et al., 1967).

In Japan, young bracken fern fronds in the fiddlehead or crosier stage of growth are used as human food. When rats were given such young bracken fern in the diet, in a proportion of one part by weight dried bracken fern to two parts of basal diet, for 4 months, all had ileal tumours such as adenomas or adenocarcinomas (Hirono et al., 1970, 1972). Young bracken fern has been used as human food after processing with wood ash, sodium bicarbonate and NaCl. Carcinogenic activity of bracken fern was markedly reduced by such treatment, but activity was still retained in the bracken fern thus prepared (Hirono et al., 1972, 1975). There have been several epidemiology studies concerning the carcinogenicity of bracken fern. Kamon and Hirayama (1975) made a survey of cancer in a mountainous area of central Japan. They reported a significantly higher risk of oesophageal cancer in people who ate hot tea gruel and bracken fern together. Pamukcu et al. (1978) studied the carcinogenicity of the milk of bracken fern-fed cows in rats and found that a significant number of rats developed intestinal or bladder tumours. They suggested milk from cows that have eaten bracken fern may thus be hazardous to humans.

Historically, isolation of the bracken fern carcinogen was difficult (Hirono and Yamada, 1987). One important reason for this was the absence of specific acute toxicity of bracken fern in small laboratory animals such as rats and mice. A number of candidate compounds have been proposed by many investigators. However, neither the causative principle of cattle bracken poisoning nor the bracken carcinogen had been successfully isolated. In 1983–1984, Hirono et al. isolated a novel norsesquiterpene glucoside of the illudane type (Figure 1.1), ptaquiloside, from bracken fern by fractionation of the aqueous extract of bracken (Niwa et al., 1983; Hirono et al., 1984a). Ptaquiloside was an unstable compound, which broke down to pterorsin B and D-glucose in both acidic and basic aqueous solutions at room temperature (Hirono and Yamada, 1987). Carcinogenicity of ptaquiloside was also tested by Hirono et al., (1984a) in female CD rats and its tumorigenicity in mammary gland and ileum was apparent indicating that ptaquiloside was the causative principle of cattle bracken poisoning. Thrombocytopenia, as well as leukocytopenia, were also induced in cattle by exposure to ptaquiloside (Hirono et al., 1984b). Ptaquiloside was found to induce neurotoxicity in mice (Fujimoto et al., 1987) and sheep (Hirono et al., 1993). This agent elicits a strong genotoxicity to mammalian hepatocytes (Mori et al., 1985a) and mutagenicity to Drosophila melanogaster (Sato et al., 1991).

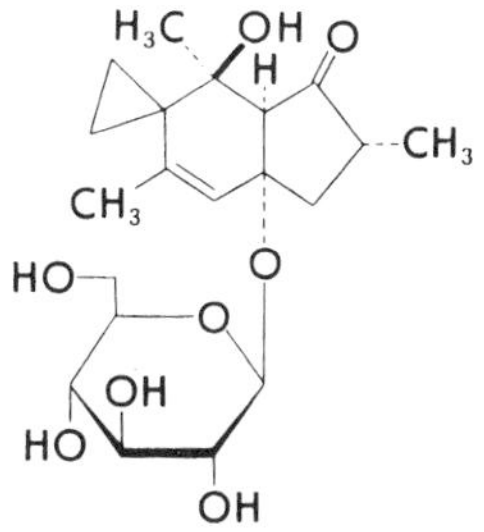

Figure 1.1 The molecular structure of ptaquiloside.

PYRROLIZIDINE ALKALOIDS

Pyrrolizidine alkaloids were first isolated from the *Senecio* genus and found in over 100 species of *Compositae*. Later, they were detected in many other genera such as in *Cynoglossum, Lindelofia* and *Heliotropium*. Over 200 pyrrolizidine alkaloids have been isolated from these plants. A disease known under different names such as Pictow disease in Canada and Winton disease in New Zealand, has been reported to be derived from the consumption of plants containing toxic pyrrolizidine alkaloids (Furuya *et al.*, 1987). About 30 pyrrolizidine alkaloids have been shown to be hepatotoxic. Coltsfoot (*Tussilago farfara*), comfrey (*Symphytum officinale*) and petasites (*Petasites japonicus*) are widely used as herbal remedies or food, and they were also demonstrated to possess hepatotoxic activity (Culvenor *et al.*, 1976; Yamada *et al.*, 1976).

The structure of pyrrolizidine alkaloids is composed of two parts, necine and necic acid. The basic structure of necine consists of 7-hydroxy-1-methylpyrrolizidine, and necic acid represents a variety of C5–C10 branched-chain acids. In most alkaloids these necines and necic acids form an ester structure. Based on the combination of necines and necic acids, the esters can be divided into four types: (i) non-esters; (ii) monoesters; (3) acyclic diesters; and (iv) macrocyclic diesters of pyrrolizidine alkaloids. Necines can be classified into four groups, i.e. a trachelanthamidine group of monohydroxylated derivatives, a retronecine group of dihydroxylated derivatives, a rosmarinecine group of trihydroxylated derivatives, and an otonecine (Furuya *et al.*, 1987). Pyrrolizidine alkaloids are metabolised via a number of different pathways. The alkaloids are easily converted into N-oxides and the reaction is readily reversed by reducing agents. Pyrrole derivatives of the alkaloids are considered to be responsible for some or all of the toxic effects of the pyrrolizidine alkaloids. Pyrrolic derivation of the pyrrolizidine alkaloids has been studied extensively by Mattocks (1970). The derivatives of the toxic pyrrolizidine alkaloids are chemically dihydropyrrolizidine esters, in which the ester group may readily be lost, leaving the positively charged dihydro-pyrrolizidine moiety (Mattocks, 1968; Schoental,

1970). Schoental (1970) suggested that epoxidation of the crucial C1,2-double bond in the dehydro-pyrrolizidine moiety, rather than pyrrolic derivatives, is probably an essential step in the biological action of pyrrolizidine alkaloids.

To date, at least six species of plants containing high levels of pyrrolizidine alkaloids, i.e. *Senecio longilobus* (Harris and Chen, 1970), *Petasites japonicus* Maxim. (Hirono *et al.*, 1973), *Tussilago farfara* L. (Hirono *et al.*, 1976), *Symphytum officinale* (Hirono *et al.*, 1978), *Farfugium japonicus* (Hirono *et al.*, 1983b) and *Senecio cannabifolis* (Hirono *et al.*, 1983b) are known to have carcinogenic activity. *Petasites japonicus* Maxim., is a form of coltsfoot and herb in the family of *Compositae*. *Petasites* is widely cultivated for use as food in Japan, and its carcinogenicity in rats was demonstrated by Hirono *et al.*, (1973). The responsible carcinogen component of petasites was later found to be petasitenine (fukinotoxin). *Tussilago farfara* L. is also used as a cough medicine in China and Japan. *Symphytrum officinale* L. is a herb of the family *Borginaeae* and is called comfrey or Russian comfrey and cultivated for use in Japan as a green vegetable or tonic. As in the case of *Petasites*, it was reported that rats fed *Tussilago* or *Symphitum* for long periods had a high incidence of liver cell adenomas or haemangioendothelial sarcomas (Hirono, 1981; Furuya *et al.*, 1987). Eight pyrrolizidine alkaloids, i.e. isatidine (Schoental *et al.*, 1954), retrorsine (Schoental *et al.*, 1954), petasitenine (Hirono *et al.*, 1977), senkirkine (Hirono *et al.*, 1979), clivoline (Kuhara *et al.*, 1980), monocrotaline (Newberne and Rogers, 1973), lasiocarpine (Svoboda and Reddy, 1972) and symphytine (Hirono *et al.*, 1979) have been shown to be carcinogenic. Tumorigenicity of the carcinogenic pyrrolizidine alkaloids is manifested predominantly in the liver. However, dehydroretronecine and monocrotaline induce local rhabdomyosarcomas and widely dispersed tumours respectively, following subcutaneous injection (Allen *et al.*, 1975).

The hazard of pyrrolizidine alkaloids and its possible relationship to human neoplasms, especially liver cell tumours, is not yet clear. In Africa and other regions, plants containing carcinogenic pyrrolizidine alkaloids are consumed as herbal remedies or foods; these plants include some species of *Senecio* which contain isatiodine, retrosine and monocrotaline. The consumption of foods and herbal remedies contaminated with pyrrolizidine alkaloids result in acute veno-occlusive lesions which progress to liver cirrhosis. The Budd–Chiari syndrome, which is manifested by hepatic vein occlusion in the native South African population, appears to be related to the consumption of bread containing *Senecio* flour (McLean, 1970). Tandon *et al.* (1978) reported epidemic data on veno-occlusive disease of the liver in Afganistan where approximately 7800 people in a population 35 000 were affected. The above authors reported that the cause was probably consumption of wheat flour heavily contaminated with the seeds of a plant of the *Heliotropium* species. Therefore, it was suggested that consumption of large amounts of pyrrolizidine alkaloids or the alkaloid-containing plants may be related to the occurrence of liver neoplasms and other human diseases.

Mutagenicity of pyrrolizidine alkaloids was first demonstrated in *Drosophila melanogaster* (Clark, 1959). Heliotrine and lasiocarpine were reported to be mutagenic in a methionine-dependent strain of *Aspergillus* (Alderson and Clark, 1966). Chromosomal aberrations caused by some pyrrolizidine alkaloids in the root-tip cells of *Allium cepa* is known (Avanzi, 1961). Yamanaka *et al.* (1979) studied the mutagenicity in 13 pyrrolizidine alkaloids in *Salmonella typhimurium* TA 100, in the presence of liver S9 mix, and found that heliotropine, lasiocarpine, petasitenine, ligularidine, senkirkine and LX201 were positive. Another systematic survey of the genotoxicity of the pyrrolizidine alkaloids was performed in the hepatocyte primary culture/DNA repair test using 17 pyrrolizidine alkaloids (Mori *et al.*, 1985b). In this study, 11 pyrrolizidine alkaloids, i.e. senecionine, seneciphylline, jacobine, epoxyseneciphylline, senecicannabine, acetylfukinotoxin, syneilesine, ligularidine, neoligularidine, dihydroclivorine and ligularizine, whose carcinogenicity was not yet known, were found to be positive. Retronecine, a pyrrolizidine alkaloid lacking necic acid, and ligularinine, lacking the C1,2 double bond in the pyrrolizidine ring, were negative, indicating a close relationship between genotoxicity and molecular structure.

SAFROLE

Safrole is one of the many allylic and benzene-derivatives with ring methoxy and/or ring methylenedioxy substituents which occur naturally in plants and are contained in various foods including herbs and vegetables. Hepatotoxicity following the ingestion of large amounts of sassafras oil by humans is established. The carcinogenic activity of safrole in rodents was demonstrated by Homburger *et al.* (1961) and Long *et al.* (1963), and the use of this agent as an oil and food additive was banned in the US. Safrole is a major component of sassafras oil which has been used for medicinal purposes as a topical antiseptic, pediculicide and carminative as well as a food additive such as flavouring agent for soft drinks. Pure safrole is a colourless or slightly yellow liquid with an odour of sassafras. Dietary exposure to safrole induces liver neoplasms in mice and rats (Enomoto, 1987).

Local sarcomas at the injection site of related compounds or possible metabolites of safrole have also been observed (Borchert *et al.*, 1973; Wislocki *et al.*, 1973). These studies suggested that 1′-hydroxysafrole, an allylic alcohol metabolite, is a proximate carcinogen of safrole and any ester formed *in vivo* could be an ultimate carcinogen of safrole. Miller and Miller (1983) and Miller *et al.* (1982) pointed to the 1′-carbon atom of the allyl group of safrole and related chemicals as the site of formation of metabolic allylic and benzylic esters. Esters of this type, like the pyrrole metabolites of the hepatocarcinogenic pyrrolizidine alkaloids, had been implicated as the reactive alkylating form of these alkaloids (Mattocks, 1968). The formation of DNA adducts *in vivo* and *in vitro* by derivatives of safrole and estragole and the characterisation of the major hepatic DNA adducts have been also studied extensively by the Miller group (Phillips *et al.*, 1981). They compared the nucleoside adducts derived by the enzymic hydrolysis of hepatic DNA from mice injected with these tritiated carcinogens, and adducts formed *in vitro* by reaction of deoxynucleosides with acetoxy and epoxy derivatives. These studies indicated the metabolic activation of 1'-hydroxy-2'3'-dehydroestragole through the formation of an electrophilic 1'-ester in mouse liver *in vivo* (Swanson *et al.*, 1979).

Although the mutagenic activity of safrole itself was not confirmed in *Salmonella typhimurium* TA1513, TA100 and TA98, 1'-hydroxysafrole was reported to be mutagenic, especially in the presence of liver-activating enzymes (Swanson *et al.*, 1979).

CARRAGEENAN

Carrageenan is a sulphated polysaccharide extracted from various red seaweeds and consisting mainly of varying amounts of the ammonium, calcium, magnesium, potassium or sodium salts of sulphate esters of galactose and 3,6-anhydrogalactose copolymers. The principal copolymers are designated kappa-, lambda-, epsilon-, and differ both in structure and in their ability to form gels upon the addition of potassium ions to dilute solutions of carrageenan (National Research Council, 1981). Native carrageenan is used in food, cosmetics, pharmaceuticals and other products in which its ability to stabilize mixtures, emulsify ingredients and thicken or gel solutions is exploited. Degraded carrageenan has been produced from extracts of *Eucheuma spinosum*, the principal component of which is iota-carrageenan, by treatment with dilute hydrochloric acid. Degraded carrageenan has long been used as an antipeptic agent in Europe (Hirono, 1987b).

It has been reported that oral administration of degraded carrageenan induced hyperplastic mucosal changes in the rabbit colon (Watt and Marcus 1970a), as well as ulcerative lesions of the large intestine in guinea pigs (Watt and Marcus, 1971), rabbits (Watt and Marcus, 1970b), rats (Marcus and Watt, 1971) and rhesus monkeys (Benitz *et al.*, 1973). Degraded carrageenan also induced colorectal squamous metasplasia and colon adenomatous polyps (Fabian *et al.*, 1973). Van Der Waaij *et al.* (1978) reported that ulcerative lesions of the large intestine induced by degraded carrageenan in guinea pigs were significantly mitigated by selective elimination of aerobic Gram-negative intestinal microflora. However, Hirono *et al.* (1981b) studied the role of intestinal bacterial flora in the degradation of carrageenan by comparing germ-free and conventional rats fed carrageenan, and concluded that bacterial flora are not essential for the manifestation of the biological effects of degraded carrageenan (Hirono *et al.*, 1981b). It is known that subcutaneous injection of native carrageenan induces sarcomas at the injection site (Cater, 1961) and dietary exposure to carrageenan enhances incidence of colonic tumours induced by azoxymethane or *N*-methylnitrosourea in rats (Watanabe *et al.*,

1978). Investigation of the degraded carrageenan in rats revealed that it induces ulcerative lesions, squamous metaplasia and tumours such as squamous cell carcinoma, adenoma and adenocarcinoma in the colon and rectum (Wakabayashi *et al.*, 1978).

Dextran sulphate sodium is a synthetic sulphated polysaccharide composed of dextran with sulphated glucose, whereas the carrageenans contain sulphated galactose and anhydrous galactose moieties. The biological effects of dextran sulphate sodium were investigated by Hirono *et al.* (1981a) following oral administration. They found that dextran sulphate sodium gives rise to colorectal tumours such as adenoma, adenocarcinoma and squamous cell carcinoma as well as ulcerative changes and squamous metaplasia in the colon and rectum. The biological effects of dextran sulphate were virtually the same as those of degraded carrageenan. Dextran sulphate sodium is known to potentiate 1,2-dimethylhydrazine-induced colorectal carcinogenesis (Hirono *et al.*, 1983a). However, this agent, as well as degraded carrageenan, lacks bacterial mutagenicity (Nagoya *et al.*, 1981) and genotoxicity in mammalian hepatocytes (Mori *et al.*, 1984).

MUSHROOM HYDRAZINES

Hydrazines and their derivatives are well known in organic chemistry and some of these synthetic hydrazines were found to have carcinogenic potential in rodents. Agaritine (β-N-(γ-L (+)-glutamyl)-4-hydroxymethylphenylhydrazine) was isolated from the pressed juice of a basidimycetes (Natori, 1987), *Agaricus bisporus*, the commonly eaten cultivated mushroom in North America and Europe, and characterised as the first example of naturally occurring hydrazines in the course of studies on non-protein amino acid metabolism (Levenberg, 1961). Carcinogenicity of methylhydrazine, a biosynthetic compound from gyromitrin was first reported by Toth (1972). Exposure to this compound in the drinking water induced lung adenomas in mice and malignant histiocytomas in the liver in hamsters. Carcinogenicity of N-methyl-N-formylhydrazine, the hydrolysis product of gyromitrin, was confirmed in mice (Toth and Nagel, 1978). Carcinogenicity testing of the major constituent of the false morel mushroom, gyromitrin, was carried out by intragastric instillation to mice, and the treatment induced tumours in the lung, preputial gland, forestomach and clitoral glands (Toth *et al.*, 1981). In the case of agaritine, the tumorigenic effect was first studied using 4-methylphenylhydrazine which was postulated to be a metabolite of 4-(hydroxymethyl)-phenylhydrazine, a hydrolysis product of agaritine. Subcutaneous administration of this compound induced lung tumours and blood vessel tumours in mice (Toth *et al.*, 1977). Furthermore, another related compound, 4-(hydroxymethyl)benzenediazonium was shown to be carcinogenic to mice (Toth *et al.*, 1981). However, carcinogenicity of agaritine itself to experimental animals has not yet been demonstrated. It appears that agaritine itself is rather unstable and can be removed by cooking, but the remaining metabolites cannot. Gyromitrin, like agaritine, is also destroyed by cooking before eating, but the possibility of human exposure to gyromitrin and its metabolites can not be completely excluded (International Agency for Research on Cancer, 1983).

Naturally occurring non-carcinogenic toxicants in food

NATURALLY OCCURRING TOXICANTS IN PLANT FOOD

Carbohydrates

Inborn errors in carbohydrate metabolism cause diseases such as galactos-aemia, fructose intolerance and congenital disaccharide intolerance which, with the exception of lactose intolerance, are rare. Hereditary fructose intoler-ance, an autosomal recessive disease, is usually characterised by a deficiency of the enzyme fructose-1-phosphate splitting enzyme aldolase and less com-monly of 1,6-diphosphatase (Froesch et al., 1963). Patients with the former deficiency suffer from liver disease, while those with the latter deficiency develop hypoglycaemia after fructose administration as well as during episodes of inadequate glucose intake. The severity of the disease in patients with fruc-tose-1-phosphate aldolase deficiency appears to depend upon the age at which fructose is introduced into the diet (Levin et al., 1968). In children under 6 months of age, there is vomiting, jaundice, dehydration, seizures and failure to thrive. If fructose is introduced into the diet after the age of 6 months, the illness is less severe (Levin et al., 1968). As in galactosaemia, phosphate ester accu-mulates in the tissues. When fruit or foods containing fructose or sorbitol are present in the diet, the infant fails to thrive and is subject to vomiting, jaundice, hepatomegaly, amino aciduria and albuminuria.

Lipids

Lipids in the form of vegetable oils or animal fats are important constituents of the human diet. Although some oils and fats might manifest acute or high toxicity, these are either eliminated by selective diet adaptations or they are diluted to such an extent that they no longer pose any serious acute health hazards. However, new sources of oils and fats have to be generated on a large commercial scale to support the needs of the growing world populations. Some of these sources of oils, both plant and animal, in the past two to three decades have been implicated in long-term toxic effects. In some cases, toxic factors have been identified, isolated and characterised. Naturally occurring fats may be consumed unseparated and still associated with foods such as meat, fish, poultry, dairy products, cereals, nuts and seeds. Therefore, the toxic effect may or may not be a single factor and would need extensive research before any conclusions could be drawn. Sometimes the bulk material in lipids may be perfectly safe but minor compounds that are present in these lipids may prove to be toxic. A well-known example of this is the presence of the pigment gossypol in raw cottonseed oil, that has proved to be toxic to many species, including man. The use of seed meal recovered from cotton production as a protein supplement for animal and human diets has made gossypol significant as a natural hazard. Gossypol is strongly acidic for a phenol, readily oxidizable, and acts as an antioxidant. The acute oral toxicity of gossypol is not high in most animals. Frequent symptoms with cumulative gossypol or cottonseed meal toxicity are loss of appetite, weight loss, hypoprothrombinaemia, diarrhoea, hair discolouration, and degenerative changes in the liver and spleen. Commercial meal containing $< 0.05\%$ gossypol is believed to be safe as a supplement in balanced diets for chickens and pigs.

As with carbohydrates, inborn errors of metabolism in certain individuals confer toxic properties to specific dietary lipids. Refsum's syndrome (phytanic acid storage disease) is an example. This is an autosomal recessive disorder caused by the lack of conversion of phytanic acid to hydroxyphytanic acid because of absence of the enzyme phytanic acid α-hydrolase (Steinberg, 1983). As a result, a normal dietary substance accumulates in myelin phospholipids. Most patients present before the age of 20 with failing vision and weakness in the extremities manifested by unsteadiness of gait: night blindness is the earliest symptom. Improvement occurs by limitation of dietary phytanic acid intake to 2 mg daily in the adult (Eldjarn et al., 1976), but the visual and hearing disorders are not reversible (Dry et al., 1982). The major histopathological changes involve the peripheral nerves and include those of hypertrophic neuropathy (Alexander, 1966).

Following the observation that myocarditis occurs in rats fed rapeseed oil (Beare-Rogers et al., 1972), much attention has focused on the major unsaturated fatty acid rapeseed oil and the related mustard oil, erucic acid (Dhopeshwarkar, 1980). Erucic acid constitutes as much as 40% of the fatty acids of rapeseed oil triglycerides. When fed trierucin, rats and several other animal species accumulate lipids, largely composed of erucic acid, in cardiac muscle. Cetoleic acid, a homologue of erucic acid, has a similar effect but the corresponding C-22 saturated fatty acid does not. Thus, the most important causative factor in rapeseed or similar oils is the amount of docosenoic acid (Teige and Beare-Rogers, 1973). It has been suggested that deposition of dietary erucic acid in the cardiac muscle is a consequence of its weak binding to serum albumin and a decreased β-oxidation (Swarttouw, 1974).

Cyclopropenic fatty acids like sterculic and malvalic acid, found in oils such as cottonseed, kapok seed or *Sterculia foetida*, have been shown to produce a variety of toxic effects in hens, rats and other species. They also acted as tumour promoters for liver cancer in the rainbow trout (Lee et al., 1971). Cottonseed oil is a component of some human diets, but no toxicity data for these fatty acids are available. However, the synergism of cyclopropenic fatty acids with certain carcinogens was examined (Lee et al., 1968).

Proteins and amino acids

Several forms of food protein such as milk proteins cause symptoms of intolerance in certain individuals through allergic or immunological mechanisms. Specific amino acids are highly toxic in patients with certain metabolic defects such as phenylketonuria. The term 'amino acid toxicity' refers to the adverse effects which occur when one or a group of amino acids is present in marked excess in the diet: such effects have been described for the sulphur-containing amino acids and for the aromatic species. Dietary sulphur amino acids affect chemical toxicity in several ways, providing glutathione, sulphate and taurine for conjugations, S-adenosylmethionine for methylation, and protein for enzymes, including cytochromes P450 (Hathcock, 1993). Monosodium glutamate, a flavour enhancer, can cause curious sensations in the head and neck, together with weakness and palpitations (Chinese Restaurant Syndrome).

During the fermentation that takes place in cheese preparation, bacterial action leads to the release of amino acids which are to some extent further converted to amines. These substances are usually vasoactive. Several pharmacologically active amines, particularly those related to the aromatic amino acids, are found in cheese (Horwitz et al., 1964). Of these, tyramine is prominent, although significant amounts of histamine, cadaverine and putrescine are also formed. Amines are also found in other foods including meat and yeast extracts, broad beans, pickled herrings, bananas, avocados, pineapples, tomatoes and certain wines. These amines can provoke severe headache in susceptible individuals. Although monoamine oxidase in intestine and liver inactivates such amines, dangerous hypertensive episodes could occur in patients taking monoamine oxidase inhibitors, when foods rich in tyramine are ingested (Blackwell et al., 1967).

A number of enzyme inhibitors occur in vegetables. Substances which could inhibit proteolytic enzymes are found throughout the plant kingdom especially in legumes. These include trypsin inhibitors, plasmin inhibitors, kallikrein inhibitors, papain inhibitors, nicotinamide deamidase inhibitor, oxidative phosphorylation inhibitor, amylase inhibitors, phosphoglucomutase inhibitor and cholinesterase inhibitor (Salunkhe and Wu, 1997). Amylase inhibitors are also found in wheat and beans (Bowman, 1945). Many of these inhibitors are destroyed by heating.

Cyanogens and cyanogenic glycosides

Mention has already been made of the toxicity of cassava. The cyanogenic glycosides are compounds that yield hydrogen cyanide upon treatment with acid or appropriate hydrolytic enzymes. These compounds are widely distributed among the higher plants. More than 1000 species of plants are known to be cyanophoric. Hydrocyanic acid (HCN) is released when tissues of the plant are crushed or disrupted. Although the production of HCN is usually attributed to the presence in the plant of one or more of the 20 known glycosides of α-hydroxynitriles, the parent glycoside has been positively identified in fewer than 50 species.

The well-known toxicity of these cyanogenetic glycosides is due to the production of HCN, a potent respiratory inhibitor. The site of inhibition is the enzyme cytochrome oxidase, being the terminal respiratory catalyst of aerobic organisms. An aldehyde or ketone, with which the HCN is combined as a cyanohydrin, is also usually produced on decomposition of a cyanogenic glycoside. Three distinct glycosides have been identified in edible species of plants: amygdalin, dhurrin and linamarin. Amygdalin is present in the kernels of some fruits and has been isolated from the seed of bitter almond. Cyanide has also been found in the kernel of apricot (about 12 to 177 mg/100 g). Kernels of almond, lemon, lime, apple, pear, cherry, prune and plum also contain cyanogenic glucosides. Immature bamboo shoot contains 800 mg cyanide/100 g. The accidental poisoning of humans who ate bitter almonds, the pits of peaches or apricots, and other stone fruit kernels has been recorded (Sayre and Kaymakcalan, 1964).

Oestrogen

Oestrogen, a substance capable of stimulating the growth of the vagina, uterus and mammary glands, is responsible for the development of female secondary characteristics. Among fruit and vegetables, carrot, soybean, potatoes, cherry, plum, garlic, sage leaf and parsley have been reported to contain substances which elicit an oestrogenic response in experimental animals (Salunkhe and Wu, 1997). Phytooestrogens are oestrogenic chemicals produced by plants. Phytooestrogens are now known to be diverse in their chemical structures as well as in their origin (Price and Fenwick, 1985). The two major chemical classes, the coumestans and isoflavonoids, each have a number of representatives with different oestrogenic potency; they may also have different patterns of biological activity (Medlock *et al.*, 1995). The oestrogenic activity of clover was first described almost 50 years ago following the observation that sheep feeding on pastures that contained clover demonstrated hyperoestrogenization and infertility (Bennetts *et al.*, 1946). Oestrogens have beneficial and adverse effects. The major adverse activities involve reproductive, carcinogenic and developmental effects. Phytooestrogens are known to induce infertility in livestock (Price and Fenwick, 1985) and probably in quail populations (Leopold *et al.*, 1976). Phytooestrogens have similar capability of inducing developmental toxicity as do other oestrogens (Sheehan, 1995). In humans, chronic unopposed oestrogen exposure is a major risk factor for the induction of endometrial adenocarcinoma (Goddard, 1992). Phytooestrogens have also antioestrogenic effects, of interest in the prevention of breast cancer (Sheehan, 1995).

Citral

Citral (3,7-dimethyl-2,6-octadienal), a common constituent of orange oil and lemon, was found to cause damage to the vascular endothelium when fed to animals. Citral may compete with retinene in the metabolism of endothelial cells. Citral is also present in such orange products as marmalade, fruit juice flavoured with orange oil, and orange drinks made by compression of the whole fruit.

Pressor amines

Certain naturally occurring phenylethylamine derivatives such as tyramine, dopamine and norepinephrine (noradrenaline) cause a marked increase in blood pressure when administered intravenously to mammals. Amines are normally rapidly deaminated after they enter the body. Many tissues contain the mitochondrial enzyme monoamine oxidase which catalyses the oxidative deamination of most of the vasoactive amines. Serotonin and histamine are also strongly vasoactive compounds. Amines are present in numerous foods. Bananas contain relatively large quantities of both serotonin and norepinephrine. Bananas and tomatoes contain tryptamine. The widespread presence of the following amines in fruit and vegetables is established: serotonin, tryptamine, tyramine, dopamine and norepinephrine in banana peel and pulp, plantain pulp, tomato, plum, avocado, potato, spinach, grape, orange and eggplant. Tea contains significant amounts of 3,4-dimethoxyphenethylamine. The toxicity of pressor amines is not well understood. The intravenous injection of as little as 1–2 mg of histamine gives rise to headaches, although orally administered histamine is much less effective. Canavanine (2-amino-4-(guanidinooxy)butyric acid) is found in many species of *Papilionoideae*. Both seed of *Canavalia ensiformis* and purified canavanine itself are toxic when fed to mice. A considerable amount of L-3,4-dihydroxyphenylalanine (L-DOPA), either free or in the form of glycosides, is found in the pods of *Vicia faba* (the broad bean). Seeds of various *Mucuna* species contain between 6 and 9% of free L-DOPA (Bell and Jenzen, 1971). Consumption of L-DOPA causes nausea, vomiting and involuntary chewing movements (Van Woert and Bowers, 1970). The amine 5-hydroxy-L-tryptophan (5-HTP), being the precursor of 5-hydroxytryptamine, is present in free form in seeds of the West African legume, *Griffonia simplicifolia* at concentrations as high as 6 to 10%. Injection of 5-HTP results in tremor, pupillary dilation, loss of light reflex, apparent blindness, salivation, marked hyperpnoea and tachycardia, but little is known about its toxicity to humans.

Saponins

Saponins are glycosides that occur in a wide variety of plants. Their toxicity is related to their activity in lowering surface tension. The saponins are divided into two main groups, steroid or triterpenoid, depending on their chemical nature. Spinach, beetroot and asparagus contain saponins.

Plant pheonolics (including tannins)

Some plant phenolics present in human food are toxicants (Singleton, 1981). The anthraquinones of rhubarb are found mainly in the root. Human poisoning occurs mainly from eating rhubarb leaves. Daphne and Aesculus poisoning have been attributed to the coumarin glycosides, daphnin and esculin. Rhodomyrtoxin is the major toxicant of Australian finer cherry (*Rhodomyrtus macrocarpa*), which causes permanent loss of sight when consumed (Singleton, 1981). Dibenzofuran, present in immature fruit at levels of 3.5 g/kg fruit, is toxic to mice at oral doses of 30 mg/kg body weight. Toxic phenols of daphne, buckeye and buckwheat are known (O'Leary, 1964). The mayapple (*Podophyllum peltatum*) contains in the dry roots about 8% of the resin podo-phyllin, of which about 20% consists of podophyllotoxin (a lignan) as well as other related substances. The resin has irritant, cytotoxic and cathartic effects, and a medicinal dose (130 mg) causes death (Salunkhe and Wu, 1997). Podophyllotoxin has an oral LD_{50} in mice of 90 mg/kg.

Tannins are plant polyphenolic substances with a molecular weight greater than 500 Da. Tannins could be classified into two groups: hydrolyzable and the condensed tannins. Tannins have the common properties of protein binding and leather forming. Repeated subcutaneous application of tannin is believed to induce liver neoplasms. Betel nuts (*Areca cetechu*), which contain 11 to 26% condensed tannins and are used as the quid for betel chewing, cause a high incidence of buccal carcinoma in central and southeast Asian countries. Betel nuts contain several pyridine alkaloids such as arecoline, arecaidine, guvacoline and guvacine. Genotoxicity and possible carcinogenicity of the betel nut ingredients have been described (Mori *et al.*, 1979; Mori, 1987). There is some evidence of a relationship between human oesophageal cancer and food or beverage tannin intake. The most convincing evidence is the unusually high incidence of oesophageal cancer in certain areas of the Transkei in South Africa, where high-tannin sorghum is consumed. The cancer appears to result from the chronic irritation of the mucosa caused by high consumption of the grain in Bautu beer and porridge. In epxerimental animals, the growth-depressing and toxic effects of tannins were dependent upon experimental conditions.

Tangeretin

Tangeretin, nobiletin and 3,3',4,5,6,7,8-heptamethoxyflavone are found in the peel of citrus fruit such as tangerine, mandarin, orange and grapefruit. With 10 mg/kg/day of tangeretin administered subcutaneously to rats during gesta-tion, 83% of the offspring, although appearing normal, were born dead or died within 3 days (Stout *et al.*, 1964). Juice expressed from orange peel contains about 20 mg/l of nobiletin and 3 mg/l of tangeretin.

Psychoactive substances

There are innumerable toxic plant substances that exert some or all of their toxic effects on the central nervous system. Caffeine and scopolamine are examples. Caffeine is present in coffee, tea and cocoa. Scopolamine, one of the belladonna alkaloids, produces a central stimulation when consumed in small doses, but causes hallucinations and is toxic in large doses. Several accidental poisonings with scopolamine have been reported (Jacobziner and Raybin, 1961). Nicotine present in tobacco plants is a central stimulant at low doses but is extremely toxic in large doses; accidental poisoning has been reported as a result of consumption of tobacco leaves. A tropane alkaloid, dioscorpine, isolated from yams (*Dioscorea hispida* and *Discorea dumetrum*), is a central nervous system depressant with an oral LD_{50} in mice of 64 mg/kg (Pinder, 1951; Bevan *et al.*, 1956). As described in 'spices', nutmeg and mace contain about 8 to 15% of a volatile oil. About 4% of this oil is myristicin, which is a natural psychotropic and pharmacologically active agent. The hallucinogenic and medicinal properties of nutmeg and mace are attributed to the presence of this compound. Myristicin is also a weak monoamine oxidase inhibitor (Truitt and Ebersberger, 1962). A number of structurally related compounds have been isolated from various food products and condiment sources and synthetic analogues with physiological activity have been prepared (Shulgin, 1966). These include elemicin, safrole, eugenol isoeugenol, methyleugenol and parsley apiole. Most of the plants which contain these compounds belong to the Umbelliferae, a group which includes such important crops as carrot, parsley, celery and dill. Falcaranol (carotatoxin) is present in one variety of carrots at a level of approximately 10 to 20 ppm (Crosby and Aharonson, 1967). This compound is an acetylenic alcohol related to, but less toxic than, either cicutoxin from *Cicuta* or water hemlock. Symptoms are similar to those produced following acute exposure to dichlorodiphenyltrichloroethanol. Falcaranol, injected into mice, produced pronounced neurotoxic symptoms (an LD_{50} value of about 100 mg/kg) (Crosby and Aharonson, 1967).

Nitrate and nitrite

Toxicity after excessive intake of naturally occurring nitrates in foods and feeds is established (Salunkhe and Wu, 1997). The animals showed tremors, diuresis, collapse and cyanosis after feeding comstalks which contain 25% by dry weight of potassium nitrate. The symptoms could be experimentally reproduced by oral dosing of cattle with doses of potassium nitrate of about 1.3 g/ kg. Nitrite as well as nitrates were detected in the blood, bile and other tissues of these animals. Freezing could prevent the formation of nitrite in spinach. The occurrence of inorganic nitrate in vegetables has, at times, given rise to serious acute toxic effects, especially those resulting from methaemoglobin formation. There are two cases of methaemoglobinaemia in infants who consumed spinach purée. Spinach contains large amounts of nitrite (above 218 mg/100 g wet weight) and a small amount of nitrate. The amount of nitrate in vegetables is as follows: 9000 ppm in radish, 4750 ppm in kale, 6000 ppm in lettuce, 3250 ppm in celery, 4500 ppm in turnip, 2250 ppm in squash, 500 ppm in carrot, 8062 ppm in beets, 4430 ppm in eggplant, 3809 ppm in spinach, 3846 ppm in broccoli, 2222 ppm in cabbage, 2000 ppm in cauliflower and 1698 ppm in parsley (Salunkhe and Wu, 1997). Increasing nitrogen fertilization increases nitrate content of the edible parts of mustard, collards, lettuce, cabbage and snap beans. Fresh carrot juice was considered to have caused a case of infantile methaemoglobinaemia diagnosed in St. Louis in June 1972 (Keating *et al.*, 1973). The nitrite level of carrot juice at 20°C increases rapidly for several hours when bacterial levels are above 10^6 cells/ml of juice. Nitrite is produced at 5°C when bacterial level is raised to 10^8 cells/ml.

Toxic phytoalexins

Phytoalexins are compounds produced by plants in response to various exogenous stimuli. A phytoalexin, phaseollin, has been isolated and identified from beans (*Phaseolus vulgaris*) infected with *Monilinia fructicola*, *Colletotrichum lindemuthianum*, *Uromyces appendiculatus*, *Pseudomonas* species, *Fusarium phaseoli*, and *Rhizoctonia salani*. Compounds present in garden peas (*Pisum sativum* L.) which belong to the phytoalexin group are pisatin and demethylpterocarpin (Stoessl, 1972). Pisatin is produced by several tissues of the pea plant and can be induced by microoganisms, chemicals, ultraviolet light and other treatments that cause cellular injury. In a toxicity study, phaseollin, hydroxyphaseollin and medicarpin, at concentrations < 0.35 mM, caused lysis of bovine erythrocytes, while pisatin was not haemolytic at concentrations up to 0.5 mM. Pisatin could injure the plasma membranes of human erythrocytes, and uncoupled oxidative phosphorylation in rat liver mitochondria. Phaseollin was highly toxic to embryonated chick eggs and may be toxic to higher animals. The sweet potato (*Ipomea batata* L.), a member of the *Convolvulanceae* family, is grown in the warm parts of all countries. In response to stress conditions, the sweet potato produces several metabolites that normally are absent or present in only minute amounts. These stress metabolites are produced by the root under a variety of conditions including fungal infection, treatment with heavy metal salts and other compounds, and mechanical injury from slicing or weevil infestation. The toxicity of mould-damaged sweet potatoes to farm animals has been reported (Wilson *et al.*, 1970). Several metabolites were isolated from black-rotted potato, most of which contained a furan moiety with an attached side chain at the 3- or β-position. One of the most abundant of these substances is an oil called ipomeamarone, a steam-distillable furanosesqui-terpenoid. This substance produces liver necrosis in mice and other animals, when fed or injected intraperitoneally. The hydroxy derivative of ipomeamar-one, ipomeamaronol isolated from mouldy sweet potatoes is also hepatotoxic. In large-scale outbreaks of mouldy sweet potato poisoning, especially among cattle, the predominant disease sign was not liver damage as might be attrib-uted to ipomeamarone; rather, the infected animals developed lung oedema with pleural fluid and died from apparent asphyxia (Wilson *et al.*, 1970). Such condition was also caused by toxins other than ipomeamarone and ipomeamaronol (Wilson *et al.*, 1971). They include two isomeric oils, 4-ipomeanol and 1-ipomeanol, which can be isolated from certain kinds of mould-damaged sweet potatoes. Normal boiling or baking of the whole sweet potatoes cannot eliminate these four toxins if they are present in sig-nificant quantities. 6-Methoxymellein is the phytoalexin in carrot roots (80 to 500 mg/g). This compound is responsible for the bitter taste produced in carrots. The ED_{50} for the toxicity of 6-hydroxymellein and 6-methoxymellein was reported to be 128 and 90 mg/ml, respectively. Mellein and 4-hydroxy-mellein have LD_{50} values of 250 to 500 and 1000 to 1500 mg/kg, respec-tively. Formation of phytoalexins (other than glycoalkaloids) through environmental stress on potato tubers is also established. Terpenoid compounds that accumulate as a result of stress include rishitin, rishitinol, phytuberin and lubimin. Most of the terpenoid stress metabolites are toxic to various fungi, but no data are available on their toxicity to other animal species.

TOXINS IN FOODS OF MARINE ORIGIN

Puffer fish

Puffer fish belong to the family Tetraodotiddae, and certain species, for exam-ple *Arothron hispidus* (deadly death puffer), are considered a delicacy in countries such as Japan. In Japan, puffer fish are eaten after being carefully cleaned and prepared by specially trained chefs. Tetrodotoxin, a sodium channel blocker, interrupts the conduction of action potentials in the nervous system without altering the resting membrane potential. The LD_{50} of this toxin is 10 mg/kg by an intraperitoneal injection. At high concentrations, striated muscle fibres are also affected. If puffer fish organs containing large amounts of the toxin are ingested, the symptoms which develop include tingling of the lip and tongue, loss of motor coordination, numbness, nausea, vomiting and convulsions. There is a high mortality and no known antidote. Although the puffer fish is the best known source of tetrodotoxin, several related species also contain variable amounts (Hall, 1988).

Scombroid toxicity

Scombroid toxicity or histamine toxicity results from the consumption of the flesh of fish belonging to the normally edible scombroid species. Under high storage temperature, free histidine in the flesh of the fish is decarboxylated by bacteria to yield toxic levels of histamine. The presence of this toxin can be detected since a sharp peppery taste is characteristic of the toxin-containing fish. After consumption, an acute phase of intoxication lasts for 8–12 hours. The symptoms are typically those of an acute allergic response and include head-ache, dizziness, flushing and a rash with intense itching. Additional com-pounds found in the fish, such as anserine and carnosine are believed to act in conjunction with the histamine to induce these symptoms. This intoxication is not severe and recovery is generally complete.

Fish egg toxins

A number of natural toxins occur in the eggs of many fish. Puffer fish (Tetraodotidae) eggs contain tetrodotoxin which, when ingested, leads to mus-cular and respiratory paralysis. Lipoprotein toxins have been found in two marine fishes, the northern blenny (*Stichaeus grigorjewi*) of Japan and the cabezon (*Scorpaenichthys marmoratus*) of western North America. Symptoms such as dizziness, headache, nausea and vomiting are characteristic of this type of poisoning. Ingestion of the lipostichaerin of the northern blenny results in decreased total lipids, neutral lipids and cholesterol in the plasma. In addition, an increase in serum transaminases and serum lactate dehydrogenase is observed, indicating parenchymal liver cell damage, Ingestion of the cabezon roe leads to a rapid depletion of lymphocytes in the spleen, and necrosis of the liver. Another group of fish egg toxins consists of those present in the roe of many freshwater species, particularly the carp family (Cyprinidae). This group of toxins has not been completely characterized and its effects when ingested appear to be quite variable.

Paralytic shellfish poisoning

Paralytic shellfish poisoning results from the ingestion of fish or shellfish which have consumed a potent toxin derived from two species of dinoflagellate, *Gonyaulax catenella* and *Gonyaulax tamarensis*. When these organisms are present in the water in large concentrations (> 20 000/ml), a visible 'red tide' is observed. Once ingested by shellfish, the dinoflagellate poison becomes bound in the hepatopancreas which renders it harmless to the shellfish. Over a period of 1–3 weeks, the toxin is gradually destroyed and excreted. If human consumption occurs during the period prior to excretion, the toxin is readily released. It is extremely potent; 30 minutes after consuming the shellfish, numbness is felt in the fingers. This progresses to paralysis, respiratory failure and death within 2–12 hours. The toxin, saxitoxin, is neurotoxic and is believed to interfere with sodium channels, an effect similar to that of tetrodotoxin found in puffer fish. Despite public announcements, consumption of the toxin-containing shellfish does occur, often with fatal consequences.

Ciguatera toxin

As with paralytic shellfish poisoning, ciguatera poisoning is due to a toxin produced by a species of dinoflagellate, *Diplopsalis*. These organisms are consumed by herbivorous organisms which in turn become food for predatory fish. One such species is the surgeonfish (*Acanthurus glaucopareicus*); over half the cases of this type of poisoning have been ascribed to consumption of this species. The toxin is a lipid with a nitrogenous moiety; it is heat-stable and thus not destroyed by cooking. Intoxication is rarely fatal. The neurotoxic effect results in a tingling sensation around the lips, tongue and throat, followed by numbness together with various gastrointestinal symptoms.

Conclusions

The principal sources of the naturally occurring food toxicants are vegetables which may in some instances contaminate food of animal origin. Certain marine species contain highly toxic substances, and humans are usually aware of the hazards they present. In the developed countries, poisoning by naturally occurring toxins is generally uncommon, although outbreaks of paralytic shellfish poisoning do occur from time to time. In underdeveloped countries, however, some traditional foods are potentially toxic under certain circumstances. In order to elucidate the mechanisms of toxic action of naturally occurring food toxicants, the involvement of metabolism, both activating and detoxifying, should be clarified. Naturally occurring carcinogens of plant origin are unique among carcinogenic agents in the environment. They are principally metabolites contained in certain plants used as food for human consumption since ancient times. Appreciation of the mode of action and mechanisms of carcinogenicity of these agents is especially important to prevent human cancers. On the basis of the results of further studies on the biological properties of toxic food factors, protective strategies will be devised to reduce toxicant-induced pathology, complemented by a lowering of human exposure to the toxicants.

References

Alderson T and Clark AM (1966) Interlocus specificity for chemical mutagens in *Aspergillus nidurans*. *Nature*, **210**, 593–595.
Alexander WS (1966) Phytanic acid in Refsum's syndrome. *Journal Neurology Neurosurgery and Psychiatry*, **29**, 412–416.

Allen JR, Hsu IC and Carstens LA (1975) Dehydroretronecine-induced rhabdomyosarcomas in rats. *Cancer Research*, **35**, 997–1002.

Avanzi S (1961) Chromosomal breakage by pyrrolizidine alkaloids and modification of the effects by cysteine. *Caryologia*, **14**, 251–261.

Beare-Rogers JL, Nera EA and Craig BM (1972) Accumulation of cardiac fatty acids in rats fed synthesized oils containing C22 fatty acids. *Lipids*, **7**, 46–50.

Bell EA and Jenzen DH (1971) Medical and ecological considerations of L-DOPA and 5-HTP in seeds. *Nature*, **229**, 136–137.

Benitz KF, Golberg L and Coulston F (1973) Intestinal effects of carrageenans in the rhesus monkey (*Macaca mulatta*). *Food and Cosmetics Toxicology*, **11**, 565–575.

Bennetts HW, Underwood EJ and Shier FL (1946) A specific breeding problem of sheep of subterranean clover pastures in western Australia. *Australian Veterinary Journal*, **22**, 2–12.

Bevan CWL, Broadbent JL and Hirst J (1956) A convulsant alkaloid of *Discorea dumetorum*. *Nature*, **177**, 935.

Blackwell, B., Marley, M., Price, J. and Taylor, D. (1967) Hypertensive interactions between monoamine oxidase inhibitors and foodstuffs. *British Journal of Psychiatry*, **113**, 349–365.

Borchert P, Miller JA, Miller EC and Shires TK (1973) 1′-Hydroxysafrole, a proximate carcinogenic metabolite of safrole in the rat and mouse. *Cancer Research*, **33**, 590–600.

Bowman DE (1945) Amylase inhibitor of navy beans. *Science*, **102**, 358–359.

Cater, D.B. (1961) The carcinogenic action of carrageenan in rats. *British Journal of Cancer*, **15**, 607–614.

Clark AM (1959) Mutagenic activity of the alkaloid heliotrine in *Drosophila*. *Nature*, **183**, 731–732.

Committee on Food Protection (1966) *Toxicants occurring naturally in foods*. National Academy of Science, Washington, DC.

Committee on Food Protection (1973) *Toxicants occurring naturally in foods*. National Academy of Sciences, Washington, DC.

Crosby DG and Aharonson N (1967) The structure of carotatoxin, a natural toxicant from carrot. *Tetrahedron*, **23**, 465–472.

Culvenor CCJ, Edgar JA, Smith LW and Hirono I (1976) The occurrence of senkirkine in *Tussilago farfara*. *Australian Journal of Chemistry* **29**, 229–230.

Dhopeshwarker GA (1980) Naturally occurring food toxicants: toxic lipids. *Progress in Lipid Research*, **19**, 107–118.

Druckrey H (1970) Production of colonic carcinomas by 1,2-dialkyl-hydrazines and azoxyalkanes. In *Carcinoma of the Colon and Antecedent Epithelium*, Burdett, W.J. (ed) Charles C. Thomas Co. Springfield Ill, pp. 267–279.

Dry J, Pradalier A and Canny M (1982) Maladie de Refsum: dix ans de régime dietetique pauvre en acid phytanique et phytol. *Annales de Medicine Interne*, 133, 483–487.

Eldjarn L, Stokke O and Try K (1976) Biochemical aspects of Refsum's disease and principles for the dietary treatment. In *Handbook of Clinical Neurology*, Vinken, PJ, Bruyn GW and Klawans HL (eds), North Holland Publ., Amsterdam, pp. 519–541.

Enomoto M (1987) Safrole. In *Naturally Occurring Carcinogens of Plant Origin*, Hirono, I. (ed.), Kodansha, Tokyo/Elsevier, Amsterdam, pp. 139–159.

Evans IA and Mason J (1965) Carcinogenic activity of bracken. *Nature*, **208**, 913–914.

Evans WC, Evans IA, Axford RFE, Threlfall G, Humphreys DA and Thomas AJ (1961) Studies on bracken poisoning in cattle Part VII. The toxicity of bracken rhizomes. *Veterinary Record*, **73**, 852–853.

Evans WC, Patel MC and Koohy Y (1982) Acute bracken poisoning in homogastric and ruminant animals. *Prooceedings of the Royal Society of Edinburgh*, **81B**, 29–64.

Fabian RJ, Abraham R., Coulston F and Golberg L (1973) Carrageenan-induced squamous metaplasia of the rectal mucosa in the rat. *Gastroenterology*, **65**, 265–276.

Froesch ER, Wolf HP and Baitsch H (1963) Hereditary fructose intolerance. An inborn defect of hepatic fructose-1-phosphate splitting aldolase. *American Journal of Medicine*, **34**, 151–167.

Fujimoto M, Ogino H and Hirono I (1987) Influence of ptaquiloside on the development of newborn mice. *The Journal of Toxicological Sciences*, **12**, 135–145.

Furuya T, Asada Y and Mori H (1987) Pyrrolizidine alkaloids. In *Naturally Occurring Carcinogens of Plant Origin*, Hirono I (ed), Kodansha, Tokyo/Elsevier, Amsterdam, pp. 25–52.

Goddard MK (1992) Hormone replacement therapy and breast cancer, endometrial cancer and cardiovascular disease; risk and benefits. *British Journal of General Practice*, **42**, 120–125.

Hall JL (1988) Food associated intoxicants. *Progress in Food and Nutrition Sciences*, **12**, 1–43.

Harris PN and Chen KK (1970) Development of hepatic tumors in rats following ingestion of *Senecio longilobus*. *Cancer Research*, **30**, 2881–2886.

Hathcock JN (1993) The effects of sulphur amino acids on chemical toxicity. In *Food, Nutrition and Chemical Toxicity*, Parke DV, Ioannides C and Walker R (eds), Smith-Gordon/Nishimura, London/Niigata, pp. 35–41.

Hirono I (1972) Carcinogenicity and neurotoxicity of cycasin with special reference to species differences. *Federation Proceedings*, **31**, 1493–1497.

Hirono, I. (1981) Natural carcinogenic products of plant origin. *CRC Critical Reviews in Toxicology*, 11, 235–277.

Hirono I (1987a) Cycasin. In *Naturally Occurring Carcinogens of Plant Origin*, Hirono, I. (ed), Kodansha, Tokyo/Elsevier, Amsterdam, pp. 3–24.

Hirono I (1987b) Carrageenan. In *Naturally Occurring Carcinogens of Plant Origin*, Hirono, I. (ed), Kodansha, Tokyo/Elsevier, Amsterdam, pp. 121–126.

Hirono I and Yamada K (1987) Bracken fern. In *Naturally Occurring Carcinogens of Plant Origin*: Hirono, I. (ed), Kodansha, Tokyo/Elsevier, Amsterdam, pp. 87–120.

Hirono I, Shibuya C and Fushimi K (1969) Tumor induction in C57BL/6 mice by a single administration of cycasin. *Cancer Research*, **29**, 1658–1662.

Hirono I, Shibuya C, Fushimi K and Haga M (1970) Studies on carcinogenic properties of bracken, *Pteridium aquilinum*. *Journal of National Cancer Institute*, **45**, 179–188.

Hirono I, Hayashi K, Mori H and Miwa T (1971) Carcinogenic effects of cycasin in Syrian golden hamsters and the transplantability of induced tumors. *Cancer Research*, **31**, 283–287.

Hirono I, Shibuya C, Shimizu M and Fushimi K (1972) Carcinogenic activity of processed bracken used as human food. *Journal of National Cancer Institute*, **48**, 1245–1250.

Hirono I, Shimizu M, Fushimi K, Mori H, Kato K and Haga M (1973) Carcinogenic activity of *Petasites japonicus* Maxim, a kind of coltsfoot. *Gann*, **64**, 527–528.

Hirono I, Sasaoka I, Shibuya C, Shimizu M, Fushimi K, Mori H, Kato K, and Haga M (1975) Natural carcinogenic products of plant origin. *Gann Monograph on Cancer Research*, **17**, 205–217.

Hirono I, Mori H and Culvenor CCJ (1976) Carcinogenic activity of coltsfoot, *Tussilago farfara* L. *Gann*, **67**, 125–129.

Hirono I, Mori H, Yamada K, Hirata Y, Haga M, Tatematsu, H and Kanie S (1977) Carcinogenic activity of petasitenine, a new pyrrolizidine alkaloid isolated from *Petasites japonicus* Maxim. *Journal of National Cancer Institute*, **58**, 1155–1157.

Hirono I, Mori H and Haga M (1978) Carcinogenic activity of *Symphytum officinale*. *Journal of National Cancer Institute*, **61**, 856–869.

Hirono I, Haga M, Fujii M, Mastuura S, Matsbara N, Nakayama M, Furuya T, Hikichi M, Takahashi, M, Uchida E, Hosaka S and Ueno I (1979) Induction of hepatic tumors in rats by senkirkine and symphytine. *Journal of National Cancer Institute*, **63**, 469–472.

Hirono I, Kuhara K, Hosaka S, Tomizawa S and Golgerg L (1981a) Induction of intestinal tumors in rats by dextran sulfate sodium. *Journal of National Cancer Institute*, **66**, 579–583.

Hirono I, Sumi Y, Kuhara K and Miyakawa M (1981b) Effect of degraded carrageenan on the intestine in germfree rats. *Toxicology Letters*, **8**, 207–212.

HironoI, Kuhara K., Yamaji T, Hosaka S and Golberg L (1983a) Carcinogenicity of dextran sulfate sodium in relation to its molecular weight. *Cancer Letters*, **18**, 29–34.

Hirono I, Ueno I, Aiso S, Yamaji T, and Haga M (1983b) Carcinogenic activity of *Farugium japonicum* and *Senecio cannabiofolis*. *Cancer Letters*, **20**, 191–198.

Hirono I, Aiso S, Yamaji T, Mori H, Yamada K, Niwa H, Ojika MJ, Wakamatsu K, Kigoshi H, Niiyama K and Uosaki Y (1984a) Carcinogenicity in rats of ptaquiloside isolated from bracken. *Gann*, **75**, 833–836.

Hirono, I., Kono, Y., Takahashi, K., Yamada, K., Niwa, H., Ojika, M., Kigoshi, H., Niiyama, K. and Uosaki, Y. (1984b) Reproduction of acute bracken poisoning in a calf with ptaquiloside, a bracken constituent. *Veterinary Record*, **115**, 375–378.

Hirono, I and Yamada, K (1987) Bracken fern. In *Naturally Occurring Carcinogens of Plant Origin*, Hirono I (ed), Kodansha, Tokyo/Elsevier, Amsterdam, pp. 87–120.

Hirono I, Ito M, Yagyu S, Haga M, Wakamatsu K, Kishikawa T, Nishikawa O, Yamada K, Ojika M and Kigosihi H (1993) Reproduction of progressive retinal degeneration (Bright blindness) in sheep by administration of ptaquiloside contained in bracken. *Journal of Veterinary Medical Science*, **55**, 979–983.

Homburger F, Kelly Jr T, Frieder G and Russfield AB (1961) Toxic and possible carcinogenic effects of 4-allyl-1,2-methylene dioxybenzene (safrole) in rats on deficient diets. *Medicina Experimentalis*, **4**, 1–11.

Horwitz D, Lovenberg W, Engelman K and Sjoerdsma A (1964) Monoamine oxidase inhibitors, tyramine, and cheese. *JAMA*, **188**, 1108–1110.

International Agency for Research in Cancer (1983) Agaritine and gyromitrin in *IARC Monographs on the Evaluation of the Carcinogenic Risk of Chemicals to Humans*, 31, IARC Lyons, pp. 63–69, 163–170.

Jacobziner H and Raybin HW (1961) Briefs on accidental chemical poisoning in New York City. *New York Journal of Medicine*, **61**, 301.

Kamon S, Hirayama T (1975) Epidemiology of cancer of the oesophagus in Miye, Nara and Wakayama prefectures with special reference to the role of bracken fern. *Proceedings of Japanese Cancer Association*, **34**, 211.

Keating JP, Lell ME, Straus AW, Zarkowsky H and Smith GE (1973) Infantile methemoglobinemia caused by carrot juice. *New England Journal of Medicine*, **288**, 825–826.

Kuhara, K, Takanashi H, Hirono I, Furuya T and Asada Y (1980) Carcinogenic activity of clivoline, a pyrrolizidine alkaloid isolated from *Ligularia dentata*. *Cancer Letters*, **10**, 117–122.

Kurland LT and Mulder DW (1954) Epidemiologic investigations of amyotrophic lateral sclerosis. *Neurology*, **4**, 355–378.

Laquer GL, Mickelsen O, Whiting MG and Kurland LT (1963) Carcinogenic properties of nuts from *Cycas circinalis* L. indigenous to Guam. *Journal of National Cancer Institute*, **31**, 919–951.

Lee DJ, Wales JH, Ayres JL and Sinnhuber RO (1968) Synergism between cyclopropenoid fatty acids and chemical carcinogens in rainbow trout (*Salmo gairdneri*). *Cancer Research*, **28**, 2312–2318.

Lee DJ, Wales JH and Sinnhuber RO (1971) Promotion of aflatoxin-induced hepatoma growth in trout by methyl melvalate and sterculate. *Cancer Research*, **31**, 960–963.

Leopold AS, Ervin M and Browning B (1976) Phytoestrogens: adverse effects on reproduction in California quail. *Science*, **191**, 98–100.

Levenberg B (1961) Structure and enzymatic cleavage of agaritine, a phenylhydrazide of L-glutamic acid isolated from *Agaricaceae*. *Journal of the American Chemical Society*, **83**, 503–504.

Levin B, Snodgrass GJ, Oberholzer VG, Burgess EA and Dobbs RH (1968) Fructosaemia. *American Journal of Medicine*, **45**, 826–838.

Long EL, Nelson AA, Fitzhugh OG and Hansen WH (1963) Liver tumors produced in rats by feeding safrole. *Archives of Pathology*, **75**, 595–604.

Marcus R and Watt J (1971) Colonic ulceration in young rats fed degraded carrageenan. *Lancet*, **2**, 765–766.

Matsumoto H (1979) Carcinogenicity of cycasin, its aglycone methylazoxymethanol, and methylazoxymethanol-glucosiduronomic acid. In *Naturally Occurring Carcinogens-Mutagens and Modulators of Carcinogenesis*, Miller EC, Miller JA, Hirono I, Sugimara T, Takayama S *et al.* (eds), Jpn Sci. Soc. Press, Tokyo; Univ. Park Press, Baltimore, pp. 67–77.

Matsumoto H and Higa, HH (1966) Studies on methylazoxymethanol, aglycone of cycasin: methylation of nucleic acids in vitro. *Biochemical Journal*, **98**, 20c–22c.

Mattocks AR (1968) Toxicity of pyrrolizidine alkaloids. *Nature*, **217**, 723–728.

Mattocks AR (1970) Toxicity and metabolism of senecio alkaloids. In *Phytochemical Ecology*, Annual Proceedings of the Phytochemical Society 8, Harbone, JB (ed) Academic Press, London, pp. 401–402.

Mclean, EK (1970) The toxic action of pyrrolizidine (senecio) alkaloids. *Pharmacological Reviews*, **22**, 429–483.

Medlock KL, Branhamn WS and Sheehan DM (1995) Effects of coumestrol and equol on the developing reproductive tract of the rat. *Proceedings of the Society for Experimental Biology and Medicine* **208**, 67–71.

Miller JA (1964) Comments on chemistry of cycads. *Federation Proceedings*, **23**, 1361–1362.

Miller JA and Miller EC (1983) The metabolic activation and nucleic acid adducts of naturally-occurring carcinogens. Recent results with ethyl carbamate and the spice flavors safrole and estragole. *British Journal of Cancer*, **48**, 1–15.

Miller JA, Miller EC and Phillips DH (1982) The metabolic activation and carcinogenicity of alkenylbenzenes that occur naturally in many spices. In *Carcinogens and Mutagens in the Environment*, Stich HF (ed), CRC Press, Boca Raton, Florida, pp. 83–96.

Mori H (1987) Betel nut. In *Naturally Occurring Carcinogens of Plant Origin: Toxicology, Pathology and Biochemistry 2*, Hirono I (ed), Bioactive Molecules. Kodansha, Tokyo/Elsevier, Amsterdam, pp. 167–180.

Mori H, Matsubara N, Ushimaru Y and Hirono I (1979) Carcinogenicity examination of betel nuts and piper betel leaves. *Experientia*, **35**, 384–385.

Mori H, Ohbayashi F, Hirono I, Shimada T and Williams GM (1984) Absence of genotoxicity of the carcinogenic sulfated polysaccharides carrageenan and dextran sulfate in mammalian DNA repair and bacterial mutagenicity assays. *Nutrition and Cancer*, **6**, 92–97.

Mori H, Sugie S, Hirono I, Yamada K, Niwa H, Ojika M Wakamatsu K and Kigoshi H (1985a) Genotoxicity of ptaquiloside, a bracken carcinogen, in the hepatocyte primary culture/DNA-repair test. *Mutation Research*, **143**, 75–78.

Mori H, Sugie S, Yoshimi N, Asada Y, Furuya T and Williams GM (1985b) Genotoxicity of a variety of pyrrolizidine alkaloids in the hepatocyte primary culture/DNA repair test using rat, mouse and hamster hepatocytes. *Cancer Research*, **45**, 3125–3129.

Nagata Y and Matsumoto H (1969) Studies on methylazoxymethanol: methylation of nucleic acids in the fetal rat brain. *Proceedings of the Society for Experimental Biology and Medicine*, **132**, 383–385.

Nagoya T, Hattori Y and Kobayashi F (1981) Mutagenicity and cytogenicity studies of dextran sulfate. *Pharmacometrics*, **22**, 621–627.

National Research Council (1981) *Food Chemicals Codex*, 3rd ed, National Academy Press, Washington, DC, pp. 74–75.

Natori S (1987) Mushroom hydrazines. In *Naturally Occurring Carcinogens of Plant Origin*. Hirono, I. (ed), Kodansha, Tokyo/Elsevier, Amsterdam, pp. 127–137.

Newberne PM and Rogers AE (1973) Nutrition, monocrotaline and aflatoxin B1 in liver carcinogenesis. *Plant Foods for Man*, **1**, 23–31.

Nishida, K, Kobayashi A and Nagahama T (1955) Cycasin, a new toxic glycoside *Cycas revoluta* Thunb.1. Isolation and structure of cycasin. *Bulletin of Agricultural Chemistry of Japanese Society*, **19**, 77–84.

Nishida K, Kobayashi A, Nagahama T, Kojima K and Yamane M (1956) Cycasin, a new toxic glycoside of *Cycas revoluta* Thunb. IV. Pharmacology of cycasin. *Seikagaku*, **28**, 218–223.

Niwa H, Ojika M, Wakamatsu, K., Yamada, K., Ohba, S., Saito, Y., Hirono, I. and Matsushita, K. (1983) Stereochemistry of ptaquiloside, a novel norsesquiterpene glucoside from bracken, *Pteridium aquilinum* var. latiusculum. *Tetrahedron Letters*, 24, 5371–5372.

O'Leary SB (1964) Poisoning in man from eating poisonous plants. *Archives of Environmental Health*, **9**, 216–242.

Pamukcu AM, Goskoy SK and Price JM (1967) Urinary bladder neoplasms induced by feeding bracken fern (*Pteris aquilina*) to cows. *Cancer Research*, **27**, 917–924.

Pamukcu AM, Ertuk E, Yalciner S, Milli U and Bryan GT (1978) Carcinogenic and mutagenic activities of milk from cows fed bracken fern (*Pteridium aquilinum*). *Cancer Research*, **38**, 1556–1560.

Phillips DH, Miller JA, Miller EC and Adams B (1981) The N2-atom of guanine and the N6-atom of adenine residues as sites for covalent binding of metabolically activated 1′-hydroxysafrole to mouse live DNA in vivo. *Cancer Research*, **41**, 2664–2671.

Pinder AR (1951) An alkaloid of *Dioscorea hispida*, Dennst. *Nature*, **168**, 1090.

Price KR and Fenwick GR (1985) Naturally occurring oestrogens in foods – A review. *Food Additives and Contaminants*, **2**, 73–106.

Radeleff RD (1970) *Veterinary Toxicology*, Lea & Febiger, Philadelphia, pp. 74–77.

Rosenberger G (1971) Nature, manifestations, cause and control of chronic enzootic haematuria in cattle. *Veterinary Medicine Reviews*, No. **2/3**, 189–206.

Rosenberger, G. and Heeschen, W. (1960) Adlerfan (*pteris aquilina*)-die Ursache des sog. Stallrotes der Rinder (Haematuria vesicalis bovis chronica). *Deutsche Tierarztlich Wochenschrift*, **67**, 201–208.

Salunkhe DK and Wu MT (1997) Toxicants in plant products. *CRC Critical Review in Food Science and Nutrition*, **9**, 37–51.

Sato T, Inaba H, Kawai K, Furukawa H, Hirono I and Miyazawa T (1991) Low level chemiluminescence from *Drosophila melanogaster* fed with chemical mutagens, polycyclic aromatic hydrocarbon quinones and a carcinogenic bracken fern. *Mutation Research*, **251**, 91–97.

Sayre JW and Kaymakcalan S (1964) Cyanide poisoning from apricot seeds among children in central Turkey. *New England Journal of Medicine*, **270**, 1113–1115.

Schoental R (1970) Hepatotoxic activity of retrorsine, senkirkine and hydrosenkirkine in new-born rats, and the role of epoxides in carcinogenesis by pyrrolizidine alkaloids and aflatoxins. *Nature*, **227**, 401–402.

Schoental R, Head MA and Peacock PR (1954) Senecio alkaloids, primary liver tumours in rats as a result of treatment with (i) a mixture of alkaloids from *S. jacobaea* Lin; (ii) retrorsine; (iii) isatidine. *British Journal of Cancer,* **8**, 458–465.

Sheehan DM (1995) The case for expanded phytoestrogen research. *Proceedings of the Society for Experimental Biology and Medicine,* **208**, 3–5.

Shulgin AT (1966) Possible implication of myristicin as a psychotropic substance. *Nature,* **210**, 380–384.

Sieber SM, Correa P, Dalgard DW, McIntire KR and Adamson RH (1980) Carcinogenicity and hepatotoxicity of cycasin and its aglycone methylazoxymethanol acetate in nonhuman primates. *Journal of National Cancer Institute,* **65**, 177–189.

Singleton VL (1981) Naturally occurring food toxicants: phenolic substances of plant origin common in food. *Advances in Food Research,* **27**, 149–242.

Smith DWE (1966) Mutagenicity of cycasin aglycone (methylazoxymethanol), a naturally occurring carcinogen. *Science,* **152**, 1273–1274.

Spatz M (1964) Carcinogenic effect of cycad meal in guinea pigs. *Federation Proceedings,* **23**, 1384–1385.

Spatz M, Smith DWE, McDaniel EG and Laqueur GL (1967) Role of intestinal microorganisms in determining cycasin toxicity. *Proceedings of the Society for Experimental Biology and Medicine,* **124**, 691–697.

Stanton MF (1966) Hepatic neoplasms of aquarium fish exposed to *Cycas circinalis. Federation Proceedings,* **25**, 661,

Steinberg D (1983) Phytanic acid storage diesease (Refsum's disease). In *The Metabolic Basis of Inherited Disease,* Stanbury, JB, Wyngaarden, JB, Fredrickson DS, Goldstein JL and Brown MS (eds), McGraw-Hill, New York, pp. 731–747.

Stoessl A (1972) Inermin associated with pisatin in peas inoculated with the fungus *Monilinia fructicola. Canadian Journal of Biochemistry,* **50**, 107–108.

Stout MG, Reich H and Huffman MH (1964) Neonatal lethality of offspring of tangeretin-treated rats. *Cancer Chemotherapy Reports,* **36**, 23–24.

Svoboda DJ and Reddy JK (1972) Malignant tumour in rats given lasiocarpine. *Cancer Research,* **32**, 908–913.

Swanson AB., Chambliss DD, Blomquist JC, Miller EC and Miller JA (1979) The mutagenicities of safrole, estragole, trans-anethole, and some of their known or possible metabolites for *Salmonella typhimurium* mutants. *Mutation Research,* **60**, 143–153.

Swarttouw MA (1974) The oxidation of erucic acid by rat heart mitochondria. *Biochimica et Biophysica Acta,* **337**, 680–689.

Tandon HD, Tandon BN and Mattocks AR (1978) An epidemic of veno-occlusive disease of the liver in Afghanistan. *American Journal of Gastroenterology,* **70**, 607–613.

Teas HJ and Dyson JG (1967) Mutation in *Drosophila* by methylazoxymethanol, the aglycone of cycasin. *Proceedings of the Society for Experimental Biology and Medicine,* **125**, 988–990.

Teige B and Beare-Rogers JL (1973) Cardiac fatty acids in rats fed marine oils. *Lipids,* **8**, 584–587.

Toth B (1972) Hydrazine, methylhydrazine and methylhydrazine sulfate carcinogenesis in Swiss mice. Failure of ammonium hydroxide to interfere in the development of tumors. *International Journal of Cancer,* **9**, 109–118.

Toth B and Nagel D (1978) Tumors induced in mice by *N*-methyl-*N*-formylhydrazine of the false morel *Gyromitra esculenta. Journal of National Cancer Institute,* **60**, 201–204.

Toth B, Tompa A and Patil K (1977) Tumorigenic effect of 4,3-methylphenylhydrazine hydrochloride in Swiss mice. *Zeitschrift fur Krebsforschung,* **89**, 245–252.

Toth R, Smith JW and Patil KD (1981) Cancer induction in mice with acetaldehyde methylformylhydrazone if the false morel mushroom. *Journal of National Cancer Institute*, **67**, 881–887.

Truitt EB Jr and Ebersberger EM (1962) Evidence of monoamine oxidase inhibition by myristicin and nutmeg *in vivo*. *Federation Proceedings*, **21**, 418.

Van Der Waaij D, Cohen B and Anver M (1978) Mitigation of experimental inflammatory bowel disease in guinea pigs by selective elimination of the aerobic gram negative intestinal microflora. *Gastroenterology*, **74**, 521–526.

Van Woert MH and Bowers MB Jr (1970) The effect of L-dopa on monoamine metabolites in Parkinson's disease. *Experientia*, **26**, 161–163.

Wakabayashi K, Inagaki T, Fujimoto Y and Fukuda Y (1978) Induction by degraded carrageenan of colorectal tumors in rats. *Cancer Letters*, **4**, 171–176.

Watanabe K, Iwashima H, Muta K, Hamada Y and Hamada K (1975) Hepatic tumors of rabbits induced by cycad extract. *Gann*, **66**, 335–339.

Watanabe K, Reddy BS, Wong CQ and Weisburger JH (1978) Effect of dietary undegraded carrageenan on colon carcinogenesis in F344 rats treated with azoxymethane or methylnitrosourea. *Cancer Research*, **38**, 4427–4430.

Watt J, and Marcus R (1970a) Hyperplastic mucosal changes in the rabbit colon produced by degraded carrageenan. *Gastroenterology*, **59**, 760–768.

Watt J and Marcus R (1970b) Ulcerative colitis in rabbits fed degraded carrageenan. *Journal of Pharmacy and Pharmacology*, **22**, 130–131.

Watt J and Marcus R (1971) Carrageenan-induced ulceration of the large intestine in the guinea pig. *Gut*, **12**, 164–171.

Williams GM, Laspia MF, Mori H and Hirono I (1981) Genotoxicity of cycasin in the hepatocyte primary culture/DNA repair test supplemented with β-glucosidase. *Cancer Letters*, **12**, 329–333.

Wilson BJ, Yang DTC and Boyd MR (1970) Toxicity of mould-damaged sweet potatoes (*Ipomoea batatas*). *Nature*, **227**, 521–522.

Wilson BJ, Boyd MR, Harris TM and Yang DTC (1971) A lung oedema factor from mouldy sweet potatoes (*Ipomola batatas*). *Nature*, **231**, 52–53.

Wislocki PG, Miller EC, Miller JA, McCoy EC and Rosenkranz HS (1973) Carcinogenic and mutagenic activities of safrole, 1'-hydroxysafrole and some known or possible metabolites. *Cancer Research*, **37**, 1883–1891.

Yamada K, Tatematsu H, Suzuki M, Hirata Y, Haga M and Hirono I (1976) Isolation and the structure of two new alkaloids, petasitenine and neopetasitenine from *Petasites japonicus* Maxim. *Chemistry Letters*, 461–464.

Yamanaka H, Nagao M, Sugimura T, Furuya T, Shirai A and Matsushima T (1979) Mutagenicity of pyrrolizidine alkaloids in the *Salmonella*/mammalian-microsome test. *Mutation Research*, **68**, 211–216.

Zedeck MS, Sternberg SS, Poynter RW and McGowan J (1970) Biochemical and pathological effects of methylazoxymethanol acetate, a potent carcinogen. *Cancer Research*, **30**, 801–812.

2 Toxicants in Food: Fungal Contaminants

Jia-Sheng Wang, Thomas W Kensler and John D Groopman

Department of Environmental Health Sciences, School of Hygiene and Public Health, Johns Hopkins University, Baltimore, MD 21205, USA

Introduction

Food normally provides the essential nutrients for human growth, development and maintenance; however, a variety of toxic chemical contaminants, both naturally occurring and synthetic, are routinely present in the food supply. In addition to food toxicants of plant and animal origin (see Chapters 1 and 3), bacterial and fungal toxins can enter the food chain at every stage of food production, processing and storage. Toxic fungal metabolites, mycotoxins, are structurally diverse and commonly present in animal feed and human food ingredients. Mycotoxins induce many adverse biological effects when consumed in sufficient quantities over time. The three major genera of mycotoxin-producing fungi are *Aspergillus, Fusarium* and *Penicillium* (Council for Agricultural Science and Technology, 1989). Members of the *Aspergillus* and *Pencillium* species typically do not invade intact grain prior to harvest (Tuite, 1979), whereas the field (preharvest) fungal species of the *Fusarium* and *Alternaria* genus do penetrate grain. Unfavourable agricultural conditions such as drought or damage to seeds by insects or mechanical harvesting can exacerbate mycotoxin production during growth, harvest and storage. Mycotoxin production occurs over a wide range of moisture content (10–33%), relative humidity (>70%) and ambient storage temperatures (4–35°C), and growth is species/strain specific (Ciegler *et al.*, 1981). The major crops affected by mycotoxins are corn, peanuts, cotton, wheat, rice and the processed food from these crops.

Spurred by the discovery of the aflatoxins in 1960, the search for mycotoxins in food during the past three decades has led to the identification of more than 100 toxigenic fungi and more than 300 mycotoxins worldwide (Sharma and

Nutrition and Chemical Toxicity. Edited by Costas Ioannides. © John Wiley & Sons Ltd. ISBN 0 471 97453 6

Salunkhe, 1991; Miller and Trenhol, 1994), and several new mycotoxins are discovered each year. Most mycotoxins have not been implicated in any toxic syndromes in animals or people, but their occurrence in the food supply invokes cause for concern because so many have been shown to be potent toxic agents. The aflatoxins, certain trichothecenes, fumonisins and ochratoxins have been implicated in highly lethal episodic outbreaks of mould poisoning in exposed animals and/or human populations (Busby and Wogan, 1981, 1984; Beardall and Miller, 1994). To date, mycotoxins with carcinogenic potency in experimental animal models include aflatoxins, sterigmatocystin, ochratoxin, fumonisin, patulin and penicillic acid. Recently, aflatoxin B_1 has been classi-fied as a category I known human carcinogen by the International Agency for Research on Cancer (IARC, 1993). Finally, teratogenic effects in experimental models have been described for aflatoxins, ochratoxin, T-2 toxin, diacetoxy-scirpenol, rubratoxin, sterigmatocystin and zearalenone (Council for Agricultural Science and Technology, 1989).

Under current trade policy, virtually all countries engaged in international commerce have enacted or proposed regulations for mycotoxins in food and feed (FAO, 1996). There are many factors that influence the establishment of tolerances for mycotoxins, such as the availability of toxicological data, the availability of data on dietary exposure, the distribution of mycotoxins across commodities, legislation of other countries with which trade contacts exist, and the availability of specific and sensitive methods of analysis. In practice, only a few countries have formally presented the rationale for the need to regulate or for the selection of a particular maximum tolerated level of different mycotox-ins. The toxicity of the mycotoxins represents a major economic concern for the agriculture and veterinary communities. In particular, their carcinogenic effects drive the public health risk assessment debate. The objective of this chapter is briefly to review the occurrence, biological effects, mechanistic interactions with DNA and other macromolecular targets and, where available, epidemio-logical associations of dietary exposure to major mycotoxins with human dis-ease outcomes. Since there are well over 10 000 articles on mycotoxins in the scientific literature, no one chapter can be comprehensive, but the references cited herein will provide a starting point for more in depth examination of the literature.

Aflatoxins

CHEMISTRY

The aflatoxins (AFs) were discovered as the causative agent in turkey X disease in Britain during the early 1960s. This syndrome resulted in the death of thou-sands of turkey poults, ducklings and chicks that were fed diets containing *Aspergillus flavus*-contaminated peanut meal (Wogan, 1965). Chemically, the AFs are highly substituted coumarin structures containing a fused dihydrofurofuran moiety. The four major AFs are B_1, B_2, G_1 and G_2 and are produced by *A. flavus* and *A. parasiticus*. AFB_1 and AFB_2 were named because of their strong blue fluorescence under ultraviolet light, whereas AFG_1 and AFG_2 fluoresced greenish-yellow. These physical properties permitted the very fast development of screening methods for the detection of AFs in grains and other commodities (Castegnaro *et al.*, 1980; Cole and Cox, 1981). The B toxins were found to have a fusion of the cyclopentenone ring to the lactone ring of the coumarin structure whereas the G toxins contained an additional fused lactone ring. AFB_1, and to a lesser extent AFG_1, were responsible for the toxicological potency of AF-contaminated grains and crude fractions derived from toxigenic fungi cultures in a number of test systems. These two toxins possess an unsaturated bond on the terminal furan ring. AFB_2 and AFG_2 are essentially biologically inactive unless metabolically oxidised to AFB_1 and AFG_1 *in vivo*. AFM_1 is a ring hydroxlation metabolite of AFB_1, originally found in the milk of AFB_1-exposed dairy animals.

Many analytical methods have been developed for the measurement of AFs in foods and feeds. These techniques include chromatographic separations following solvent extraction, such as the minicolumn, thin-layer and high-pressure liquid chromatography (Groopman and Donahue, 1988), and immunological assays using specific antibodies or antisera, such as enzyme-linked immunosorbent assays, radioimmunoassay and immunoaffinity chromatography (Chu *et al.*, 1987; Trucksess *et al.*, 1991). Each of these methodologies has unique characteristics as regards specificity and sensitivity. In addition, some methods are adequate for qualitative analysis while other techniques are quantitative. To date, many commercial assays for the measurement of AFS have been devised and rigorously tested by regulatory agencies and these data are then used in assessment analyses (Koeltzow and Tanner, 1990; Pohland *et al.*, 1990).

OCCURRENCE IN AGRICULTURAL COMMODITIES

Commodities most often found to contain AFs are peanuts, various other nuts, cottonseed, corn and rice. Human exposure can occur by consumption of AFs from these sources and the products derived from them as well as from tissues, eggs and the milk (AFM_1) of animals that consume contaminated feeds. The requirements for AF production are relatively non-specific, since the moulds can produce AFs on almost any foodstuff. Contamination with AFB_1 generally predominates in nature; dietary foodstuffs typically contain AFB_1 and AFB_2 in molar ratios of 1.0 to 0.1 and when all four aflatoxins occur, AFB_1, AFB_2, AFG_1 and AFG_2 in a proportion of 1.0 : 0.1 : 0.3 : 0.03, respectively (Ciegler *et al.*, 1981). While contamination by the moulds may be universal within a given geographical area, the levels or final concentrations of AFs in the grain product can vary from less than 1 μg/kg (1 ppb) to > 12 000 μg/kg (12 ppm) (Ellis *et al.*, 1991). For this reason, the measurement of human consumption of AF by sampling foodstuffs is extremely imprecise. Further, obvious contamination of a commodity with A. flavus or A. parasiticus does not necessarily demonstrate the presence of AFs, and the appearance of a sound, uninfected sample of commodity dos not preclude the existence of significant quantities of AFs.

Widespread concern regarding the toxic effects of AFs in humans and animals and possible transfer of residues from animal tissues and milk to humans has led to regulatory actions governing the interstate as well as global transport and consumption of AF-contaminated food and feed commodities. The United States Food and Drug Administration (FDA) has set action levels for AF in corn and other feed commodities. For feeding mature non-lactating animals the action level is 100 ppb; for commodities destined for human consumption and interstate commerce, 20 ppb; and for milk (AFM_1) 0.5 ppb.

TOXIC EFFECTS ON ANIMALS

AFs are potent liver toxins, and their effects in animals vary with dose, length of exposure, species, breed and diet or nutritional status (reviewed in Eaton and Groopman, 1994). These toxins may be lethal when consumed in large doses; sublethal doses can induce chronic toxicity, and low levels of chronic exposure can result in neoplasia, primarily liver cancer, in many animal species (Wogan and Newberne, 1967; Wogan, 1969, 1973; Busby and Wogan, 1984). AFB_1, the most potent and commonly occurring AF, is acutely toxic (LD_{50} 0.3–9.0 mg/kg) to all species of animals, birds and fish tested. Sheep and mice are the most resistant whereas cats, dogs, rats and rabbits are the most sensitive species. Acute effects include death with or without signs of anorexia, depression, ataxia, dyspnoea, anaemia and haemorrhage from body orifices. In subchronic cases icterus, hypoprothrombinaemia, haematomas and gastroenteritis are common. Chronic aflatoxicosis is characterised histologically by bile duct proliferation, periportal fibrosis, icterus and cirrhosis of the liver. Prolonged exposure to low levels of AFB_1 leads to hepatoma, cholangiocarcinoma, hepatocellular carcinoma and other tumours. In addition, AFB_1 inhibits DNA synthesis, DNA-dependent RNA polymerase activity, messenger RNA synthesis and protein synthesis (Busby and Wogan, 1984; McLean and Dutton, 1995). Inhibition of protein synthesis may be related to several lesions and signs of aflatoxicosis including fatty liver (failure to mobilise fats from the liver), coagulopathy (inhibition of prothrombin synthesis) and reduced immune function. AFs also affect immune responses in the animals, including reduced response in both cellular responses and humoral factors.

ACUTE AFLATOXICOSIS IN HUMANS

Data confirming clinical indications of acute aflatoxicosis in humans have accumulated in the literature, often anecdotally and usually in subpopulations of developing countries (Shank et al. 1972). Among the first demonstration of direct AF exposure in people, Campbell *et al.* (1970) detected AFM_1 in the urine of Filipinos ingesting peanut butter contaminated with approximately $500 \mu g$ AFB_1/kg. It was estimated that 14% of the ingested aflatoxin was excreted at this metabolite. Suggestive evidence of acute aflatoxicosis in humans has been reported from Taiwan and Uganda (Shank, 1981). Vomiting, abdominal pain, pulmonary oedema and fatty infiltration and necrosis of the liver characterised this syndrome. More extensive documentation of an outbreak of putative aflatoxin poisoning was provided in 1974 from Western India (Krishnamachari *et al.*, 1975a,b). Unseasonal rains and the scarcity of food prompted the consumption of heavily moulded corn (five specimens analysed contained 6 to 16 mg Af/kg (ppm) corn) by people in over 200 villages. Of the 994 patients examined, there were at least 97 fatalities, with death in most instances due to gastrointestinal haemorrhage. The illness was not infectious and occurred only in households where mould-contaminated corn was consumed. Histopathology of liver specimens revealed extensive bile duct proliferation, a lesion often noted in experimental animals following acute AF exposure. The possibility of a concurrent presence of other mycotoxins was not investigated and multifactorial aetiologies were not ruled out in these cases. An incident of acute aflatoxicosis in Kenya (Ngindu *et al.*, 1982) was also associated with consumption of maize highly contaminated with AF. There were 20 hospital admissions with a 20% mortality rate.

A disease of children in Thailand with symptoms similar to those of Reye's syndrome was conjecturally associated with aflatoxin exposure (Shank, 1981). Vomiting, convulsions, coma and death with cerebral oedema and fatty involvement of the liver, kidney and heart characterised the disease. AF poisoning was suggested as a possible cause, because the symptoms of Reye's syndrome in humans are similar to those observed with acute aflatoxicosis in monkeys. Subsequently, AFB_1 was found in the liver, brain, kidney, bile and gastrointestinal tract contents in 22 out of 23 of these fatalities, and AFB_1 levels were higher than in other samples from deceased patients from other causes. In a recent report (Lye *et al.*, 1995), the consumption of AF-contaminated noodles resulted in acute hepatic encephalopathy in children in Malaysia. Up to 3 mg of AF was suspected to be present in a single serving of these contaminated noodles.

MUTAGENICITY AND CARCINOGENICITY IN EXPERIMENTAL MODELS

Mutagenicity of AFB_1 has been demonstrated using many model systems including; HeLa cells, *Bacillus subtilis*, *Neurospora crassa*, *Salmonella typhimurium* (reverse and forward mutation) and Chinese hamster ovary (CHO) cells. AFB_1 is a potent carcinogen in many species of animals, including rodents, non-human primates and fish (Busby and Wogan, 1984). Generally, the liver was the primary target organ affected; however, under certain circumstances, dependent on such variables such as animal species and strain, dose, route of administration and dietary factors, significant numbers of tumours were induced at other sites such as kidney and colon. Most of the published information on AFB_1 carcinogenicity has been obtained from studies in rats, which are highly susceptible to the toxin. Dietary concentrations during prolonged feeding as low as 2 ppb induced cancers. There is an increasing literature in recent years on the carcinogenic responses of the rainbow trout (an even more sensitive species than the rat) and various monkey species (some of whom are possibly more appropriate models for human risk estimation). Such experiments have often examined dose–response characteristics and the influences of such parameters as a route of administration, size and frequency of dose, and the sex, age and strain of the test animal (see Eaton and Groopman, 1994).

AFB_1 has been demonstrated to induce liver tumours in two species of lower primates fed a diet containing 2 mg AFB_1/kg: the tree shrew (*Tupaia glis*) (Reddy *et al.*, 1976) and the marmoset (*Saguinus oedipomidas*) (Lin *et al.*, 1974). All liver tumours in the tree shrew were hepatocellular carcinomas and they developed in a manner similar to those observed in the rat. In contrast, the marmoset histological data revealed an association of cirrhotic changes with liver tumour development. Rhesus monkeys have also been found to be susceptible to AFB_1-induced cancers. In three reports in single animals, two cases of hepatocellular carcinoma (Adamson *et al.*, 1973; Tilak, 1975) and one cholangiocarcinoma was observed in animals treated with AFB_1 for 5.5 to 6 years by an oral or a mixed oral and intramuscular dosing regimen. Data from 47 monkeys, representing three species (rhesus, cynomolgus and African green) receiving AFB_1 by intraperitoneal and/or oral routes for periods greater than 2 months, have been published (Sieber *et al.*, 1979). Primary liver tumour incidence was 19% (5/26) in animals surviving for longer than 6 months and total tumour incidence was 50% (13/26). The five primary liver tumours included two hepatoceullar carcinomas and three haemangioendothelial sarcomas. There were also six gallbladder or bile duct carcinomas that in five cases extended to the liver parenchyma. Thus, there are extensive biological data demonstrating the high potency of AFB_1 as a toxin and carcinogen for a wide variety of animal species.

METABOLISM

Metabolism is critical for the biological activity and disposition of the AFs. AFB_1 undergoes cytochrome P450 (CYP)-catalysed oxidation to various hydroxylated derivatives as well as to two unstable, highly reactive epoxide isomers. Detoxication of AFB_1 is accomplished by enzymic conjugation of the hydroxylated metabolites with moieties such as a glucuronic acid to form glucuronide esters excreted in urine or bile. An alternative route for removal of AFB_1 from the organism involves glutathione *S*-transferase-catalysed reactions of the epoxide metabolites with glutathione and its subsequent excretion in the urine and bile. In the course of AFB_1 metabolism, the reactive electrophilic epoxides can covalently react with various nucleophilic centres in cellular macromolecules such as DNA, RNA, histones and albumin. The consequence of this activation process poses a biological hazard for the cell or organism and constitutes a putative mechanism through which AFB_1 exerts toxic, carcinogenic and genotoxic effects. Initial reports by Shimada and Guengerich (1989) found that CYP3A4 was a major human hepatic cytochrome P450 involved in the bioactivation of AFB_1 to its genotoxic epoxide. Liver samples with increasing levels of CYP3A4 also produced higher amounts of the DNA adduct, AFB_1-N^7-guanine *in vitro*. Using cells expressing five forms of human CYP450 cDNA, Aoyama *et al.* (1990) found that CYP1A2, 2A3, 2B7, 3A3 and 3A4 activated AFB_1 to mutagenic metabolites as assessed by the production of histidine revertants of *Salmonella typhimurium* in the Ames test. These CYPs also catalysed conversion of radiolabelled AFB_1 to DNA-bound derivatives. Seven other human CYPs, 2C8, 2C9, 2D6, 2E1, 2F1, 3A5 and 4B1, did not significantly activate AFB_1 as measured by both the Ames test and the DNA-binding assay. In another report, metabolism of AFB_1 was examined using microsomes derived from human lymphoblastoid cell lines expressing transfected CYP1A2 or CYP3A4 cDNAs and in microsomes prepared from human liver donors (Crespi *et al.*, 1990; Eaton and Gallagher, 1994). Only CYP1A2-expressing lymphoblast microsomes activated AFB_1 to an aflatoxin-8,9-epoxide at both low ($16 \mu M$) and high ($128 \mu m$) AFB_1 concentrations, whereas activation of AFB_1 to the epoxide in CTP3A4-expressing lymphoblast microsomes was detected only at high substrate concentrations. These results suggest that CYP1A2 is a high-affinity P450 enzyme principally responsible for the bioactivation of AFB_1 at low substrate concentrations associated with dietary exposure, whereas CYP3A4 is a relatively low affinity for AFB_1 epoxidation.

Despite the controversies about the specific role of individual human cytochrome P450s in the metabolism of aflatoxin to its 8,9-epoxide, there is no doubt that this epoxide is the critical metabolic step for genotoxic damage. The initial finding supporting this pathway was the identification of the major AFB_1-DNA adduct by Essigmann *et al.* (1977) as 8,9-dihydro-8-(N^7-guanyl)-9-hydroxy-AFB_1 (AFB_1-N^7-guanine). Its presence was subsequently confirmed *in vivo* (Croy *et al.*, 1978). This adduct could lead to subsequent formation of a repair-resistant adduct, depurination or error-prone DNA repair, resulting in single-strand breaks, base pair substitution or frameshift mutations (Hsieh, 1986). Mispairing of the adduct induces both transversion and transition mutations. Such interactions may also result in the activation of oncogenes and/or inactivation of tumour suppressor genes in target organs. The investigation of the interactions and biological consequences of AFB_1 with DNA has been an intensive area of study, since DNA adduct formation is probably a requisite event in the initiation of cancer by AFB_1.

RELATIONSHIP WITH HUMAN HEPATOCELLULAR CARCINOMA

Human hepatocellular carcinoma (HCC) is one of the leading causes of cancer mortality in Asia and Africa. In the People's Republic of China (PRC), this disease accounts for at least 150 000 deaths per year with an incidence rate in some areas of the country approaching 100 cases per 100 000 per year. This malignancy is the third leading cause of cancer mortality in males behind cancer of the oesophagus and stomach as reported by the National Cancer Office of the Ministry of Public Health, PRC (1980). This cancer varies world-wide by at least 100-fold. Over the past 30 years there have been extensive efforts to investigate the association between AF exposure and human HCC. Many epidemiological studies have found that increased AF ingestion correspond to increased HCC incidence (Groopman et al., 1988, 1996; Wogan, 1992; IARC, 1993; Wang, et al., 1996), though several other investigations have not (Campbell et al., 1990; Srivatanakul et al., 1991).

Studies by Yeh and Shen (1986) on the epidemiology of HCC in the Guangxi Autonomous Region of China investigated the interaction between hepatitis B virus (HBV) infection and dietary AF exposure. The staple food of people living in this region during the 1960s and 1970s was corn, which was often contaminated with high levels of AFB_1. In some heavily contaminated areas, AFB_1 content ranged from 53.8 to 303 ppb, while the lightly contaminated regions showed AFB_1 levels in grains of less than 5 ppb. After five to eight years of follow-up, HCC incidence was determined for these two regions of heavy and light AF contamination. Those individuals who were hepatitis B surface antigen (HBsAg)-positive and found to have heavy AF exposure had an HCC incidence of 649 cases per 100 000 compared with 66 cases per 100 000 in AF lightly contaminated areas. Those people who were HBsAg negative and eating heavily contaminated AF diets had an HCC rate of 99 per 100 000 compared with no cases detected in the light contaminated area (Yeh et al., 1989).

Several recent studies have used newly developed molecular biomarkers for AF to confirm these putative interactions between AF exposure and HBV infection in the causation of HCC. A nested case-control study initiated in 1986 in Shanghai collected 18 244 urine samples from healthy males between the ages of 45 and 64. In the subsequent seven years, 50 of these individuals developed HCC. The urine samples for these cases were age- and residence-matched with 267 controls and analysed for both AF biomarkers and HBsAg status. The data revealed a statistically significant increase in the relative risk (RR) = 3.4 for those HCC cases where urinary AFs was detected. For HBsAg-positive people only, the RR = 7, but for individuals with both urinary AFs and positive HBsAg status, RR = 59 (Ross et al., 1992; Qian et al., 1994). These results show a causal relationship between the presence of two specific biomarkers (AFT and HBsAg) and HCC risk.

In Qidong, Jiangsu Province, PRC, liver cancer accounts for 10% of all adult deaths and both HBV and AF exposures are common (Wang, JS et al., 1996). A nested case-control study within a cohort has followed (Kuang *et al.*, 1996) 804 healthy HBsAg-positive individuals (728 male, 76 female) aged 30–65 years. Between 1993 and 1995, 38 of these individuals developed HCC, and age, gender, residence and time of sampling matched serum samples from 34 of these cases to 170 controls. AFB_1-albumin adduct levels were determined by radioimmunoassay. The relative risk for HCC cases among AFB_1-albumin-positive individuals was 2.4 (95% confidence interval (C.I.), 1.2, 4.7). Two other studies have been carried out in Taiwan. In a cohort of 8068 men followed-up for three years, 27 cases of HCC were identified and matched with 120 healthy controls. Serum samples were analysed for AFB_1-albumin adducts by ELISA and AFB_1-DNA adducts were identified by immunohistochemical detection (Yu *et al.*, 1995; Lunn *et al.*, 1997). The proportion of subjects with detectable serum AFB_1-albumin adducts was higher for HCC cases (74%) than matched controls (66%), giving an odds ratio of 1.5. There was also a statistically significant association between detectable levels of AFB_1-albumin adduct and HCC risk among men younger than 52 years old, showing a multivariant-adjusted odds ratio of 5.3.

Wang, L *et al.* (1996) examined 56 cases of HCC in Taiwan diagnosed between 1991 and 1995. Age, sex, residence and date of recruitment from 200 healthy controls from a large cohort study individually matched these cases. Blood samples were analysed for hepatitis B and C viral markers and for aflatoxin-albumin adduct, and urine was tested for aflatoxin metabolites. HBsAg carriers had a significantly increased risk for HCC and after adjustment for HBsAg serostatus, the matched odds ratio was significantly elevated for subjects with high levels of urinary AF metabolites. When stratified into tertiles, a dose–response relationship with HCC was observed. HBsAg-seropositive subjects with high AF exposure had a higher risk than subjects with high AF exposure only or HBsAg seropositivity only. In male HBsAg-seropositive subjects, adjusted odds ratio was 2.8 (95% C.I. = 0.9–9.1) for detectable compared with non-detectable AF-albumin adducts and 5.5 (C.I. = 1.3–23.4) for high compared with low urinary AF metabolite levels. These results strongly suggest that environmental AF exposure enhances the hepatic carcinogenic potential of HBV.

The relationship between AF exposure and development of HCC is further highlighted by the recent molecular biological studies on the p53 tumour suppressor gene, the most common mutated gene detected in many human cancers (Harris, 1995, 1996). Initial results came from three independent studies of p53 mutations in HCCs occurring in populations exposed to high levels of dietary AF and found high frequencies of G→T transversions, with clustering at codon 249 (Bressac *et al.*, 1991; Hsu *et al.*, 1991; Li *et al.*, 1993). In contrast, studies of p53 mutations in HCCs from Japan and other areas where there is little exposure to AF found no mutations at codon 249 (Ozturk *et al.*, 1991). These studies provide a circumstantial linkage between this signature mutation of p53 and AF exposure in HCC from China and Southern Africa.

Fujimoto *et al.* (1994) further examined HCC tissues obtained from two different areas in China: Qidong, where exposure to HBV and AFB_1 is high; and Beijing, where exposure to HBV is high but that of AFB_1 is low. They analysed these tumour tissues for mutations in the p53 gene and loss of heterozygosity for the p53, Rb and APC genes. The frequencies of mutation, loss and aberration of the p53 gene in 25 HCC specimens from Qidong were 60, 58 and 80%, respectively. The frequencies in nine HCC specimens from Beijing were 56, 57 and 78%; however, the frequency of a $G{\rightarrow}T$ transversion at codon 249 in HCCs from Qidong and Beijing were 52 and 0%, respectively. These data show distinct differences in the pattern of p53 mutations at codon 249 between HCCs in Qidong and Beijing and suggest that AFB_1 and/or other environmental carcinogens may contribute to this difference.

The observation of the codon 249 mutation in p53 with AF exposure is not limited to only China and Southern Africa. Senegal is a country where HCC incidence is one of the highest in the world and where people are exposed to high levels of AFs. Fifteen HCC tissues from this country were examined for mutation at codon 249 of the p53 gene (Coursaget *et al.*, 1993) Mutations at codon 249 of the p53 gene were detected in 10 of the 15 tumour tissues tested (67%). This frequency of mutation in codon 249 of the p53 gene is the highest described to date in the literature. Aguilar *et al.* (1994) examined the role of AFB_1 and p53 mutations in HCCs and in normal liver samples from the United States, Thailand and Qidong, China where AFB_1 exposures are negligible, low and high, respectively. The frequency of the $AGG{\rightarrow}AGT$ mutation at codon 249 paralleled the level of AFB_1 exposure, which further supports the hypothesis that AF has a causative and probably early role in human hepatocarcinogenesis.

Results derived from experimental studies have also linked AF as a causative agent in the described p53 mutations. Previous work had shown that AFB_1 exposure causes almost exclusively $G{\rightarrow}T$ transversions in bacteria (Foster *et al.*, 1983) and that AF-epoxide can bind to the particular codon 249 of p53 in a plasmid *in vitro* (Puisieux *et al.*, 1991). Further study (Aguilar *et al.*, 1993) examined the mutagenesis of codons 247–250 of p53 gene by rat liver microsome-activated AFB_1 in human HepG2 cells and found that AFB_1 preferentially induced the transversion of $G{\rightarrow}T$ in the third position of codon 249; however, AFB_1 also induced $G{\rightarrow}T$ and $C{\rightarrow}A$ transversions into adjacent codons, albeit at lower frequencies. Cerutti *et al.* (1994) studied the mutability of codons 247–250 of p53 with AFB_1 in human hepatocytes using the same strategy and found that AFB_1 preferentially induced $G{\rightarrow}T$ transversion in the third position of codon 249, generating the same mutation which is found in a large fraction of HCCs from regions of the world with AFB_1-contaminated food. These experimental results support a role for AFB_1 as an aetiological factor for HCCs in heavily AFB_1-contaminated areas.

Fumonisins

OCCURRENCE IN AGRICULTURAL COMMODITIES

The fumonisins are a family of mycotoxins produced by *Fusarium moniliforme*, a fungus that is a ubiquitous contaminant of corn around the world. Fumonisins are also found at high levels in milk and cereal products (Scott, 1993). Six fumonisins have been isolated and characterized from *F. moniliforme* (Gelderblom *et al.*, 1992b), designated as fumonisin $B_1(FB_1), B_2, B_3, B_4, A_1$ and A_2. Only FB_1 and FB_2 appear to be toxicologically significant (Thiel *et al.*, 1992) and have been studied to any extent. FB_1 and FB_2 were first isolated in 1988; invariably they occur together, with FB_2 at levels of 15–35% those of FB_1. Levels of FB_1 vary yearly, but are consistently in the 0.5 to 2 ppm range in US cornmeal, and have been reported as high as 150 ppm in corn destined for human consumption in South Africa (Binkerd *et al.*, 1993; Scott, 1993; Doko and Visconti, 1994; Visconti and Doko, 1994). Switzerland has a regulatory limit of fumonisins of 1 ppm in human food (FAO, 1996).

TOXICITY

F. moniliforme-contaminated corn has been linked to several human and animal diseases including luekoencephalomalacia in horses, pulmonary oedema in swine, and hepatotoxicity in horses, swine and rats (Thiel *et al.*, 1992). Both culture materials from *F. moniliforme*-inoculated corn and pure FB_1 are capable of producing similar effects in animals (Kellerman *et al.*, 1990; Wilson *et al.*, 1990; Diaz and Boermans, 1994). Neurotoxic and hepatotoxic syndromes may occur singly or together in horses. Neurotoxic symptoms, including loss of feed consumption, lameness, ataxia, oral and facial paralysis and recumbency begin within days after initial consumption of mouldy corn or by direct administration of FB_1 and can be rapidly followed by seizures and morbidity. Focal malacia and liquefaction of cerebral white matter with peripheral haemorrhage is the common pathology. Centrilobular necrosis, fibrosis and bile duct proliferation with increased mitosis, acute inflammation and fatty degeneration of the liver are also characteristic histological findings.

Administration of FB_1 to swine induces pulmonary oedema, especially at higher doses. At lower doses, slowly progressive hepatic disease is most prominent (Thiel *et al.*, 1992). Hepatotoxicity and renal toxicity have been observed following treatment of rats or mice with FB_1. Feeding of FB_2 at dietary levels of 0.05 to 0.1% induced early liver lesions in rats similar to those induced by FB_1 (Gelderblom *et al.*, 1992a).

Recent studies have provided some possible insights into the mechanisms of toxicity (Wolf, 1994). The fumonisins have structural similarity to the long-chain (sphingoid) base backbones of sphingolipids. Wang *et al.* (1991) demonstrated that incubation of rat hepatocytes with fumonisins inhibited incorporation of serine into the sphingosine moiety of cellular sphingolipids with an IC_{50} of

0.1 μM for FB_1. In contrast, FB_1 increased the amount of the biosynthetic intermediate sphinganine, which suggests that fumonisins inhibit the conversion of sphinganine to N-acyl-sphinganines. Consistent with this mechanism, FB_1 inhibited the activity of sphingosine N-acyltransferase (ceramide synthase) in rat liver microsomes and reduced the conversion of sphingoside to ceramide by intact hepatocytes. It was subsequently shown, using mouse cerebellar neurons in culture, that FB_1 inhibited ceramide synthase in mouse brain microsomes with a competitive-like kinetic behaviour with respect to both sphinganine and stearoyl-CoA (Merrill et al., 1993). Thus, disruption of the de novo pathway of sphingolipid biosynthesis may be a critical event in the diseases that have been associated with consumption of fumonisins. The increase in intracellular sphinganine coupled with the concomitant decrease in ceramides may induce apoptosis in these tissues.

CARCINOGENICITY IN ANIMALS

When rats were fed a diet supplemented with the same maize contaminated with F. moniliforme that had caused an outbreak of luekoencephalomalacia in horses, all rats developed hepatic nodules, cholantiofibrosis of cholangiocarcinomas within six months (Wilson et al., 1985). Lifetime studies in rats fed diets containing maize that had been inoculated with F. moniliforme yielded a high incidence (16/20) of liver tumours, while no lesions were seen in control animals. Gelderblom et al. (1991, 1992a) have directly assessed the carcinogenicity of FB_1 in a study where a semi-purified corn-based diet containing 50 mg/kg of pure (> 90%) FB_1, isolated from culture material of F. moniliforme strain MRC 826, was fed to rats over a period of 26 months. The liver was the main target organ in the FB_1-treated rats and the hepatic pathological changes were identical to those previously reported in rats fed culture material of F. moniliforme. All FB_1-treated rats that died or were killed from 18 months onwards suffered from a micro- and macro-nodular cirrhosis and had large expansible nodules of cholangiofibrosis at the hilus of the liver. Ten out of 15 FB_1-treated rats (66%) developed primary HCC. Chronic interstitial nephritis was present in the kidneys of FB_1-treated rats killed after 26 months. No lesions were observed in the oesophagus, heart or forestomach of FB_1-treated rats, which is contrary to previous findings when culture material of the fungus was fed to rats. It appears that FB_1 is responsible for the hepatocarcinogenic and the hepatotoxic effects, but not all the other toxic effects associated with ingestion of food contaminated with F. moniliforme.

Although FB_1 is hepatocarcinogenic, it lacks mutagenic activity in Salmonella mutagenicity tests (Gelderblom et al., 1992b). Both FB_1 and FB_2 lack genotoxic effects in in vivo and in vitro DNA repair assays in primary hepatocytes (Norred et al., 1992). Several rat studies in vivo, in which putative initiated cells were promoted with 2-acetylaminofluorene/carbon tetrachloride treatment, indicated that FB_1 was a poor cancer initiator. FB_1 does exert strong effects on post-initiation events, with primary actions on tumour promotion and selection of initiated cells. Enhanced expression of γ-glutamyltranspeptidase-positive foci is seen following feeding of FB_1 (0.1%) for four weeks to rats initiated with diethylnitrosamine. FB_1 inhibits growth in hepatocytes *in vitro* and *in vivo*. The principal effect of FB_1 in normal and transformed human cells is anti-proliferative, resulting from increased apoptotic cell death as opposed to decreased cell proliferation.

HEALTH EFFECT ON HUMANS

Several ecological studies have examined the relationship between exposure to *Fusarium* toxins and oesophageal cancer. Interpretation of these studies is complicated by the presence of many toxins from many species of fungi in the foodstuffs surveyed. An initial study conducted by Marasas *et al.* (1988) in high-risk and low-risk regions of Transkei (South Africa) for oesophageal cancer, found a correlation between the proportion of kernels in both mouldy and healthy maize samples infected by *F. moniliforme* and oesophageal cancer. In a follow-up study (Marasas *et al.*, 1991), the mean proportion of maize kernel infected with *F. moniliforme* in both healthy and mouldy maize samples from households in the high-incidence oesophageal cancer area were significantly higher (42% and 68%, respectively) than those in the low incidence area (8% and 35%, respectively). FB_1 and FB_2 levels in healthy maize samples from the low-risk area were approximately 20 times lower than those in healthy samples from high-risk areas (Sydenham *et al.*, 1990). Thiel *et al.* (1992) estimated that naturally poisoned horses consumed levels of fuminisins equivalent to those shown to be toxic experimentally, and that humans in high oesophageal cancer risk areas can potentially consume levels higher than those shown to be carci-nogenic in rats.

A number of surveys have been conducted in Henan Province in Northern China. Zhen *et al.* (1984) cultured and isolated fungal strains from samples of wheat, corn, dried sweet potato, rice and soya beans in five counties with a high incidence of oesophageal cancer and three with a low incidence. The frequency of contamination by *F. moniliforme* was significantly higher in food samples from high-risk areas, although the frequency of contamination by all other fungi analysed was also significantly higher in samples from the high-risk counties. A small sampling of corn was collected in 1989 in Linxian and Shangqiu Counties in Henan Province, high- and low-risk areas, respectively, for oesophageal cancer. The incidence of fumonisin contamination of Linxian corn (48%) was about two-fold higher than that of Shangqiu corn (25%). The former samples were frequently co-contaminated with trichothecenes. Of the fumonisin-positive samples, the mean levels in Linxian corn were found to be 872 ng/g for FB_1 and 448 ng/g for FB_2, while the corn from Shangqiu had 890 ng/g for FB_1 and 330 ng/g for FB_2 (Yoshizawa *et al.*, 1994). While these studies, as well as those conducted in South Africa, demonstrate correlations between high oesophageal cancer rates and contamination of foods, primarily corn, with *F. moniliforme*, the specific role of the fumonisins or other related toxins in the aetiology of this cancer remains to be firmly established.

Ochratoxins

OCCURRENCE IN AGRICULTURAL COMMODITIES

Ochratoxins are a group of structurally related metabolites that are produced by *A. ochraceus* and related species, as well as *P. viridicatum* and certain other *Penicillium* species (Kuiper-Goodman and Scott, 1989). The major mycotoxin in this group is ochratoxin A (OA) which appears to be the only one of major toxicological significance. Chemically, OA contains an isocoumarin moiety linked by a peptide bond to phenylalanine. OA has been detected in many food commodities throughout the world, but is found primarily in grains (barley, oats, rye, corn and wheat) grown in northern temperate areas, and results in the contamination of bread and cereal products. In addition to cereals, animal products such as pig's kidneys, blood sausage and coffee beans can be significant human dietary sources of OA. While OA has been found in many foodstuffs in many countries, the highest frequency of OA contamination in foods ($\sim 10\%$) was found in Croatia where Balkan endemic nephropathy (BEN) was prevalent (Plestina *et al.*, 1990). Moreover, average concentrations are higher in foods from nephropathic regions, often exceeding 2 mg/kg (Pepljnjak and Cvetnic, 1985). As of 1995, thirteen countries have established regulatory limits for OA. The acceptable level ranges from 1 to 50 µg/kg for food and from 100 to 1000 µg/kg for animal feeds (FAO, 1996). Current analytic limits of detection are about 1 µg/kg; however, the scientific basis for the promulgated regulatory limits does not appear to have been clearly established (van Egmond, 1991).

TOXICITY

The toxicity of OA varies considerably with dose across animal species (Galtier, 1991). Species also vary in their susceptibility to acute poisoning by OA, oral LD_{50} values ranging from 0.2 to 50 mg/kg body weight as OA are nephrotoxic. Dogs and pigs are most sensitive (0.2 and 1 mg/kg body weight, respectively). Synergistic effects of OA with other mycotoxins, such as citrinin and penicillic acid, in terms of LD_{50} were seen in mice (Sansing *et al.*, 1976). The presence of OA in feed is believed to be the most important cause of spontaneous mycotoxic porcine and poultry nephropathy (Elling *et al.*, 1975; Krogh, 1978). OA induces haematological changes in rats and mice at high dose and produces hepatic toxicity, particularly at higher doses. Administration of an LD_{50} dose (20 mg/kg) of OA to rats induces periportal liver necrosis. OA is teratogenic in mice, rats and hamsters, the major target in the foetus being the developing central nervous system. OA is also immunosuppressive at low doses, affecting immune function at both the level of antibody synthesis and natural killer cell activity (Kuiper-Goodman and Scott, 1989). One toxic mechanism of OA is the inhibition of protein synthesis by competition with phenylalanine in the phenylalanyl-tRNA synthetase-catalysed reaction. OA also inhibits other enzymes that use phenylalanine as a substrate such as phenylalanine hydroxylase. The effect of OA on protein synthesis is followed by an inhibition of RNA synthesis, which might affect proteins with a higher turnover. OA also lowers the level of phosphoenolpyruvate carboxykinase, a key enzyme in gluconeogenesis; this inhibition is reported to be due to a specific degradation of mRNA that codes for this enzyme. Recently, OA was also found to enhance lipid peroxidation both *in vitro* and *in vivo* (IARC, 1993).

CARCINOGENICITY AND MUTAGENICITY

OA has been tested for carcinogenicity by oral administration, employing several protocols, in three strains of mice and one strain of rats. The kidney, in particular, the tubular epithelial cells, was the major site for OA-induced lesions. In male ddY and DDD mice, atypical hyperplasia, cystadenomas and carcinomas of the renal tubular cells were induced, as were neoplastic nodules and hepatocyte tumours of the liver (Kanisawa, 1984). In these strains, mice were fed 50 mg OA/kg diet for 30 weeks followed by basal diet for 40 weeks or 25 mg OA/kg diet for 70 weeks, respectively. No renal tumours were seen in the control animals from either experiment. In B6C3F1 mice, tubular-cell adenomas and carcinomas of the kidneys were induced in male mice and the incidences of hepatocellular adenomas and carcinomas were increased in male and female mice (Bendele *et al.*, 1985). These mice were fed a diet supplemented with crude OA (84%) at 0, 1 or 40 mg/kg diet for two years. While no kidney tumours were seen in the control or low-dose groups, hepatocellular tumours were seen in both the low- and high-dose OA groups. In male and female F344 rats, OA induced non-neoplastic (degeneration, karyomegaly, proliferation, cytoplasmic alteration, hyperplasia) and neoplastic effects (adenomas, and carcinomas with metastases) in the kidneys; the incidence of fibroadenomas of the mammary glands was also increased in female rats (Boorman, 1989). These animals received 0, 21, 70 or 210 μg/kg body weight of pure OA by gavage, five days a week for 2 years. Kidney tumours increased in a dose-related manner in animals of each sex.

OA is genotoxic in *E. coli* by means of induction of the SOS DNA-repair activity and is mutagenic in NIH3T3 cells expressing selected cytochrome P450s and carrying a shuttle vector containing the bacterial *lacZ* gene as a reporter gene (IARC, 1993). Increases in sister chromatid exchange rates have been observed in CHO cells in the presence of S9 mixture, and in peripheral human lymphocytes cultured in a conditioned medium. OA was also mutagenic in several *Salmonella* tester strains when this conditioned medium from OA-treated hepatocytes was used. By contrast, OA is not mutagenic in standard Ames assays, with or without S9. OA induced DNA single-strand breaks in cultured mouse and CHO cells, and formed DNA adducts in mouse kidney and to a lesser extent in liver and spleen (Dirheimer and Creppy, 1991).

HEALTH EFFECT ON HUMANS

It has been suggested for several decades that excessive exposure to OA plays a substantive role in the development of BEN (Krogh 1974). BEN is a bilateral, non-inflammatory, chronic nephropathy in which the kidneys are extremely reduced in size and weight, and show diffuse cortical fibrosis (Radovanovic, 1991; Vukelic *et al.*, 1991). Functional impairment is characterised by progressive hypercreatininaemia, hyperuraemia and hypochromic anaemia. In an endemic region of Croatia (Sostaric and Vukelic, 1991), about 14 villages and approximately 10 000 people are estimated to be at high risk. Evidence of an extremely high incidence of urinary tract tumours in the endemic areas for BEN, particularly of urothelial tumours of the pelvis and ureter has been described, suggesting a common causative agent. In Bulgaria, 16 cases of urinary tract tumours were reported among 33 autopsied patients with BEN. Other case-control studies have indicated lower, but consistent associations between nephropathies in the endemic areas and urinary tract tumours. A survey of the geographical distribution of BEN and urinary tract tumours was carried out in the early 1970s in central Serbia. This study indicated that the annual incidence of cancer of the renal pelvis and ureter was 39 per 100 000 in counties affected by BEN and 15 per 100 000 in the non-endemic counties. A study of Croatia using records of urinary tract tumours collected between 1974 and 1989 reported significantly more tumours of the renal pelvis and ureter in areas of the County of Slavonski Brod in endemic as opposed to non-endemic areas. More urinary tract tumour cases were seen in women than men in these endemic areas. Smaller differences in the incidence of bladder cancer were seen between the two areas.

A causal relationship between exposure to OA and these human diseases are suggested by: (i) similarities in the morphological and functional renal impairment induced by OA in animals and those observed in BEN; and (ii) the finding that foods from the endemic areas are more heavily contaminated with OA than foods from disease-free areas. The presence of OA in human blood has been suggested as an indicator for indirect assessment of exposure to this nephrotoxic agent. In several countries, therefore, human blood has been collected with the purpose of obtaining more information on the intake of OA. Analysis of serum samples in European countries from nearly a dozen studies revealed that blood from healthy humans was contaminated with OA at concentrations of 0.1–40 ng/ml. The frequency of contamination of human sera, which ranged from 4 to 57%, seems to indicate continuous, widespread exposure of humans to OA (Petova-Bocharova and Castegnaro, 1991).

Petkova-Bocharova *et al.* (1988) reported, in a study conducted in Bulgaria, the association between BEN and/or urinary tract tumours and OA content in blood samples taken from 187 subjects living in endemic villages and 125 individuals in non-endemic villages. Among 61 patients with BEN and/or urinary tract tumours, 14.8% had levels of 1–2 ng/ml and 11.5% had more than 2 ng/ml OA in their blood. This proportion was significantly higher than that in a control group of 63 individuals from unaffected families in the endemic villages (7.9% and 3.2%, respectively). A significantly larger proportion of blood samples collected from patients with BEN and/or urinary tract tumours (26.7%) contained OA than those from healthy people living in the same endemic area (12.1%) or from healthy people living in non-endemic areas of Bulgaria. Analysis of OA contamination of home-produced, home-stored beans and corn indicated that significantly more samples from the endemic area than the non-endemic area contained detectable levels of OA (54% versus 12%).

A recent case-control study provides some molecular evidence for the possible role of ochratoxin in the development of urinary tract tumours in Bulgaria (Pfohl-Leszkowicz *et al.*, 1993). Tumour tissues from three kidneys and five bladders of Bulgarian patients undergoing surgery for cancer, and from three non-malignant kidneys collected from French subjects were analysed for DNA adducts. Several adducts with the same rate of flow values as those obtained from mouse kidney after treatment with OA were detected, mainly in kidney but also in bladder tissues from Bulgaria. No adducts were detected in French kidney tissues. Prospective, nested-case control studies would be useful to more fully characterise the role of ochratoxins in urinary tract tumours in the high-risk areas of Europe. Many of the fungi that produce ochratoxins also produce other mycotoxins. Currently, it is not possible to estimate the risk to human health from ochratoxin exposure, but this is an area of a very active research investigation.

Trichothecenes

The trichothecenes are a family of over 150 structurally related compounds (National Research Council, 1983; Grove, 1988; Beasley, 1989) produced by several fungal genera (*Fusarium, Cephalosporium, Myrothecium, Stachybotrys* and *Trichoderma*). Chemically, they are sesquiterpenes characterised by a double bond at position C-9, an epixode ring at C-12, and various patterns of hydroxy and acetoxy substitutions at position C-3, C-4, C-15, C-7 and C-8. There are four major naturally occurring trichothecene mycotoxins (deoxynivalenol, nivalenol, T-2 toxin and diacetoxyscirpenol) produced in food and fed by *Fusarium* species. Despite the extensive literature on the trichothecenes that focuses on their agricultural significance, there is not a comparable epidemiological database that can be used to assess human health impact from exposure to these compounds.

DEOXYNIVALENOL

Deoxynivalenol (DON) is probably the most widely distributed *Fusarium* mycotoxin. Its occurrence in foods in North America, Japan and Europe is common, but the concentrations are generally low (Tanaka *et al.*, 1988; Scott, 1989, 1990; WHO, 1990); however, its contamination in cereals in some developing countries, particularly in southern China (Luo, 1988) and parts of South America and Africa, is usually high during most years. In 1980 and 1981 in Canada and 1982 in the United States, DON was found in wheat as the result of severe infestations with the wheat scab fungus, *F. graminearum*. In both countries, the soft winter wheats were most severely affected. In Canada, dried corn was found to contain higher levels of DON. Currently, several countries have set the guidelines or official tolerance levels for DON in food and feed (FAO, 1996). The range varies from 0.005 to 4 mg/kg. Acute mycotoxicosis affecting fairly large numbers of people and caused by ingestion of DON-contaminated food have been reported in China, India and some other countries (Luo, 1988; Bhat *et al.*, 1989; WHO, 1990; Miller, 1991). The toxicology of this agent was recently reviewed by Rotter *et al.* (1996).

T-2 TOXIN

T-2 toxin is produced primarily by *F. sporotrichioides* and has been reported in many parts of the world (Ueno, 1983; Scott, 1989; WHO, 1990). It is formed in large quantities under the usual circumstance of prolonged wet weather at harvest. Natural contamination of foods and feeds by T-2 toxin in the United States has been reported in only one incident involving heavily moulded corn. An official tolerance level of 0.1 mg/kg was established for T-2 toxin in grains in Russia (FAO, 1996).

T-2 toxin, as a representative trichothecene, has been well studied for its toxic effects in many animal models and has been reviewed in detail (Ueno, 1983, 1987; Beasley, 1989). General signs of toxicity in animals include weight loss, decreased feed conversion, feed refusal, vomiting, bloody diarrhoea, severe dermatitis, haemorrhage, decreased egg production, abortion and death. Histological lesions consist of necrosis and haemorrhage in proliferating tissues of the intestinal mucosa, bone marrow, spleen, testis and ovary. T-2 toxin can alter haemostatis and affect cellular immune response in animals, as well as a strong inhibitor of protein and DNA synthesis. T-2 toxin is also teratogenic to mice and rats. As the major trichothecene mycotoxin, T-2 toxin has been implicated in a variety of animal and human toxicoses, such as alimentary toxic aleukia, Msleni joint disease, scabby grain toxicosis and Kashin–Beck disease (Beardall and Miller, 1994).

Other mycotoxins

The following briefly describes a number of mycotoxins that have been extensively studied in field and laboratory investigations. The brevity of their review should not be equated with toxicological significance, but only reflects the limited space available in this chapter. Since contamination of food by these mycotoxins varies greatly from year to year, there is every reason to believe that in the future one of these agents will be viewed as a major public health problem.

ZEARALENONE

Zearalenone (ZEN) is produced primarily by *F. graminearum* and is among the most widely distributed *Fusarium* mycotoxins. It is associated mainly with maize but occurs in modest concentrations in wheat, barley, sorghum and other commodities (Kuiper-Goodman *et al.*, 1987). An official tolerance level of 1 mg/kg ZEN in grains, fats and oils was established in Russia. Proposed levels in other countries are 0.2 mg/kg ZEN in maize in Brazil and 0.03 mg/kg in all food in Romania. ZEN has oestrogenic effects in domestic pigs and experimental animals (Prelusky *et al.*, 1994). F-2 toxicosis and hyperoestrogenism are two diseases in pigs caused by ZEN. ZEN is teratogenic to mice and rats and induces chromosomal anomalies in cultured rodent cells. Its carcinogenicity was tested by administration through the diet in one experiment in mice and in two experiments in rats. An increased incidence of hepatocellular adenomas was observed in female mice and of pituitary adenomas in mice of both sexes. No increase in the incidence of tumours was observed in rats (IARC, 1993). Given the recent concerns about the significance of human environmental oestrogen exposure, the hormonal activity of this mycotoxin warrants a risk assessment study.

STERIGMATOCYSTIN

Several species of *Aspergillus, Penicillium luteum* and a *Bipolaris* species produce sterigmatocystin. Chemically, sterigmatocystin resembles the AFT and is a precursor in the biosynthesis of AFT. It has been detected at low concentrations in green coffee, mouldy wheat and in the rind of hard Dutch cheese. Sterigmatocystin is a hepatotoxin, but is less potent than aflatoxin B_1. It was mutagenic in the Ames test, the *Rec* assay, and the *Bacillus subtilis* assay (Berry, 1988). It can bind covalently to DNA and form DNA adducts. It has been established that sterigmatocystin is carcinogenic to rats and mice, mainly inducing liver tumours. The DNA adduct formation of sterigmatocystin was recently reviewed by McConnell and Garner (1994).

CITREOVIRIDIN

Citreoviridin, also called yellow rice toxin, was originally isolated from cultures of moulds obtained from rice associated with a disease called cardiac beriberi that had occurred for three centuries in Japan (Ueno, 1974). The disease is characterised by palpitation, nausea, vomiting, rapid and difficult breathing, cold and cyanotic extremities, rapid pulse, abnormal heart sounds, low blood pressure, restlessness and violent mania leading to respiratory failure and death. Citreoviridin induced some signs resembling cardiac beriberi in experimental animals, such as paralysis, dyspnoea, cardiovascular disturbances and loss of eyesight. The natural occurrence of citreoviridin in corn and other foods and feedstuffs has also been observed (Council for Agricultural Science and Technology, 1989). Several species of *Penicillium* and a single species of *Aspergillus* have been reported to produce this toxin. Cirreoviridin and afla-toxin were found to occur simultaneously in corn; however, it is not clear if there is any enhanced toxicity from simultaneous exposure to these agents.

CITRININ

Citrinin is a yellow-coloured mycotoxin that is produced by several *Penicillium* and *Aspergillus* species. Citrinin has been found to occur in cereal grains such as wheat, barley, corn and rice. Concentrations found in these grains are often several times higher than for accompanying OA (Scott, 1994). Citrinin binds *in vitro* to human serum protein, however, no evidence could be obtained of interaction with DNA (Barber *er al.*, 1987). Like OA, citrinin causes kidney damage in laboratory animals similar to swine nephropathy, and may interact synergistically with OA in cases of swine nephropathy in Denmark (Kroch, 1978).

PATULIN

Patulin is produced primarily by *P. expansum*, though other *Pencillium* and *Aspergillus* species can also act as patulin producers (Scott, 1994). Commodities found contaminated with patulin are mainly fruit and fruit juices in Europe and North America. Patulin is chemically stable in apple and grape juices, and may constitute a potential threat to humans. Currently, 11 countries have set regulatory limits for patulin in fruit juice, the levels ranging from 30 to 50 μg/l (FAO, 1996). The toxicity of patulin has been studied in many experimental models including chicken, quail, cat, cattle, rabbit, mice and rats. The toxic effects on these animals were found to be oedema and haemorrhage in brain and lungs, capillary damage in the liver, spleen and kidney, paralysis of motor nerves, and convulsions (Beardall and Miller, 1994). Patulin is also an immunosuppressive agent that inhibits multiple aspects of macrophage function (Pestka and Bondy, 1994).

CYCLOPIAZONIC ACID

Cyclopiazonic acid (CPA) is produced by several species of *Penicillium* and *Aspergillus*, and was found to occur naturally in corn, peanuts, cheese and in kodo millet that was implicated in natural human intoxication in India (Rao and Husain, 1985). CPA is toxic to the gastrointestinal tract, liver, heart, kidney and skeletal muscle in experimental animals (Voss *et al.*, 1990).

TREMORGENIC MYCOTOXINS

These mycotoxins, including penitrems, paspalitrems, lolitrems, aflatrem and fumitremorgens, are produced by several species of *Penicillium, Aspergillus, Claviceps* and *Acremonium.* Tremorgenic mycotoxins are found to occur in corn, mouldy silage, cream cheese, walnuts, hamburger bun and beer, and have been implicated in the aetiology of several tremorgenic syndromes (staggers syndromes) in cattle, dog and human (Cole and Dorner 1986; Hocking *et al.*, 1988). Typically, irritability, muscle tremor, uncoordinated movements and a general weakness in the legs characterise these intoxications. More severely affected animals are not able to stand. The toxic effects are aggravated when animals are forced to move. Deaths are indirect, usually from dehydration, pneumonia or drowning. An anectodal case of human intoxication happened to a physician who became actually ill approximately 4 hours after consuming about 30 ml of mouldy beer contaminated with penitrem A and *P. crustosum.* Self-described symptoms included tremor, throbbing frontal headache, feverish feeling, nausea, vomiting, double vision, weakness and bloody diarrhoea. All symptoms in this individual disappeared, with no apparent residual effects, after 30 hours (Council for Agricultural Science and Technology, 1989).

Summary

This chapter has briefly reviewed a number of the mycotoxins that are of concern to toxicologists in both the regulatory and experimental setting. This review is dominated by aflatoxin, which is overwhelmingly the most highly studied mycotoxin. Aflatoxin is a human carcinogen and its presence constitutes a major economic and health problem worldwide; however, it is by no means the singular toxic mycotoxin that is found in foods. Some of the major mycotoxins, such as the fumonisins, have only recently been discovered. Critically, in experimental models, the toxicological impact from mycotoxins ranges from acute toxicity to immune suppression to cancer, and very few studies to date have examined the potential increased toxicological interactions from multiple mycotoxin exposure. Thus, in the future a more generic approach to the study of these compounds is required is to fulfil the needs of the risk assessment community that is trying to promulgate the regulatory framework required to limit the health impacts of these naturally occurring toxins.

Acknowledgements

Financial support for the authors was provided in part by USPHS grants P30 ES03819, P01 ES06052 and R01-CA39416.

References

Adamson RH, Correa P and Dalgard DW (1973) Occurrence of a primary liver carcinoma in a Rhesus monkey fed aflatoxin B1. *Journal of National Cancer Institute*, **50**, 549–553.

Aguilar F., Hussain SP and Cerutti P (1993) Aflatoxin B_1 induces the transversion of G→ T in codon 249 of the p53 tumor suppressor gene in human hepatocytes. *Proceedings of National Academy of Science, USA*, **90**, 8586–8590.

Aguilar F, Harris CC, Sun T, Hollstein M and Cerutti P (1994) Geographic variation of p53 mutational profile in nonmalignant human liver. *Science*, **264**, 1317–1319.

Aoyama T, Yamano S, Guzelian PS, Gelboin HV and Gonzalez FJ (1990) Five of 12 forms of vaccinia virus-expressed human hepatic cytochrome P450 metabolically activate aflatoxin B1. *Proceedings of National Academy of Science, USA*, **87**, 4790–4793.

Barber J, Cornford JL, Howard TD and Sharples D (1987) The structure of citrinin *in vivo*. *Journal of Chemical Society, Perkins Transactions*, **1**, 2743–2744.

Beardall JM and Miller JD (1994) Diseases in humans with mycotoxins as possible causes. In *Mycotoxins in Grain: Compounds Other Than Aflatoxins*, Miller JD and Trenholm HL (eds), Eagan Press, St. Paul, MN, pp. 487–539.

Beasley VR (1989) *Trichothecene Mycotoxicosis: Pathophysiologic Effects*, Vols I and II, CRC Press, Boca Raton, Florida.

Bendele AM, Carlton WW, Krogh P and Lillehoj EB (1985) Ochratoxin A carcinogenesis in the (C57B1/6J x C3H)F1 mouse. *Journal of the National Cancer Institute*, **75**, 733–742.

Berry C (1988) The pathology of mycotoxins. *Journal of Pathology*, **154**, 301–311.

Bhat RV, Beedu SR, Ramakrishna Y and Munshi KL (1989) Outbreak of trichothecene mycotixocosis associated with consumption of mould-damaged wheat products in Kashmir Valley, India, *Lancet*, **i**, 35–37.

Binkerd KA, Scott DH, Everson RJ, Sullivan JM and Robinson FR (1993) Fumonisin contamination of the 1991 Indian corn crop and its effects on horses. *Journal of Veterinary Diagnosis and Investigation*, **5**, 653–655.

Boorman G (1989) NTP technical report on the toxicology and carcinogenesis studies of ochratoxin A in F344/N rats (gavage studies). *National Institute of Health Publication*, No. 88, 2813.

Bressac B, Kew M, Wands J and Ozturk M (1991) Selective G to T mutations of p53 gene in hepatocellular carcinoma from Southern Africa. *Nature*, **350**, 429–431.

Busby WF and Wogan GN (1981) Trichothecenes. In *Mycotoxins and N-Nitro-Compounds: Environmental Risks*, Vol. II, Shank RC (ed), CRC Press, Boca Raton, Florida, pp. 29–45.

Busby WF and Wogan GN (1984) Aflatoxins. In *Chemical Carcinogenesis*, Searle CE (ed), American Chemical Society, Washington, DC, pp. 945–1136.

Campbell TC, Caedo JP Jr, Bulatao-Jayme J, Salamat L and Engel RW (1970) Aflatoxin M1 in human urine. *Nature*, **227**, 403–404.

Campbell TC, Chen JS, Liu CB, Li JY, and Parpia B (1990) Nonassociation of aflatoxin with primary liver cancer in a cross-sectional ecological survey in the People's Republic of China. *Cancer Research*, **50**, 6882–6893.

Castegnaro M, Hunt DC, Sansone EB, Schuller PL, Siriwardana MG, Telling GM, van Egmond HP and Walker EA (1980) *Laboratory Decontamination and Destruction of Aflatoxins B1, B2, G1, G2 in Laboratory Wasters*, IARC Scientific Publications No. 37, IARC, Lyon France.

Cerutti P, Hussain P, Pourzand C and Aguilar F (1994) Mutagenesis of the H-ras proto-oncogene and the p53 tumor suppressor gene. *Cancer Research*, **54**, 1934S–1938S.

Chu FS, Fan TS, Zhang GS, Xu YC, Faust S and McMahon PL (1987) Improved enzyme-linked immunosorbent assay for aflatoxin B1 in agricultural commodities. *Journal of The Association of Official Analytical Chemists*, **70**, 854–857.

Ciegler A, Burmaister HR, Vesonder RF and Hesseltine CW (1981) Mycotoxins: Occurrence in the environment. In *Mycotoxins and N-Nitro-Compounds: Environmental Risks*. Vol. I, Shank RC (ed), CRC Press, Boca Raton, Florida, pp. 1–50.

Cole RJ and Cox RH (1981) *Handbook of Toxic Fungal Metabolites*, Academic Press, Inc., New York.

Cole RJ and Dorner JW (1986) Role of fungal tremorgens in animal disease. In *Mycotoxins and Phycotoxins*, Steyn PS and Vleggaar R (eds), Elsevier Scientific Publishing Co., Amsterdam, The Netherlands, pp. 501–511.

Council for Agricultural Sciences and Technology (1989) Mycotoxins: Economic and health risks, Report No. 116, Ames, Iowa, pp. 1–70.

Coursaget P, Depril N, Chabaud M, Nandi R, Mayelo V, LeCann P and Yvonnet B (1993) High prevalence of mutations at codon 249 of the p53 gene in hepatocellular carcinomas from Senegal. *The British Journal of Cancer*, **67**, 1395–1397.

Crespi CL, Steimel DT, Aoyama T, Gelboin HV and Gonzalez FJ (1990) Stable expression of human cytochrome P450IA2 cDNA in a human lymphoblastoid cell line: role of the enzyme in the metabolic activation of aflatoxin B1, *Molecular Carcinogenesis*, **3**, 5–8.

Croy RG, Essigmann JM, Reinhold VN and Wogan GN (1978) Identification of the principal aflatoxin B1-DNA adduct *in vivo* in rat liver. *Proceedings of National Academy of Science, USA*, **75**, 1745–1749.

Diaz GJ and Boermans HJ (1994) Fumonisin toxicosis in domestic animals: a review. *Veterinary and Human Toxicology*, **36**, 548–555.

Dirheimer G and Creppy EE (1991) Mechanism of action of ochratoxin A. In *Mycotoxins, Endemic Nephropathy and Urinary Tract Tumors*, Castegnaro M, Plestina R, Dirheimer G, Chernozemsky IN and Bartsch H (eds), IARC Scientific Publication No. 115, IARC, Lyon, France, pp. 145–151.

Doko MB and Visconti A (1994) Occurrence of fumonisins B1 and B2 in corn and corn-based human foodstuffs in Italy. *Food Additives and Contamination*, **11**, 433–439.

Eaton DL and Gallagher EP (1994) Mechanisms of aflatoxin carcinogenesis. *Annual Review of Pharmacology and Toxicology*, **34**, 135–172.

Eaton DL and Groopman JD (1994) *The Toxicology of Aflatoxins: Human Health, Veterinary, and Agricultural Significance*, Academic Press, Inc., San Diego.

Elling F, Hald B, Jacobsen C and Krogh P (1975) Spontaneous toxic nephropathy in poultry associated with ochratoxin A. *Acta Pathologica et Microbiologica Scandinavica*, Section A, **83**, 739–741.

Ellis WO, Smith JP, Simpson BK and Oldham JH (1991) Aflatoxin in food: occurrence, biosynthesis, effects on organisms, detection, and methods of control. *Critical Review of Food Science and Nutrition*, **30**, 403–439.

Essigmann JM, Croy RG, Nadzan AM, Busby WF Jr, Reinhold VN, Buchi G and Wogan GN (1977) Structural identification of the major DNA adduct formed by aflatoxin B1 in vitro. *Proceedings of National Academy of Science, USA*, **74**, 1870–1874.

Food and Agricultural Organization of The United Nations (1996) *Worldwide Regulations for Mycotoxins*, FAO, Rome.

Foster PL, Eisenstadt E and Miller JH (1983) Base substitution mutation induced by metabolically activated aflatoxin B$_1$. *Proceedings of National Academy of Science, USA*, **80**, 2695–2698.

Fujimoto Y, Hampton LL, Wirth PJ, Wang NK, Xie JP and Thorgeirsson SS (1994) Alterations of tumor suppressor genes and allelic losses in human hepatocellular carcinoma in China. *Cancer Research*, **54**, 281–285.

Galtier P (1991) Pharmacokinetics of ochratoxin A in animals. In *Mycotoxin, Endemic Nephropathy and Urinary Tract Tumors*, Castegnaro M, Plestina R, Dirheimer G, Chernozemsly IN, and Bartsch H (eds), IARC Scientific Publications No. 115, Lyon, France, pp. 187–200.

Gelderblom WC, Kriek NP, Marasas WF and Thiel PG (1991) Toxicity and carcinogenicity of the Fusarium moniliforme metabolite, fumonisin B1, in rats. *Carcinogenesis*, **12**, 1247–1251.

Gelderblom WC, Semple E, Marasas WF and Farber E (1992a) The cancer-initiating potential of the fumonisin B mycotoxins. *Carcinogenesis*, **13**, 433–437.

Gelderblom WC, Marasas WF, Vleggaar R, Thiel PG and Cawood ME (1992b) Fumonisins: isolation, chemical characterization and biological effects. *Mycopathologia*, **117**, 11–16.

Groopman JD and Donahue KF (1988) Aflatoxin, a human carcinogen: determination in foods and biological samples by monoclonal antibody affinity chromatography. *Journal of The Association of Official Analytical Chemists*, **71**, 861–867.

Groopman JD, Cain LG and Kensler TW (1988) Aflatoxin exposure in human populations and relationship to cancer. *CRC Critical Review of Toxicology*, **19**, 113–145.

Groopman JD, Wang J-S and Scholl PF (1996) Molecular biomarkers for aflatoxins: from adducts to gene mutations to human liver cancer. *Canadian Journal of Physiology and Pharmacology*, **74**, 203–209.

Grove JF (1988) Non-macrocyclic trichothecenes. *Natural Products Reports*, **15**, 187–209.

Harris CC (1995) Deichman Lecture-p53 tumor suppressor gene: at the crossroads of molecular carcinogenesis, molecular epidemiology and cancer risk assessment. *Toxicology Letters*, **82/83**, 1–7.

Harris CC (1996) p53 tumor suppressor gene: from the basic research laboratory to the clinic – an abridged historical perspective. *Carcinogenesis*, **17**, 1187–1198.

Hocking AD, Holds K and Tobin NF (1988) Intoxication by tremorgenic mycotoxin (Penitrem A) in a dog. *Australian Veterinary Journal*, **65**, 82–85.

Hsieh DPH (1986) Genotoxicity of mycotoxins. In *New Concepts and Developments in Toxicology*, Chambers PL, Gebring P and Sakai F (Eds), Elsevier, New York, pp. 251–259.

Hsu IC, Metcalf RA, Sun T, Wesh JA, Wang NJ and Harris CC (1991) Mutational hotspot in the p53 gene in human hepatocellular carcinomas. *Nature*, **350**, 427–428.

IARC Working Group on the Evaluation of Carcinogenic Risks to Humans (1993) *Some Naturally Occurring Substances: Food Items and Constituents, Heterocyclic Aromatic Amines and Mycotoxins*, Vol. 56, IARC, Lyon, France.

Kanisawa M (1984) Synergistic effect of citrinin on hepatorenal carcinogenesis of ochratoxin A in mice, In *Toxigenic Fungi, Their Toxins and Health Hazard*, Kurata H and Ueno Y (eds), Japanese Association of Mycotoxicology, Tokyo, Japan, pp. 245–254.

Kellerman TS, Marasas WF, Thiel PG, Gelderblom WC, Cawood M and Coetzer JA (1990) Leukoencephalomalacia in two horses induced by oral dosing of fumonisin B1. *Onderstepoort Journal of Veterinary Research*, **57**, 269–275.

Koeltzow DE and Tanner SN (1990) Comparative evaluation of commercially available aflatoxin test methods. *Journal of the Association of Official Analytical Chemists*, **73**, 584–589.

Krishnamachari KAVR, Bhat RV, Nagarajan V and Tilak TBG (1975a) Investigations into an outbreak of hepatitis in parts of Western India. *The Indian Journal of Medical Research*, **63**, 1036–1049.

Krishnamachari KAVR, Nagarajan V, Bhat RV and Tilak TBG (1975b) Hepatitis due to aflatoxicosis. An outbreak in Western India. *Lancet*, **i**, 1061–1062.

Krogh P (1974) Mycotoxin porcine nephropathy: a possible model for Balkan endemic nephropathy. In *Endemic Nephropathy*, Puchlev A, Dinev IV, Milev B and Doichinov D (eds), Bulgarian Academy of Sciences, Sofia, Bulgaria, pp. 266–270.

Krogh P (1978) Causal associations of mycotoxin nephropathy. *Acta Pathologica et Microbiologica Scandinavica*, Section A, supplement **269**, 7–28.

Kuang S-Y, Fang X, Lu P-X, Zhang Q-N, Wu Y, Wang J-B, Zhu Y-R, Groopman JD, Kensler TW and Qian G-S (1996) Aflatoxin-albumin adducts and risk for hepato-cellular carcinoma in residents of Qidong, People's Republic of China. *Proceedings of American Association for Cancer Research*, **37**, 1714.

Kuiper-Goodman T and Scott PM (1989) Risk assessment of the mycotoxin ochratoxin A. *Biomedical and Environmental Sciences*, **2**, 179–248.

Kuiper-Goodman T, Scott PM and Watanabe H (1987) Risk assessment of the mycotoxin zearalenone. *Regulatory Toxicology and Pharmacology*, **7**, 253–306.

Li D, Gao Y, He L, Wang NJ and Gu J (1993) Aberrations of p53 gene in human hepatocellular carcinoma from China. *Carcinogenesis*, **14**, 169–173.

Lin JJ, Liu C and Svoboda DJ (1974) Long term effects of aflatoxin B1 and viral hepatitis on marmoset liver (a preliminary report). *Laboratory Investigation*, **30**, 267–278.

Lunn, RM, Zhang Y-J, Wang L-Y, Chen C-J, Lee P-H, Lee C-S, Tsai W-Y and Santella RM (1997) p53 mutations, chronic hepatitis B virus infection, and aflatoxin exposure in hepatocellular carcinoma in Taiwan. *Cancer Research*, **57**, 3471–3477.

Luo Y (1988) Fusarium toxins contamination of cereals in China. In *Proceedings of the 7th International IUPAC Symposium on Mycotoxins and Phycotoxins*, Aibara K, Kumagai S, Ohtsubo K and Yoshizawa T (eds), Japanese Association of Mycotoxicology, Tokyo, Japan, pp. 97–98.

Lye MS, Ghazali A, Mohan J, Alwin N and Nair RC (1995) An outbreak of acute hepatic encephalopathy due to severe aflatoxicosis in Malaysia. *American Journal of Tropical Medicine and Hygiene*, **53**, 68–72.

Marasas WFO, Jaskiewicz K, Venter FS and van Schalkwyk DJ (1988) *Fusarium moniliforme* contamination of maize in oesophageal cancer areas in Transkei. *South African Medical Journal*, **74**, 110–114.

Marasas WFO, Wehner FC, van Rensburg SJ and van Schalkwyk DJ (1991) Mycoflora of corn produced in human esophageal cancer areas in Transkei, southern Africa. *Phytopathology*, **71**, 792–796.

McConnell IR and Garner RC (1994) DNA adducts of aflatoxins, sterigmatocystin and other mycotoxins. *IARC Scientific Publications*, **125**, 49–55.

McLean M and Dutton MF (1995) Cellular interactions and metabolism of aflatoxin: an update. *Pharmacology and Therapeutics*, **65**, 163–192.

Merrill AH Jr, van Echten G, Wang E and Sandhoff K (1993) Fumonisin B1 inhibits sphingosine (sphinganine) N-acyltransferase and *de novo* sphingolipid biosynthesis in cultured neurons *in situ*. *The Journal of Biological Chemistry*, **268**, 27299–27306.

Miller JD (1991) Significance of grain mycotoxins for health and nutrition. In *Fungi and Mycotoxins in Stored Products (ACIAR Proceedings 36)*, Champ BR, Highley E, Hocking AD and Pitt JL (eds), Australian Center for International Agriculture Research, Canberra, pp. 126–135.

Miller JD and Trenholm HL (1994) *Mycotoxins in Grain: Compounds Other Than Aflatoxins*, Eagan Press, St. Paul, MN.

National Cancer Office of the Ministry of Public Health, PRC (1980) *Studies on mortality rates of cancer in China*. People's Publishing House, Beijing, PRC.

National Research Council (1983) *Protection Against Trichothecene Mycotoxins*. National Academy Press, Washington, DC.

Ngindu A, Johnson BK, Kenya PR, Ngira JA, Ocheng DM, Nandwa H, Omondi TN, Jansen AJ, Ngare W, Kaviti JN, Gatei D and Siongok TA (1982) Outbreak of acute hepatitis caused by aflatoxin poisoning in Kenya *Lancet*, **i**, 1346–1348.

Norred WP, Plattner RD, Vesonder RF, Bascon CW and Voss KA (1992) Effects of selected secondary metabolites of *Fusarium moniliforme* on unscheduled synthesis of DNA by rat primary hepatocytes. *Food and Chemical Toxicology*, **30**, 233–237.

Ozturk M and collaborators (1991) p53 mutation in hepatocellular carcinoma after aflatoxin exposure. *Lancet*, **338**, 1356–1359.

Pepljnjak S and Cvetnic Z (1985) The mycotoxicological chain and contamination of food by ochratoxin A in the nephropathic and non-nephropathic areas in Yugoslavia. *Mycopathologia*, **90**, 147–153.

Pestka JJ and Bondy GS (1994) Immunotoxic effects of mycotoxins. In *Mycotoxins in Grain: Compounds Other Than Aflatoxins*, Miller JD and Trenholm HL (eds), Eagan Press, St. Paul, MN, pp. 339–358.

Petkova-Bocharova T and Castegnaro M (1991) Ochratoxin A in human blood in relation to Balkan endemic nephropathy and urinary tract tumors in Bulgaria. In *Mycotoxin, Endemic Nephropathy and Urinary Tract Tumors*, Castegnaro M, Plestina R, Dirheimer G, Chernozemsky IN and Bartsch H (eds), IARC Scientific Publications, No. 115, Lyon, France, pp. 135–137.

Petkova-Bocharova T, Chernozemsky IN and Castegnaro M (1988) Ochratoxin A in human blood in relation to Balkan endemic nephropathy and urinary system tumors in Bulgaria. *Food Additives and Contamination*, **5**, 299–301.

Pfohl-Leszkowicz A, Grosse Y, Castegnaro M, Nicolov IG, Chernozemsky IN, Bartsch H, Betbeder AM, Creppy EE and Dirheimer G (1993) Ochratoxin A-related DNA adducts in urinary tract tumors of Bulgarian subjects. IARC Scientific Publications, No. 117, pp. 141–148.

Plestina R, Ceovic S, Gatenbeck S, Habazin-Vovak V, Hult K, Hokby E, Krogh P and Radic B (1990) Human exposure to ochratoxin A in areas of Yugoslavia with endemic nephropathy. *Journal of Environmental Pathology, Toxicology and Oncology*, **10**, pp. 145–148.

Pohland AE, Thorpe CW and Nasheim S (1990) Mycotoxin methodology. *Journal of Environmental Pathology, Toxicology and Oncology*, **10**, 110–119.

Prelusky DB, Rotter BA and Rotter RG (1994) Toxicology of mycotoxins. In *Mycotoxins in Grain: Compounds Other Than Aflatoxins*, Miller JD and Trenholm HL (eds), Eagan Press, St. Paul, MN, pp. 359–403.

Puisieux A, Lim S, Groopman JD and Ozturk M (1991) Selective targeting of p53 gene mutational hotspots in human cancers by etiologically defined carcinogens. *Cancer Research*, **51**, 6185–6189.

Qian G-S, Yu MC, Ross R, Yuan J-M, Gao Y-T, Wogan GN and Groopman JD (1994) A follow-up study of urinary markers of aflatoxin exposure and liver cancer risk in Shanghai, P.R.C. *Cancer Epidemiology, Biomarkers and Prevention*, **3**, 3–11.

Radovanovic Z (1991) Epidemiological characteristics of Balkan endemic nephropathy in eastern regions of Yugoslavia. In *Mycotoxin, Endemic Nephropathy and Urinary Tract Tumors*, Castegnaro M, Plestina R, Dirheimer G, Chernozemsky IN, and Bartsch H (eds), IARC Scientific Publications, No. 115, Lyon, France, pp. 11–20.

Rao BL and Husain A (1985) Presence of cyclopiazonic acid in kodo millet (*Paspalum scrobiculatum*) causing Akodua poisoning in man and its production by associated fungi. *Mycopathology*, **89**, 177–180.

Reddy JK, Svoboda DJ and Rao MS (1976) Induction of liver tumors by aflatoxin B1 in the tree shrew (Tupaiaglis), a nonhuman primate. *Cancer Research*, **36**, 151–160.

Ross R, Yuan J-M, Yu MC, Wogan GN, Qian G-S, Tu J-T, Groopman JD, Gao Y-T and Henderson BE (1992) Urinary aflatoxin biomarkers and risk of hepatocellular carcinoma. *Lancet*, **339**, 943–946.

Rotter BA, Prelusky DB and Pestka JJ (1996) Toxicology of deoxynivalenol (vomitoxin). *Journal of Toxicology and Environmental Health*, **48**, 1–34.

Sansing GA, Lillehoj EB, Detroy RW and Miller MA (1976) Synergistic toxic effects of citrinin, ochratoxin A and penicillic acid in mice. *Toxicon*, **14**, 213–220.

Scott PM (1989) The natural occurrences of trichothecenes. In *Trichothecene Mycotoxicosis: Pathophysiologic Effects*, Vol. I, Beasley VR (ed), CRC Press, Boca Raton, Florida, pp. 1–26.

Scott PM (1990) Trichothecenes in grains. *Cereal Foods World*, **35**, 661–669.

Scott PM (1993) Fumonisins. *International Journal of Food Microbiology*, **18**, 257–270.

Scott PM (1994) Penicillium and Aspergillus toxins. In *Mycotoxins in Grain: Compounds Other Than Aflatoxins*, Miller JD and Trenholm HL (eds), Eagan Press, St. Paul, MN, pp. 261–285.

Shank RC (1981) Environmental toxicoses in humans. In *Mycotoxins and N-Nitro-Compounds: Environmental Risks*, Vol. I. Shank RC (ed), CRC Press, Boca Raton, FL, pp. 107–140.

Shank RC, Gordon JE, Wogan GN, Nandasuta A and Subhamani B (1972) Dietary aflatoxins and human liver cancer. III. Field survey of rural Thai families for ingested aflatoxin. *Food and Cosmetics Toxicology*, **10**, 71–84.

Sharma RP and Salunkhe DK (1991) *Mycotoxins and Phytoalexins*, CRC Press. Boca Raton, FL.

Shimada T and Guengerich FP (1989) Evidence for cytochrome pp-450$_{NF}$, the nifedipine oxidase, being the principal enzyme involved in the bioactivation of aflatoxins in human liver. *Proceedings of National Academy of Science, USA*, **86**, 462–465.

Sieber SM, Correa P, Dalgard DW and Adamson RH (1979) Induction of osteogenic sarcomas and tumors of the hepatobiliary system in nonhuman primates with aflatoxin B1. *Cancer Research*, **39**, 4545–4554.

Sostaric B and Vukelic M (1991) Characteristics of urinary tract tumors in the area of Balkan endemic nephropathy in Croatia. In *Mycotoxin, Endemic Nephropathy and Urinary Tract Tumors*, Castegnaro M, Plestina R, Dirheimer G, Chernozemsky IN and Bartsch H (eds), IARC Scientific Publications, No. 115, Lyon, France, pp. 29–35.

Srivatanakul P, Parkin DM, Jiang YZ, Khlat M, Kao-Ian UT, Sontipong S and Wild C. (1991) The role of infection by *Opisthorchis viverrini*, hepatitis B virus, and aflatoxin exposure in the etiology of liver cancer in Thailand: A correlation study. *Cancer*, **68**, 2411–2417.

Sydenham EW, Thiel PG, Marasas WFO, Shephard GS, van Schalkwyk DJ and Koch KR (1990) Natural occurrence of some Fusarium mycotoxins in corn from low and high esophageal cancer prevalence areas of the Transkei, Southern Africa. *Journal of Agriculture and Food Chemistry*, **38**, 1900–1903.

Tanaka T, Hasegawa A, Yamamoto S, Lee, U-S, Sugiura Y and Ueno Y (1988) Worldwide contamination of cereals by the Fusarium Mycotoxins nivalenol, deoxynivalenol and zearalenone. I. Survey of 19 countries. *Journal of Agriculture and Food Chemistry*, **36**, 979–983.

Tiel PG, Marasas WFO, Sydenham EW, Shephard GS and Gelderblom WCA (1992) The implications of naturally occurring levels of fumonisins in corn for human and animal health. *Mycopathologia*, **117**, 3–9.

Tilak TB (1975) Induction of cholangiocarcinoma following treatment of a rhesus monkey with aflatoxin. *Food and Cosmetics Toxicology*, **13**, 247–249.

Trucksess MW, Stack ME, Neshei S, Page AW and Albert RH (1991) Immunoaffinity column coupled with solution fluorometry or liquid chromatography postcolumn derivatization for determination of aflatoxins in corn, peanuts, and peanut butter: Collaborative study. *Journal of the Association of Official Analytical Chemists*, **74**, 81–88.

Tuite J (1979) Field and storage conditions for the production of mycotoxins and geographic distribution of some mycotoxin problems in the United States. In *Interactions of Mycotoxins in Animal Production*, National Academy of Sciences Press, Washington, DC, pp. 19–42.

Ueno Y (1974) Citreoviridin from *Penicillium citreoviridae* Biourge. In *Mycotoxins*, Purchase IFH (ed), Elsevier Scientific Publishing Co., New York, pp. 283–302.

Ueno Y (1983) General toxicology. In *Trichothecenes: Chemical, Biological and Toxicological Aspects*, Ueno Y (ed), Elsevier, New York, pp. 135–146.

Ueno Y (1987) Trichothecenes in food. In *Mycotoxins in Food*, Krogh P (ed), Academic Press, London, pp. 123–147.

van Egmond HP (1991) Worldwide regulations for ochratoxin A. In *Mycotoxins, Endemic Nephropathy and Urinary Tract Tumors*, Castegnaro M, Plestina R, Dirheimer G, Chernozemsky IN and Bartsch H (eds), IARC Scientific Publication No. 115, IARC, Lyon, France pp. 331–336.

Visconti A and Doko MB (1994) Survey of fumonisin production by Fusarium isolated from cereals in Europe. *Journal of the Assoication of Official Analytical Chemists*, **77**, 546–550.

Voss KA, Norred WP, Hinton DM, Cole RJ and Dorner JW (1990) Subchronic oral toxicity of cyclopiazonic acid (CPA) in male Sprague-Dawley rats. *Mycopathologia*, **110**, 11–18.

Vukelic M, Sostaric B and Fuchs R (1991) Some pathomorphological features of Balkan endemic nephropathy. In *Mycotoxin, Endemic Nephropathy and Urinary Tract Tumors*, Castegnaro M, Plestina R, Dirheimer G, Chernozemsky IN, and Bartsch H (eds), IARC Scientific Publications, No. 115, Lyon, France, pp. 37–42.

Wang E, Norred WP, Bacon CW, Riley RT and Merril AH Jr (1991) Inhibition of sphingolipid biosynthesis by fumonisins. Implications for diseases associated with *Fusarium moniliforme*. *The Journal of Biological Chemistry*, **266**, 14486–14490.

Wang J-S, Qian G-S, Zarba A, He X, Zhu Y-R, Zhang B-C, Jacobson L, Gange SJ, Munoz A, Kensler TW and Groopman JD (1996) Temporal patterns of aflatoxin-albumin adducts in hepatitis B surface antigen-positive and antigen-negative residents of Daxin, Qidong county, People's Republic of China. *Cancer Epidemiology, Biomarkers & Prevention*, **5**, 253–261.

Wang L, Hatch M, Chen C, Levin B, You S, Lu S, Wu M, Wu WP, Wang LW, Wang Q, Huang G, Yang P, Lee H and Santella RM (1996) Aflatoxin exposure and risk of hepatocarcinoma in Taiwan. *International Journal of Cancer*, **67**, 602–625.

WHO (1990) *Selected Mycotoxins: Ochratoxins, Trichothecenes, Ergot*, Environmental Health Criteria 105, Geneva.

Wilson TM, Nelson PE and Kenpp CR (1985) Hepatic neoplastic nodules, adenofibrosis, and cholangicarcinomas in Fischer 344 rats fed corn naturally contaminated with *Fusarium moniliforme*. *Carcinogenesis*, **6**, 1155–1160.

Wilson TM, Ross PF, Rice LG, Osweiler GD, Nelson HA, Owens DL, Plattner RD, Reggiardo C, Noon TH and Pickrell JW (1990) Fumonisin B1 levels associated with an epizootic of equine leukoencephalomalacia. *Journal of Veterinary Diagnosis and Investigation*, **2**, 213–216.

Wogan GN (1965) Chemical nature and biological effects of the aflatoxin. *Bacteriological Review*, **30**, 460–478.

Wogan GN (1969) Naturally occurring carcinogens in foods. *Progress in Experimental Tumor Research*, **11**, 134–162.

Wogan GN (1973) Aflatoxin carcinogenesis. In *Methods in Cancer Research*, Busch H (ed), Academic Press, New York, pp. 309–344.

Wogan GN (1992) Aflatoxins as risk factors for hepatocellular carcinoma in humans. *Cancer Research*, **52**, (Suppl.), 2114S–2118S.

Wogan GN and Newberne PM (1967) Dose-response characteristics of aflatoxin B1 carcinogenesis in the rat. *Cancer Research*, **27**, 2370–2376.

Wolf G (1994) Mechanism of the mitogenic and carcinogenic action of fumonisin B1, a mycotoxin. *Nutrition Review*, **52**, 246–247.

Yeh F-S and Shen K-N (1986) Epidemiology and early diagnosis of primary liver cancer in China. *Advances in Cancer Research*, **47**, 297–329.

Yeh F-S, Yu MC, Mo C, Luo S, Tong MJ and Henderson BE (1989) Hepatitis B virus, aflatoxins, and hepatocellular carcinoma in southern Guangxi, China. *Cancer Research*, **49**, 2506–2509.

Yoshizawa T, Yamashita A and Luo Y (1994) Fumonisin occurrence in corn from high- and low-risk areas for human esophageal cancer in China. *Applied and Environmental Microbiology*, **60**, 1626–1629.

Yu M-W, Chen C-J, Wang L-W and Santella RM (1995) Aflatoxin B1 adduct level and risk of hepatocellular carcinoma. *Proceedings of American Association for Cancer Research*, **36**, 1644.

Zhen Y, Yang S, Ding L, Han F, Yang W and Liu Q (1984) The culture and isolation of fungi from cereals in five high and three low incidence counties of esophageal cancer in Henan province. *Chinese Journal of Oncology*, **6**, 27–29.

3 Toxicants in Food: Generated During Cooking

Kerstin I Skog[1] and Margaretha Jägerstad[2]

[1]*Department of Applied Nutrition and Food Chemistry, Centre for Chemistry and Chemical Engineering, Lund University, PO Box 124, SE-221 00 Lund, Sweden*
[2]*Department of Food Science, Swedish University of Agricultural Sciences, PO Box 7051, SE-750 07, Uppsala, Sweden*

Introduction

During the past decades, several new classes of genotoxic food-borne compounds have been identified and quantified in heat-treated foods. Their occurrence in foods is very much dependent on the cooking conditions and the presence of precursors and modifiers. One of the first reports of food toxicants generated by cooking was published by Widmark (1939), who prepared organic solvent extracts of grilled horse meat and repeatedly painted them on the skin of mice, resulting in tumours in the mammary glands.

During the 1960s and 1970s, much interest was focused on two new classes of chemicals producing tumours in long-term animal studies – polycyclic aromatic hydrocarbons (PAHs) and N-nitroso compounds. These compounds are present in some cooked foods, particularly fried, grilled or barbecued, meat and fish products. Exposure to these compounds also results from: (i) food processing, e.g. curing, drying, smoking, roasting, refining and fermentation; (ii) occupational exposure, and (iii) air pollution. N-nitroso compounds are also formed endogeneously in the body (IARC, 1973, 1983, 1985).

In the late 1970s, a new, highly mutagenic class of compounds, heterocyclic amines (HAs), was identified in meat extract and grilled or broiled meat and fish (Nagao *et al.*, 1977; Sugimura *et al.*, 1977). These workers used the Ames test and were able to identify several heterocyclic amines which showed extremely high mutagenic potency; 100 to 100 000-fold higher than PAHs and N-nitroso compounds. Long-term animal studies showed, however, that these new

Nutrition and Chemical Toxicity. Edited by Costas Ioannides. © John Wiley & Sons Ltd. ISBN 0 471 97453 6

compounds were moderately active in inducing tumours. In contrast to PAHs, the heterocyclic amines are formed not only during barbecuing, deep-fat frying, smoking and grilling but also during pan frying, and roasting/baking.

Toxic lipid oxidation products, particularly cholesterol oxide products (COPs), constitute another group of compounds causing concern. Reliable data have been reported during the past decade which show these compounds to be especially common in foods exposed to severe cooking conditions, e.g. deep-fat frying and pan frying following long-term storage in a freezer or in dehydrated form. COPs have been reported to be both atherogenic (risk factor for causing coronary heart disease) and carcinogenic (Paniangvait et al., 1995; Dutta et al., 1996).

Following a number of evaluations, the International Agency for Research on Cancer (IARC) has come to the conclusion that several of these food-borne mutagens are probably or possibly carcinogenic to humans, based on both high-dose, long-term animal studies and in vitro genotoxicity tests. Yet, there is insufficient scientific evidence that these mutagens really cause human cancer, and no limits have been set for their presence in cooked foods. However, the relevant authorities in most Western countries recommend minimising their occurrence. This chapter provides a brief overview of the state-of-the-art research on these compounds with respect to their formation, occurrence, exposure, risk evaluation and ways of minimising their levels in foods using improved cooking methods and developments in food technology. For more extensive discussions, we recommend recent reviews (Walker, 1990; Lijinsky, 1991; Tricker and Kubachi, 1992; Sugimura et al., 1993; Eisenbrand and Tang, 1993; Gangolli et al., 1994; Paniangvait et al., 1995; Felton et al., 1997; Gooderham et al., 1997; Skog et al., 1988).

Polycyclic aromatic hydrocarbons

CHEMISTRY AND FORMATION

Polycyclic aromatic hydrocarbons (PAHs) are composed mainly of compounds consisting of three or more fused benzene rings without any acyclic groups. Figure 3.1 shows structures of the most commonly detected PAHs in cooked foods, of which benzo[a]pyrene (B[a]P) is regarded as the most carcinogenic (IARC, 1983; Lijinsky, 1991).

PAHs are produced from organic compounds by condensation of smaller units at high temperatures, forming stable polynuclear aromatic compounds. The mechanism of formation of PAHs is not fully understood, but two principal pathways are considered to be involved, pyrolysis and pyrosynthesis. At high temperatures, organic compounds are easily fragmented into smaller compounds, mostly free radicals, which may then recombine to form a number of relatively stable PAHs. At temperatures below 400°C, only small amounts of

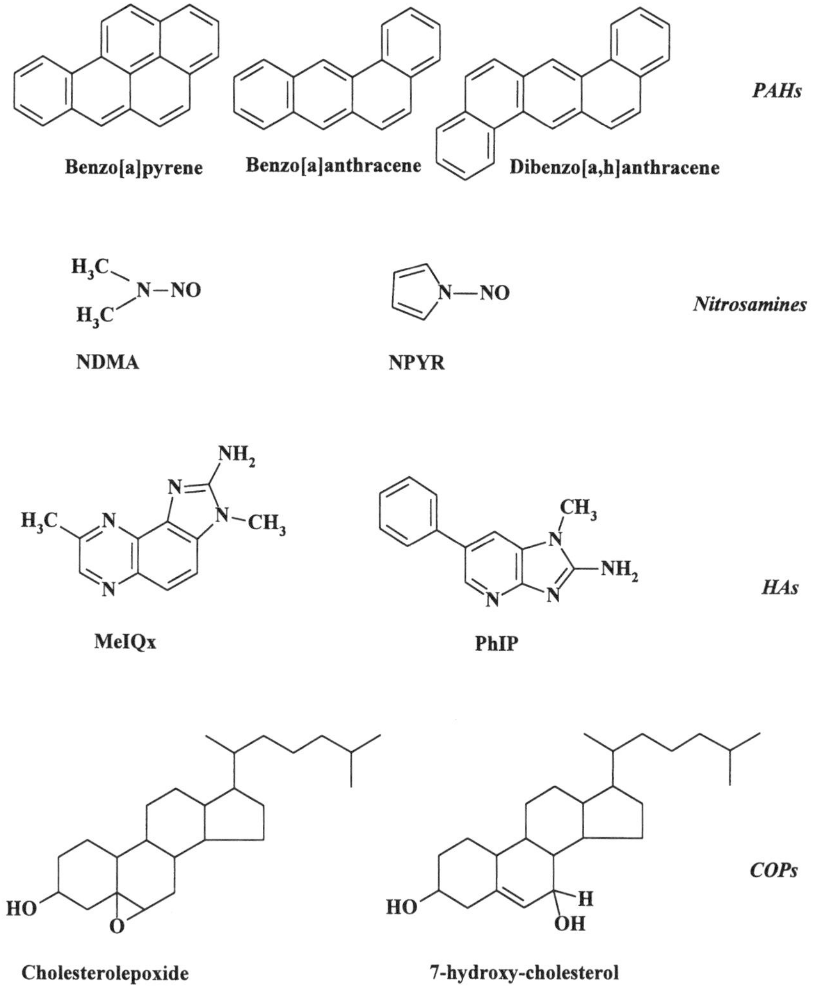

Figure 3.1 Structures of the major forms in cooked foods of polyaromatic hydrocarbons (PAHs), nitrosamines, heterocyclic amines (HAs) and cholesterol oxide products (COPs).

PAHs are formed. However, the amounts of PAHs increase linearly in the range 400 to 1000°C (IARC, 1983; Lijinsky, 1991).

OCCURRENCE OF PAHs IN COOKED FOOD

The level of PAHs in cooked foods varies and is of minor importance at the cooking temperatures used during normal frying conditions, where the heat is transferred to the food via conduction. The use of gas grilling or electrical broiling, where the heat is transferred mainly via radiation, yields detectable, but normally very low, levels of PAHs. Charcoal, being a pyrolysed fuel, produces only small amounts of PAHs, while in contrast, exposure of foods to combustion fumes, especially from pine or spruce cones, will lead to markedly increased levels of PAHs. Particularly high levels can be expected when food is grilled over a log fire, in direct contact with the flames. On the other hand, when flames no longer emerge, the embers of a log fire emit only moderate amounts of PAHs (for references, see Larsson, 1986; Lijinsky, 1991).

The fat content is another important factor in the formation of PAHs in grilled foods, and its propensity to melt and drip onto the heat source, where it is pyrolysed, gives rise to PAHs. The PAHs formed in this way may contaminate the food as the combustion fumes pass over the food. This source of PAHs was first recognised by Linjinsky and Shubik (1964). Fatty meats yield more fat drippings than lean meat and consequently higher PAHs levels are formed in fatty products. The influence of fat is more evident when the contribution from the fuel itself is small, as is the case in charcoal grilling. Cooking time, cooking temperature and distance between the food and the heat source affect the level of PAHs. The impact of a hot source on the levels of B[a]P in grilled frankfurters is shown in Table 3.1.

OTHER DIETARY SOURCES

The major contribution to the PAH content in food is contamination from various combustion processes. Burning of fossil fuels, wood or other organic material emits PAHs into the environment. Foods from agricultural crops may thus be contaminated primarily through surface adsorption of airborne particles. Consequently, leafy vegetables, fruit and cereals grown close to major roads and/or highly industrialised areas may be contaminated by PAHs. Only a minor part of this contamination originates from the uptake of PAHs via the soil, unless the level of PAHs in the soil exceeds 1 mg/kg. Tea and coffee may

Table 3.1 Levels of benzo[a]pyrene (B[a]P) in frankfurters grilled by different techniques

Grilling method	Number of samples	B[a]P(µg/kg) average	Range
Ungrilled	2	0.2	0.1–0.3
Frying pan	5	0.1	ND–0.2
Electric oven	2	0.2	0.1–0.3
Charcoal fire	13	0.3	ND–1.0
Cone fire	7	18	2–31
Log fire	17	54	6–212
Log fire embers	9	8	<1–25

ND, not detected.
From Larsson *et al.* (1983).

contain PAHs from air pollution, but more importantly from the roasting and drying processes. However, only minute amounts of PAHs are transferred into the beverage during the brewing of coffee and tea.

In the past, smoked meat and fish could contain very high amounts of PAHs, depending on the source of smoke, for instance if cones from pine and spruce were used. Nowadays, the use of external smoke generators offers the possibility of cleaning the smoke by cooling, spraying or filtering it before it enters the smoking chamber. A significant reduction in soot and PAHs in treated smoke has been reported (Toth and Blaas, 1972).

PAHs are mainly located in the outer layer of the food product, which means that in smoked fish, most are found in the skin. In a study by Larsson (1982), the flesh of smoked herring was found to contain 0.2–2.7 μg B[a]P per kg, while the skin contained between 10 and 60 μg B[a]P/kg. According to the literature, the amounts of B[a]P in smoked fish range from non-detectable to a few μg per kg, but the total PAH content is generally 20 to 100-fold higher.

The presence of PAHs in vegetable oils has been observed in the past. Here, also improved refining techniques using activated charcoal, and evaporation of PAHs in the deodorisation process have led to the removal of most of the PAHs. However, deodorisation has only a marginal effect on high-molecular weight PAHs, of which several are classified as carcinogens.

EXPOSURE TO PAHs

The intake of PAHs in Europe, USA and Japan has been estimated to be around 1 mg per person per year. Most data are for B[a]P, with values in the range 0.01 to 0.61 mg per person per year. Thus, a daily average intake of 2–3 μg PAHs per person seems reasonable, of which B[a]P constitutes 0.5–5%. Figure 3.2 illustrates the estimated contribution of various food groups in an average Swedish diet to the intake of nine commonly reported PAHs in food. The major part of the PAHs intake is due to contamination through air pollution and only about 25–30% of the PAHs originate from cooking, mainly grilled or smoked foods.

RISK EVALUATION

PAHs are covalently bound to DNA through epoxides. B[a]P, benz[a]anthracene and dibenz[a,h]anthracene have been considered *probably* carcinogenic to humans on the basis of data obtained from animal experiments and *in vitro* test systems. In addition, experimental data indicate that other such compounds may *possibly* be carcinogenic to humans (IARC, 1973, 1983).

There is no conclusive evidence concerning a possible relationship between ingestion of PAH-contaminated food and human cancer. A few studies (for references, see Chu and Chen, 1985) have suggested a link between an

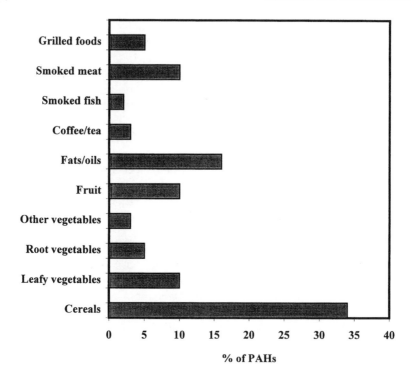

Figure 3.2 Estimated contribution (in %) of various food groups in an average Swedish diet to the total dietary intake of nine PAHs (fluoranthene, pyrene, benz[a]anthracene, chrysene/triphenylene, benzo[b]fluoranthene, benzo[j]fluoranthene/benzo[k]fluoranthene, benzo[e]pyrene, benzo[a]pyrene and indeno[1,2,3-cd]pyrene. Reproduced by permission from Larsson (1986).

increased incidence of stomach cancer and frequent consumption of smoked food. However, as smoked food may contain other potentially carcinogenic substances, such as nitrite and nitrosamines, the observed effects cannot be ascribed definitively to PAHs.

The Committee on Diet, Nutrition and Cancer, appointed by the National Research Council of the USA, stated in their report that of those PAHs occurring in the average American diet, only three, namely B[a]P, benz[a]anthracene and dibenz[a,h]anthracene, have been found to be carcinogenic in animals following oral administration. The Committee concluded that 'Since studies in animals have shown that PAHs are carcinogenic when administered orally, and occupational exposure to substances containing PAHs have been associated with skin and lung cancer, it would be prudent to minimize the dietary exposure to PAHs' (Chu and Chen, 1985).

METHODS OF MINIMISING EXPOSURE TO PAHs FROM COOKED FOODS

When barbecuing or smoking foods, the smoke from the combustion of wood or fossil fuels should be prevented from coming into direct contact with the food, unless the smoke is purified with regard to PAHs. Cooking over a log fire in direct contact with the flames should be avoided. It is important to wait until the log fire has turned into embers. In addition, the use of special grills, designed to prevent melted fat from dripping onto the heat source, reduces the PAHs contamination significantly.

In some countries, legislative limits have been set for PAHs in certain foods, with the aim of minimising the intake of PAHs. In Germany, Poland and Austria a limit of 1 μg/kg is currently imposed for B[a]P in smoked meat products.

N-Nitroso compounds

CHEMISTRY AND FORMATION

N-Nitroso compounds is the general term covering all substances with N-nitroso-groups. Currently, several hundred such compounds are known (for references, see IARC, 1985; Tricker and Preussman, 1991; Tricker and Kubachi, 1992). A large group of N-nitroso compounds occurring in food are the volatile carcinogenic N-nitrosamines: NDMA (*N*-nitrosodimethylamine), NDEA (*N*-nitrosodiethylamine), NPYR (*N*-nitrosopyrrolidine) and NPIP (*N*-nitrosopiperidine). However, the main forms of N-nitroso compounds in food are non-volatile, including a large number of compounds that could be potentially formed, e.g. proteins containing N-nitrosated peptide linkages, such as NPRO (*N*-nitrosoproline). Non-volatile N-nitroso compounds have not been reported as mutagenic or carcinogenic, but they might act as precursors to volatile carcinogenic nitrosamines. Another group of N-nitroso compounds, the nitrosamides, contains substances such as N-nitrosoureas, N-nitrosocarbamates and N-nitrosoguanidines. The structure of two nitrosamines commonly reported in cooked foods, NDMA and NPYR, is shown in Figure 3.1.

The N-nitroso compounds could either be formed in some way outside the human body or synthesised *in vivo*, which means that formation has taken place endogenously. During food processing, preservation or preparation, nitrogen oxides can react with amino compounds to produce N-nitroso compounds. Sources of nitrogen oxides (nitrosating agents) in the food are mainly added nitrate and/or nitrite, naturally occurring nitrite, or nitrogen oxides resulting from the heating and/or drying of foods with combustion gases in which molecular nitrogen can be oxidised to nitrogen oxides. For example, during the smoking of fish, the amines present in fish and the nitrogen oxides in smoking gas can react chemically to produce N-nitroso compounds.

Formation of N-nitroso compound in the body is based on reactions between for example, nitrite and amines, amides or alkyl ureas. Since N-nitrosation is acid-catalysed, generally with a pH optimum between 2 and 4 depending on the substrate, this means that conditions favouring nitrosation reactions exist in the human stomach. On the other hand, conversion of nitrate to nitrite is rather limited at low pH. In the normal (acidic) stomach, nitrite of dietary and salivary origin is utilised in the nitrosation reactions. Saliva is the major site of nitrite production in humans. In infected bladder, nitrite may be produced by bacterial reduction of urinary nitrate (Bartsch and Montesano, 1984; Magee, 1989).

Nitrosation reactions can be influenced by the presence of nitrosation inhibitors (redox compounds, such as ascorbate and vitamin E) and enhancers (metal ions, carbonyl compounds and nucleophilic anions such as Cl^-, I^- and SCN^-). In plant-based foods, phenolic compounds can enhance or inhibit nitrosation, depending on their structure.

OCCURRENCE OF N-NITROSO COMPOUNDS IN COOKED FOODS

Nitrite is added to certain foods, especially meat products, to inhibit the growth of the bacterium *Clostridium botulinum*, which can produce one of the most toxic substances known; a very small amount of the toxin can cause life-threatening neurological symptoms. When bacon or smoked belly of pork is fried, NPRO is produced through nitrosation of the amino acid proline and is then decarboxylated to NPYR, which is carcinogenic. High temperature and long frying time increase the amounts of NPYR formed. In addition, the formation of other volatile nitrosamines increases during frying of cured meat products. While uncooked cured meats may contain between not detectable to 25 ppb NPYR, fried bacon might contain up to 200 ppb (Walker, 1990). Equal parts of volatile N-nitroso compounds are found in the bacon and in the dripping after frying though, according to some reports, up to 90% of the volatile nitrosamines produced during cooking are vaporised (Österdahl, 1988; Hotchkiss, 1989; Tricker and Preussman, 1991; Tricker and Kubachi, 1992).

OTHER DIETARY SOURCES

In the past, direct drying of certain foodstuffs using combustion gases containing nitrogen oxides could result in the formation of nitrosamines. This is the reason why beer and whiskey based on dried malt were shown to contain relatively high amounts of nitrosamines. Modification of malting techniques in the brewing industry, switching from direct heating to indirect heating where the malt is not exposed to gases, has substantially reduced the amounts of N-nitroso compounds in beer by almost 90% (Walker, 1990).

During the smoking of fish, nitrogen oxides in the smoke can react with amines, i.e. diethylamine and triethylamine, present in the fish tissues and form N-nitroso compounds. In Asia, the methods used to prepare dry nitrite-salted fish result in extremely high concentrations of volatile nitrosamines. Furthermore, sausages and various cheeses have been reported occasionally to contain nitrosamines (Walker, 1990; Tricker and Preussmann, 1991).

EXPOSURE TO N-NITROSO COMPOUNDS

Table 3.2 lists the daily intakes of NDMA according to dietary surveys published 1978–1991 (Gangolli et al., 1994). For most Western countries, the average exposure to carcinogenic volatile N-nitroso compounds from the diet is generally of the order of 0.3–1.0 μg per person per day, with cured meats (cooked and uncooked) and beer as major sources. Corresponding figures for non-volatile N-nitrosoamines are estimated to be 10–100 μg per person per day. In Asia, the dietary exposure to volatile nitrosamines is much higher due to the intake of fish products derived from dried and nitrite-salted fish.

Inhalation of cigarette smoke is another significant source of N-nitrosated compounds. Estimates show that an average smoker may be exposed to more than 15 μg volatile N-nitroso compounds per day (Miller Jones, 1992). Furthermore, the endogenous formation of N-nitroso compounds is another source of great concern. One study reported urinary excretion of several μg of nitrosoproline (non-carcinogenic) per day following the ingestion of extra proline together with the ordinary diet. In addition, some individuals may be exposed occupationally to N-nitroso compounds, for example, those working in leather tanneries, rubber and tyre industries.

Table 3.2 Daily intake of nitrosodimethylamine (NDMA) in different countries

Country	NDMA intake (μg/day)	Major NDMA source
UK[a]	0.53	Cured meats (81%)
UK	0.6	Beer; cured meats
The Netherlands	0.38	Beer (71%)
The Netherlands[b]	0.10	Not evaluated
FRG (1979/1980)	1.10 (men)	Beer (65%)
FRG (1979/1980)	0.57 (women)	Cured meats (10%)
FRG (1981)	0.53 (men)	Beer (40%)
FRG (1981)	0.35 (women)	Cured meats (18%)
FRG (1989/1990)	0.28 (men)	Beer (31%)
FRG (1989/1990)	0.17 (women)	Cured meats (36%)
Japan	1.8	Dried fish (91%)
Japan	0.5	Fish products (68%); beer (30%)
Sweden	0.12	Meat products (61%); beer (32%)
Finland[c]	0.08	Smoked fish (75%)
China	No data	Marine foods
Italy	No data	Cured meats
USSR	No data	Meat and fish products

[a]Beer not included in the survey. [b]Determined by 24 h duplicate diet analysis. [c]Based on limited data.
From Gangolli et al. (1994), with permission from Elsevier Science.

RISK EVALUATION

There is overwhelming evidence that some N-nitroso compounds are carcinogenic in most animals (Bartsch and Montesano, 1984; IARC, 1985; Hotchkiss,
1989; Magee, 1989; Walker, 1990; Tricker and Preussmann, 1991). Even transplacental carcinogenesis has been observed for several N-nitroso compounds.
Nitrosamines require metabolic activation to be mutagenic/carcinogenic,
whereas nitrosamides are active without metabolism. The liver is the main
site of metabolic activation of nitrosamines, but other human tissues can also
metabolise nitrosamines, at least the simple symmetrical dialkylnitrosamines.
Interestingly, large quantitative differences in metabolic rate (up to 150-fold)
have been found to occur between individuals (for a review, see Harris et al.,
1982). The basis for the carcinogenicity of nitrosamines is their capacity to
alkylate purines and pyrimidines of DNA, resulting in single-point mutations.
Of the volatile nitrosamines most commonly found in food, NDEA appears to
be the most potent carcinogen, whereas NDMA has somewhat lower potency,
and the heterocyclic NPYR and NPIP even lower.

In epidemiological studies, positive correlations have been observed
between high intake of nitrosamine-containing products and cancer of the
oesophagus, stomach and nasal cavity. These sites of carcinogenicity correspond to the organs of experimental animals most affected by N-nitroso compounds, i.e. lung, trachea, oesophagus and nasal cavity. In Chinese studies,
several sources of evidence suggest a correlation between either dietary nitrosamines or endogenous nitrosation of dietary amines, and increased incidence
of oesophageal cancer. In addition, several studies have shown an association
between intake of salted/preserved fish and the induction of several cancer
forms: gastric cancer in Japan and Norway, cancer of the nasal cavity and
oesophagus in China, and colorectal cancer in Finland. Animal studies support
these epidemiological findings. The observed correlation between nitrosamine
exposure and cancer in smokers also supports the suggestion of a similar link
between N-nitroso compounds present in food and cancer induction.

METHODS OF MINIMISING EXPOSURE TO N-NITROSO COMPOUNDS

During recent years, the levels of N-nitroso compounds in the human diet have
decreased significantly. This is due to reductions in the levels of nitrates and
nitrites added to foods, and the simultaneous addition of ascorbic acid, which
inhibits the formation of N-nitroso compounds in cured meat products.
Recommendations have been made to fry bacon with caution, not to use lids
and not to consume the frying fat rendered out of the bacon, i.e. the pan
residue. Soaking bacon in water before frying, as well as microwave cooking
instead of using a griddle or a frying pan, significantly lowers the NPYR levels
(Österdahl, 1988).

Heterocyclic amines

CHEMISTRY

Cooked food mutagens are mutagenic/carcinogenic heterocyclic amines (HAs) formed during cooking, most notably in muscle meats. HAs are multi-site carcinogens in rodents and show potent mutagenic activity in bacterial test systems (Ames/*Salmonella* test). The first groups of mutagenic compounds to be identified are called pyrido-imidazoles, or -indoles [Trp-P-1 (3-amino,-1,4-dimethyl-5*H*-pyrido[4,3-*b*]indole), Trp-P-2 (3-amino-l-methyl-5*H*-pyrido[4,3-*b*]indole), AαC (2-amino-9*H*-pyrido[2,3-*b*]indole), MeAαC (2-amino-3-methyl-9*H*-pyrido[2,3-*b*]indole)] (for a review see Sugimura *et al.*, 1993). Other HAs are derivatives of imidazoquinolines [IQ (2-amino-3-methylimidazo[4,5-*f*]quinoline), MeIQ (2-amino-3,4-methylimidazo[4,5-*f*]quinoline)] or imidazoquinoxalines [IQx (2-amino-3- methylimidazo[4,5-*f*]quinoxaline), MeIQx (2-amino-3,8-dimethylimidazo[4,5-*f*]quinoxaline), DiMeIQx (2-amino-3,4,8, or 3,7,8 trimethylimidazo[4,5-*f*]quinoxaline)] and are commonly called IQ compounds. Another group of HAs is the imidazopyridines [PhIP (2-amino-l-methyl-6-phenylimidazo[4,5-*b*]pyridine)]. HAs have a stable aromatic structure with an exocyclic amino group. The structures of two of the most commonly detected compounds in cooked foods, MeIQx and PhIP, are shown in Figure 3.1.

FORMATION OF HAs

Fried beef, pork, chicken and fish generally contain the same group of heterocyclic amines, in similar proportions. This suggests that HAs formed during cooking all have similar precursors. Creatine, free amino acids and sugars, all occurring naturally at low levels in muscle meat, have been shown to be precursors of the IQ compounds and PhIP (for a review, see Skog, 1993; Skog *et al.*, 1998). Several reports have indicated that creatine is an essential reactant and is present in the form of creatine phosphate as an energy source only in vertebrates. When heated, amino acids and sugars participate in the Maillard reaction, which has been proposed as a major process in the formation of heterocyclic amines. The Maillard reaction involves the formation of Strecker aldehydes, while subsequent secondary reactions lead to pyrazines and pyridines. A tentative pathway for the formation of IQ compounds was suggested more than 10 years ago by Jägerstad *et al.* (1983). According to their hypothesis, creatine is converted to creatinine, forming the amino-imidazo part of the molecules. The remaining parts arise from pyridines or pyrazines, formed in the Maillard reaction between sugars and amino acids. In another possible reaction route, with the same precursors, it was suggested that creatine condenses with an aldehyde before reacting with a pyridine or a pyrazine to form IQ compounds (for a review, see Skog *et al.*, 1998). Other suggestions include the formation of pyridine and pyrazine radicals, which give pyridine and pyrazine derivatives reacting further with creatinine, or reactions between alkylpyridine and dialkylpyrazine radicals and creatinine. There are certainly other routes of formation of IQ compounds. PhIP can be formed from just two compounds, phenylalanine and creatine. No reaction rule has been suggested for pyrido-imidazoles and -indoles.

Temperature appears to be a more important factor than time in the formation of heterocyclic amines. At temperatures below 100°C, the amount of HAs formed is low, but increases with increasing cooking temperature and time (for a review, see Skog et al., 1998). There is often a dramatic increase in the amount of HAs formed when the temperature increases to 200°C and above. Oven roasting produces less HAs than pan frying. HAs have also been demonstrated in fish smoked at 80–85°C for several hours (Skog et al., 1998). The low water activity in the surface layer of the fish probably favours the Maillard reaction and thus the formation of HAs during the smoking process.

MODIFYING FACTORS

Sugars in low amounts have an enhancing effect on the formation of heterocyclic amines, while sugars in molar excess have an inhibiting effect. Meat naturally contains low amounts of glucose and the addition of glucose or lactose to minced meat before frying was found to reduce the formation of MeIQx (Skog, 1993).

Fat is easily oxidised at cooking temperatures, and may affect the Maillard reaction and influence the formation of HAs for example, through the free radicals formed. Alternatively, auto-oxidation of fats and degradation of lipid hydroperoxides may produce dicarbonyl compounds and aldehydes which can react with amino acids. When beefburgers were fried in fats with different chemical compositions, the amounts of MeIQx were found to be related to the oxidation status and antioxidant content of the frying fats (Johansson et al., 1995).

Iron is another compound in meat which can enhance the formation of heterocyclic amines. Iron is a pro-oxidant and might enhance the formation of pyrazines and pyridines through a free radical mechanism. On the other hand, some antioxidants act as free radical scavengers, thus reducing the amount of HAs formed via free radical reactions. Food additives, e.g. bisulphite, nitrite, citrate, ascorbic acid, vitamin E and liquid smoke, have been found to decrease the amount of MeIQx formed during frying of minced beef, and reducing agents were shown to be more effective than chelating agents (for a review, see Skog et al., 1998).

The importance of precursors has been demonstrated in several studies. Short microwave treatment of minced meat released a liquid containing many of the heterocyclic amine precursors. After frying, the content of MeIQx in the beef patties was markedly decreased (Felton et al., 1994). Recently, marinating has been shown to decrease the formation of HAs in fried/grilled chicken; however, the mechanism behind this decrease is not known (Tikkanen et al., 1996; Knize et al., 1997).

OCCURRENCE OF HAs

Table 3.3 lists data from the literature relating to the amounts of MeIQx and PhIP in meat and fish products cooked with common domestic methods, and in process flavours/meat extracts. Only these two HAs are considered, although additional compounds, in lower amounts, have been found in several studies (for reviews, see Layton *et al.*, 1995; Skog *et al.*, 1998). In most foods, the amounts of HAs are low, at the ng/g level; however, the amounts of HAs vary greatly, and cover a 100-fold range, depending on food composition and cooking conditions. Greater amounts are generally found in meat than in fish, and in pure meat compared with mixed meat products, e.g. meatballs or sausages. Various commercial fast-food products have been reported to contain low or undetectable amounts of HAs. Pan residues have been shown to contain heterocyclic amines; sometimes the content of MeIQx and PhIP in pan residues is as high or higher than in the corresponding piece of meat. Commercial beef flavours and meat extracts were shown to contain HAs but only low or non-detectable amounts were found in commercial bouillon cubes. Cooked foods appear to be the major source for heterocyclic amines, but some studies have shown their presence in cooking fumes, beer, wine, cigarette smoke and outdoor air.

EXPOSURE TO HAs

Human exposure to HAs has been estimated to range from a few ng/day to some μg/day, depending on dietary habits and cooking practices (Sugimura *et al.*, 1993; Wakabayashi *et al.*, 1993; Layton *et al.*, 1995). Although the consumption of these compounds is very low, several of the HAs are consumed at the same time and the combined effect has not been sufficiently invesigated. Animal studies have shown that orally administered HAs are efficiently and rapidly absorbed by the gastrointestinal tract and excreted almost completely

Table 3.3 Literature values of MeIQx and PhIP in meat and fish products, pan residues, meat extracts and beef flavours

Food	MeIQx (ng/g)	PhIP (ng/g)
Beef burger, fried	0–7	0–32
Meat balls, fried	0–0.8	0–0.6
Chicken, fried	0–3	0–70
Salmon, fried	0–5	0–23
Beef burger, pan residue	0–6	0–13
Meat extract	0–80	0–4
Beef flavour	0–20	0–4
Beef stock cube	0–0.6	0–0.3

From Skog *et al.* (1998)

through bile, urine and faeces within 72 hours. The remaining compounds are mostly retained in the liver and the kidneys (for a review, see Aeschbacher and Turesky, 1991). HAs has been detected in urine from volunteers consuming a normal diet, but not from patients receiving parenteral alimentation, suggesting that humans are normally exposed to HAs (Wakabayashi et al., 1993). Other studies have shown that MeIQx and PhIP are absorbed and rapidly metabolised by humans (Gooderham et al., 1997).

RISK EVALUATION

HAs have been found to be carcinogenic to various organs in animals following long-term oral administration (Eisenbrand and Tang, 1993; IARC, 1993; Sugimura et al., 1993). The predominant tumour sites for MeIQx and PhIP, when given to mice and rats, are liver, colon and mammary gland. It has also been shown that IQ induces liver tumours in cynomolgus monkeys (non-human primates), after chronic dosage of 10 or 20 mg/kg for five days per week. A high-fat diet has been shown to increase the carcinogenicity of low levels of IQ in several target organs in rats, especially the mammary gland (Weisburger et al., 1995). MeIQx and PhIP were excreted into the breast milk, when given to lactating rats and absorbed by their 5-day-old pups. PhIP was detected in the stomach content of suckling pups after administration to lactating mice, and transplacental transfer of PhIP to foetuses was also demonstrated. Neonatal mice are highly sensitive to test chemicals, and a two-generation study showed PhIP to increase the risk of mammary carcinoma development in the second generation (Ito et al., 1997). Moreover, heterocyclic amines, at a total dose of 5000- to 10 000-fold less than the standard chronic bioassays, have caused tumours in neonatal mice. In common with many other genotoxic compounds, HAs require metabolic activation before they can exert mutagenic or carcinogenic effects.

A common feature of many chemical carcinogens is their ability to form covalent adducts with DNA. This step is thought to be a prerequisite for the initiation of the carcinogenic process. DNA adduct formation from MeIQx has been studied at very low doses in humans and rodents (Turteltaub et al., 1997). The results showed a linear relationship between adduct levels and dose, except at high chronic doses, where a plateau was reached, and that humans form more DNA adducts per dose than rats. This indicates that linear extrapolation from high-dose animal studies may underestimate human DNA damage at low doses (Felton et al., 1997).

In the past few years, several epidemiological studies have focused on meat consumption and cancer. Carcinogenic substances are produced during cooking and some findings suggest that exposure to HAs may be involved in the development of human cancer. Conflicting data exist regarding the relative risk associated with the intake of (fried) meat, but the results of many studies have wide confidence intervals and therefore no reliable conclusions can be drawn.

However, no investigation has directly assessed the intake of HAs in relation to cancer development.

METHODS OF MINIMISING EXPOSURE TO HAs

The IARC regards some of the HAs as probably (IQ) or possibly (MeIQ, MeIQx and PhIP) carcinogenic to humans and recommends a reduced exposure to them (IARC, 1993). This could be achieved by small changes in cooking practices: discarding pan residues and preparing gravy using bouillon cubes, marinating, lowering cooking temperatures, also in combination with the addition of sugars or other colour enhancers, microwave cooking and oven roasting. Frying beefburgers using a thermostatically controlled hotplate, maintaining a low, constant cooking temperature, is another way of reducing the amounts of HAs. When optimising the conditions for various food processes, the formation of HAs should be taken into account in order to increase food quality and food safety.

Lipid oxidation products

CHEMISTRY AND FORMATION

Lipids in food consist of a broad group of compounds, e.g. triacylglycerols (triesters of glycerol with fatty acids), the structurally related phospholipids and sterols of either animal or plant origin. Of these compounds, unsaturated and polyunsaturated fatty acids are easily subjected to auto-oxidation, which is the main reaction involved in the oxidative deterioriation of lipids. This reaction proceeds via a free radical mechanism following exposure to light or metal ions (initiation). The free radical then combines with molecular oxygen to form a peroxy radical, followed by formation of hydroperoxide and another free radical. The reaction is repeated many times and is similar to a chain reaction. The chain reaction is terminated first when the free radicals are quenched by reacting with other free radicals or free radical scavengers, e.g. antioxidants (Fennema, 1996).

The primary reaction products are hydroperoxides, which are unstable and break down in several steps to produce a range of secondary breakdown products with varying toxicological significance. The secondary breakdown products include many carbonyl compounds, saturated and unsaturated acids, aldehydes, ketones and alcohols. During the later stage of lipid peroxidation, polymerisation takes place. Auto-oxidation of lipids is facilitated by many factors, in particular temperature, light, oxygen, free radical initiators, metal ions, pro-oxidants and a shortage of antioxidants (Fennema, 1996).

Cholesterol is often present in association with membrane lipids, e.g. phospholipids, rich in unsaturated and polyunsaturated fatty acids. The formation of cholesterol oxide products (COPs) is greatly accelerated by auto-oxidation of coexisting unsaturated triacylglycerols, thereby forming oxygenated forms or epoxides of cholesterol (Figure 3.1). Very recently, phytosterol oxides, which are structurally related to cholesterol oxides, have been identified and quantified in cooked or processed foods. While cholesterol oxides have been reported to be strong candidates for the development of atherosclerosis (coronary heart disease), and to be cytotoxic and mutagenic/carcinogenic, the physiological effects of oxidised phytosterols are less clear (Bösinger et al., 1993; Dutta et al., 1996).

OCCURRENCE OF LIPID OXIDATION PRODUCTS IN COOKED FOODS

Since the primary lipid oxidation products of triacylglycerols, e.g. hydroxyperoxides and free radicals, are reactive or unstable, these products are generally not monitored in the diet. Secondary lipid oxidation products are, however, present in numerous forms and are analysed in terms of peroxide value, anisidine value or rancimatic value (the degree of polarity). The reasons for analysing lipid oxidation products is due rather to off-flavour problems than toxicity, while the presence of COPs has become of increasing concern from a toxicological point of view (for references, see Bösinger et al., 1993; Paniangvait et al., 1995).

When heating butter in a shallow frying pan under conditions similar to those in domestic cooking, the presence of COPs amounting to several ppm was observed (Nourooz-Zadeh and Appelqvist, 1988; Paniangvait et al., 1995). Nourooz-Zadeh and Appelqvist (1989) investigated the presence of COPs in cooked bacon; frying bacon at 170°C for 10 minutes resulted in detectable amounts of some COPs, which increased slightly after extending the frying time to 20 minutes. No detectable amounts of COPs were observed in the lean part of the bacon or the melted-out fat remaining in the pan residue.

The effect of electric grilling of marine fish products on the oxidation of cholesterol was investigated by Shozen et al., (1995). Several kinds of salted–dried and boiled–dried marine fish products were broiled. All fish products were found to contain substantial amounts of epoxides (8–45 ppm on a dry matter basis) and oxygenated derivatives (20–50 ppm on a dry matter basis) of COPs before broiling. Only two high-fat products, e.g. Pacific round herring and Japanese whiting showed slightly increased values of COPs after grilling.

Several studies (for references, see Dutta et al., 1996) have reported the presence of COPs in deep-fat-fried products, e.g. french fries and potato chips, especially if animal fats or mixtures of vegetable oils and animal fats had been used. Park and Addis (1986) investigated french fries cooked in tallow and found between 6.8 and 58.8 ppm of derivatives of COPs. In the same study, fried chicken meat and skin did not show any quantifiable amounts of COPs. Recently, the occurrence of phytosterol oxides has been monitored in french fries cooked at 200°C in various blends of vegetable oils (rapeseed oil/palm oil, sunflower oil and high-oleic sunflower oil). The highest levels of oxidised sterols were found when using a rapeseed oil/palmoil blend, where french fries were found to contain 4 ppm of total oxidised sterols (Dutta and Appelqvist, 1997).

OTHER DIETARY SOURCES

Processing of foods, e.g. refining and hydrogenation of vegetable oils, and dehydration of milk and egg for the manufacture of milk powder and egg powder, are examples of processes which may produce oxidised phytosterols and cholesterols. Spray-drying of egg powder using indirect heating resulted generally in COP levels below the detection limits. After 12 months of storage, the COPs had increased to 5–6 ppm (based on lipids) in the egg powder, which is still acceptable from a sensory and functional point of view. According to the literature, higher values of COPs are usually found when egg powder is produced by direct heating. Egg powder is a common ingredient in many cake mixes available commercially. During storage of these products, COPs may be developed (for references, see Bösinger et al., 1993; Paniangvait et al., 1995; Dutta et al., 1996).

Usually, pasteurised milk contains COPs below the detection limit (< 1 ppm). Milk powder, cream and butter may contain ppm levels of COPs after long-term storage. A butter-oil produced in India, 'ghee', may contain extremely high concentrations of COPs, especially when used repeatedly for frying, where levels as high as 96 ppm cholesterol epoxides or expoxides of cholesterol have been reported. Another source of COPs is cheese, particularly stored dried cheese powder, grated cheese, which is a common ingredient in 'au gratin' and pasta dishes (for references, see Nourooz-Zadeh, 1988).

Raw meat and fish stored in freezers have been reported to contain some COPs. Dehydrated, complete dishes containing fatty foods, have shelf-lives up to 5 years and in such products remarkably high levels of COPs have been reported. Smoked and dried meat, for instance venison, have also been reported to contain high amounts of COPs, particularly after storage at sub-zero temperatures. Among cooked fish products, particularly those prepared from dehydrated and/or salted products, e.g. shrimps and Swedish 'lutfisk' (boiled ling previously soaked in lye) may contain considerable amounts of COPs (Nourooz-Zadeh, 1988; Bösinger et al., 1993; Paniangvait et al., 1995).

RISK EVALUATION

Humans are exposed to oxidised lipids in their diet from dairy products and edible fats, cooked meals prepared from freeze-stored fatty meat and fish, deep-fat fried foods and powdered dehydrated foods, especially after long-term storage. The relationship between long-term consumption of lipid oxidation products and human health is far from clear. The results of animal studies must be interpreted with caution, since the intake of oxidised products must be high

(10–15% w/w of diet) to produce an effect in laboratory animals, and probably does not represent an intake typical for humans. Further research is needed on the long-term effects of consuming mildly oxidised fats produced under commercial and domestic cooking conditions. In the absence of more epidemiological data, it is reasonable to assume that a moderate consumption is safe (for references, see Kubow, 1990).

Since the early 1970s, a number of reports on the health risks of certain COPs have been published (for reference, see Bösinger et al., 1993; Dutta et al., 1996). Deposition of cholesterol in arteries and the aorta, resulting in atherosclerotic plaque, was a model of plaque formation that was accepted for many years. Subsequent studies by several groups demonstrated more damaging effects of COPs resulting in arterial wall injuries, atherosclerotic plaque and aortic accumulation of calcium. Arterial cell wall injuries might be linked to the inhibitory effect of COPs on cholesterol biosynthesis, thereby decreasing cholesterol in the cell membrane, resulting in altered membrane function or disruption and premature cell death, which in turn may lead to tissue necrosis, abnormal cell proliferation and formation of atheromas. Support for involvement of COPs for atherosclerotic plaque formation comes from animal experiments showing that COPs could influence eicosanoic acid production from arachidonic acid, thereby interacting with the prostaglandin synthesis. As far as the toxicity of oxidised phytosterol products is concerned, very little has been reported so far (Bösinger et al., 1993).

METHODS OF MINIMISING EXPOSURE TO LIPID OXIDATION PRODUCTS

Several researchers have suggested that prevention of cholesterol oxidation in processed foods should be similar to procedures employed to prevent lipid oxidation. Those suggestions include: cooking and processing of foods should be conducted as far as possible in the absence of pro-oxidants, but in the presence of antioxidants; and using low temperatures or minimum temperature processing conditions. In addition, packaging and storage should exclude oxygen and light, and be conducted at low temperature.

Conclusions

There is no doubt that humans are regularly exposed to mutagens and animal carcinogens, not least from cooked foods. Exposure varies among individuals due to dietary habits and differences in cooking practice. Interestingly, the four classes of possibly carcinogenic substances occurring in cooked foods – PAHs, N-nitrosocompounds, HAs and COPs – are generally analysed separately, though it is quite clear that they might be present together in some cooked foods, e.g. nitrosamines and HAs in fried bacon, HAs and PAHs in barbecued foods, and PAHs, nitrosamines and HAs in smoked fish. In addition, oxidised lipids including COPs may be present occasionally.

The mutagenic/carcinogenic effects of these four classes of compounds have been investigated separately, but we do not know if there are any synergistic or antagonistic effects of a simultaneous exposure. Thus, future work should evaluate such combined effects in more physiological doses and also include aspects of transplacental transfer and exposure by milk during lactation. Meanwhile, it is prudent to minimise their occurrence in cooked foods.

References

Aeschbacher H-U and Turesky RJ (1991) Mammalian cell mutagenicity and metabolism of heterocyclic amines. *Mutation Research*, **259**, 235–250.

Bartsch H and Montesano R (1984) Relevance of nitrosamines in human cancer. *Carcinogensis*, **5**, 1381–1393.

Bösinger S, Luf W and Brandl E (1993) Oxysterols: their occurrence and biological effects. *International Dairy Journal*, **3**, 1–33.

Chu MML and Chen CW (1985) The evaluation and estimation of potential carcinogenic risks of polynuclear aromatic hydrocarbons (PAH). United States Environmental Protection Agency Research and Development, 1–29.

Dutta PC and Appelqvist L-Å (1997) Studies on phytosterol oxides I: Effect of storage on the content of potato chips prepared in different vegetable oils and II: Content in some vegetable oils and in french fries prepared in these oils. *Journal of the American Oil Chemists' Society*, **74**, 647–666.

Dutta PC, Przybylski R, Appelqvist L-Å and Eskin NAM (1996) Formation and analyses of oxidised sterols in frying fat. In *Deep Frying. Chemistry, Nutrition, and Practical Applications*, Perkins EG and Erickson MD (eds), AOCS Press, Champaign, Illinois, pp. 112–150.

Eisenbrand T and Tang W (1993) Food-borne heterocyclic amines. Chemistry, formation, occurrence and biological activities. A literature review. *Toxicology*, **84**, 1–82.

Felton JS, Fultz E. Dolbeare FA and Knize MG (1994) Effect of microwave pretreatment of heterocyclic aromatic amine mutagens/carcinogens in fried beef patties. *Food and Chemical Toxicology*, **32**, 897–903.

Felton JS, Malfatti MA, Knize MG, Salmon CP, Hopmans EC and Wu R (1997) Health risks of heterocyclic amines. *Mutation Research*, **376**, 37–41.

Fennema OR (1996) *Food Chemistry*, 3rd ed, Marcel Dekker Inc., New York.

Gangolli SD, van den Brandt PA, Feron VJ, Janzowsky C, Koerman JH, Speijers GJA, Spiegelhalder B, Walker R and Wishnok JS (1994) Nitrate, nitrite, and N-nitroso compounds. *European Journal of Pharmacology. Environmental Toxicology and Pharmacology*, **292**, 1–38.

Gooderham NJ, Murray, S. Lynch, AM, Yadollahi-Farsani M, Zhao K, Rich K, Boobis AR and Davies DS (1997) Assessing human risk to heterocyclic amines. *Mutation Research*, **376**, 53–60.

Harris CC, Grafstrom JF, Lechner JF and Autrup H (1992) Metabolism of N-nitrosamines and repair of DNA damage in cultured human tissues and cells. In *Nitrosoamines and Human Cancer*, Magee PN (ed), Cold Spring Harbor, NY, pp. 121–139.

Hotchkiss JH (1989) Preformed N-nitroso compounds in foods and beverages. *Cancer Survey*, **8**, 295–321.

IARC (1973) International Agency for Research on Cancer: Monographs on the Evaluation of Carcinogenic Risk of Chemicals to Humans. Certain polycyclic aromatic hydrocarbons and heterocyclic compounds, Vol. 3, Lyon, France.

IARC (1983) International Agency for Research on Cancer: Monographs on the Evaluation of Carcinogenic Risk of Chemicals to Humans. Polynuclear aromatic compounds, Part 1, Chemical, Environmental and Experimental Data, Vol. 32, Lyon, France.

IARC (1985) International Agency for Research on Cancer: Monographs on the evaluation of the carcinogenic risk of chemicals to humans. Tobacco habits other than smoking: betal-quid and areca-nuit chewing; and some related nitrosamines, Vol. 37, Lyon, France.

IARC (1993) International Agency for Research on Cancer: Monographs on the Evaluation of Carcinogenic Risk to Humans: Some Naturally Occurring Aromatic Amines and Mycotoxins, Vol. 56, Lyon, France, pp. 163–242.

Ito N, Hasegawa R, Imaida K, Tamano S, Hagiwara A, Hirose M and Shirai T (1997) Carcinogenicity of 2-amino-l-methyl-6-phenyl[4,5-b]pyridine (PhIP) in the rat. *Mutation Research*, **376**, 107–114.

Jägerstad M, Laser Reuterswärd A, Öste R, Dahlqvist A, Olsson K, Grivas S and Nyhammer T (1983) Creatinine and Maillard reaction products as precursors of mutagenic compounds formed in fried beef. In *The Maillard Reaction in Foods and Nutrition*, Waller G and Feather M (eds), Washington, DC, pp. 507–519.

Johansson, M, Fredholm L, Bjerna I and Jägerstad M (1995) Influence of frying fat on the formation of heterocyclic amines in fried beefburgers and pan residues. *Food and Chemical Toxicology*, **33**, 993–1004.

Knize MG, Salmon CP, Mehta SS and Felton JS (1997) Analysis of cooked muscle meats for heterocyclic aromatic amine carcinogens. *Mutation Research*, **376**, 129–134.

Kubow S (1990) Toxicity of dietary lipid peroxidation products. *Trends in Food Science and Technology*, **September**, 67–71

Larsson BK (1982) Polycyclic aromatic hydrocarbons in smoked fish. *Zeitschrift für Lebensmittel-Untersuchung und Forschung*, **174**, 101–107.

Larsson BK (1986) Polycyclic aromatic hydrocarbons in Swedish foods. Aspects on analysis, occurrence and intake. PhD Thesis, Swedish University of Agricultural Science, Uppsala, Sweden.

Larsson BK, Sahlberg GP. Eriksson AT and Busk L (1983) Polycyclic aromatic hydrocarbons in grilled food. *Journal of Agricultural and Food Chemistry*, **31**, 867–873.

Layton DW, Bogen KT, Knize MG, Hatch FT, Johnson VM and Felton JS (1995) Cancer risk of heterocyclic amines in cooked foods: an analysis and implications for research. *Carcinogenesis*, **16**, 39–52.

Lijinsky W (1991) The formation and occurrence of polynuclear aromatic hydrocarbons associated with food. *Mutation Research*, **259**, 251–261.

Lijinsky W and Shubik P (1964) Benzo(a)pyrene and other polynuclear hydrocarbons in charcoal-broiled meat. *Science*, **145**, 53–55.

Magee PN (1989) The experimental basis for the role of nitroso compounds in human cancer. *Cancer Survey*, **8**, 207–239.

Miller Jones J (1992) In *Food Safety*, Eagan Press, St. Paul, US, pp. 244–257.

Nagao M, Honda M, Seino Y, Yahagi T and Sugimura T (1977) Mutagenicities of smoke condensates and the charred surface of fish and meat. *Cancer Letters*, **2**, 221–226.

Nourooz-Zadeh J (1988) Cholesterol oxides in foods and food safety aspects. Analytical methods, levels in some Swedish foods and food safety aspects. PhD Thesis, The Swedish University of Agricultural Science, Uppsala, Sweden.

Nourooz-Zadeh J and Appelqvist, L-Å (1988) Cholesterol oxides in Swedish foods and food ingredients: butter and cheese. *Journal of the American Oil Chemists' Society*, **65**, 1635–1641.

Nourooz-Zadeh J and Appelqvist, L-Å (1989) Cholesterol oxides in Swedish foods and food ingredients: lard and bacon. *Journal of the American Oil Chemists' Society*, **66**, 586–592.

Österdahl B-G (1988) Volatile nitrosamines in foods on the Swedish market and estimation of their daily intake. *Food Additives and Contaminants*, **5**, 587–595.

Paniangvait P, King AJ, Jones AD and German BG (1995) Cholesterol oxides in foods of animal origin. A critical review. *Journal of Food Science*, **60**, 1159–1174.

Skog K, Johansson M and Jägerstad M (1998) Carcinogenic heterocyclic amines in model systems and cooked foods. A review on formation, occurrence and intake. *Food and Chemical Toxicology*, in press.

Park SW and Addis PB (1986) Identification and quantitative estimation of oxidised cholesterol derivatives in heated tallow. *Journal of Agricultural and Food Chemistry*, **34**, 653–659.

Shozen K, Oshima T, Ushio H and Koizumi C (1995) Formation of cholesterol oxides in marine fish products induced by grilling. *Fisheries Science*, **61**, 817–821.

Skog K (1993) Cooking procedures and food mutagens: a literature review. *Food and Chemical Toxicology*, **31**, 655–675.

Sugimura T, Nagao M, Kawachi T, Honda M, Yahagi T, Seino Y, Sato S, Matsukara N, Shirai A, Sawamura M and Matsumoto H (1977) Mutagens-carcinogens in food, with special reference to highly mutagenic pyrolytic products in broiled foods. In *Origins of Human Cancer*, Hiatt HH, Watson JD and Winsten JA (eds), Cold Spring Harbour Laboratory Press, New York, pp. 1561–1577.

Sugimura T, Wakabayashi K, Nagao M and Esumi H (1993) A new class of carcinogens: heterocyclic amines in cooked food. In *Food, Nutrition and Chemical Toxicity*, Parke DV, Ioannides, C and Walker R (eds), Smith-Gordon and Nishimura Ltd, pp. 259–276.

Tikkanen LM, Latva-Kala KJ and Heiniö R-L (1996) Effects of commercial marinades on the mutagenic activity, sensory quality and amount of heterocyclic amines in chicken grilled under different conditions. *Food and Chemical Toxicology*, **34**, 725–730.

Toth L and Blaas W (1972) Einfluss der Räuchhertechnologie auf den Gehalt von geräucherten Fleischwaren an cancerogenen Kohlenwasserstoffen. I. Einfluss verschiedener Räuchervefahren. *Fleischwirtschaft*, **52**, 1121–1124.

Tricker AR and Kubachi SJ (1992) Review of the occurrence and formation of non-volatile N-nitroso compounds in foods. *Food Additives and Contaminants*, **9**, 39–69.

Tricker AR and Preussmann R (1991) Carcinogenic N-nitrosamines in the diet: occurrence, formation, mechanisms and carcinogenic potential. *Mutation Research*, **259**, 277–289.

Turteltaub KW, Mauthe RJ, Dingley KH, Vogel JS, Franz C, Garner RC and Shen N (1997) MeIQx-DNA adduct formation in rodent and human tissues at low doses. *Mutation Research*, **376**, 243–252.

Wakabayashi K, Ushiyama H, Takahashi M, Nukaya H, Kim S-B, Hirose M, Ochiai M, Sugimura T and Nagao M (1993) Exposure to heterocyclic amines. *Environmental Health Perspectives*, **99**, 129–133.

Walker R (1990) Nitrates, nitrites and N-nitrosocompounds: a review of the occurrence in food and diet and the tocicological implications. *Food Additives Contaminants*, **7**, 717–768.

Weisburger JH, Rivenson A, Kingston DGI, Wilkins TD, Van Tassell RJ, Nagao M, Sugimura T and Hara Y (1995) Dietary modulation of the carcinogenicity of the heterocyclic amines. In *Heterocyclic Amines in Cooked Foods: Possible Human Carcinogens*, Adamson RH, Gustafsson J-Å, Ito N, Nagao M, Sugimura T, Wakabayashi K, and Yamazoe Y (eds), Princeton Scientific Publishing Co., Inc., Princeton, NJ, pp. 240–250.

Widmark EMP (1939) Presence of cancer-producing substances in roasted food. *Nature*, **143**, 984.

4 Toxicants in Food: Food Allergens

Gerald Reese and Samuel B Lehrer

Department of Medicine, Section of Allergy and Clinical Immunology, Tulane University School of Medicine, New Orleans, USA

Adverse reactions to foods

Adverse reactions to foods, although caused by different mechanisms, can be confused with one another since they elicit similar symptoms (Sampson and Metcalfe, 1991). In the broadest terms, an adverse reaction to a food is defined as a clinically abnormal response attributed to exposure to foods or food additives. This includes both immunologic and non-immunologic reactions (Table 4.1). 'True' food allergy, or food hypersensitivity, is an immunologically mediated adverse reaction and occurs only in specifically sensitised individuals. Most food allergies are mediated by IgE antibodies and have a rapid onset, typically within minutes of exposure (Sampson and Metcalfe, 1991). Allergens, as any other antigens, are able to induce a specific humoral and/ or cellular immune response. However, allergens induce a Th-2 rather than a Th-1 lymphocyte response, thus resulting in the production of allergen-specific IgE. IgE antibodies bind to specific receptors on mast cells or basophils (the effector cell) and when allergen reaches the sensitised mast cell, it cross-links surface-bound IgE ('bridging') triggering the release of preformed and newly synthesised mediators. These mediators, in turn, elicit the clinical signs and symptoms of allergic diseases including asthma, eczema, hay fever and anaphylaxis (Geha, 1984; Roitt *et al.*, 1985). There is evidence for genetic control of IgE antibody production to specific allergens (Marsh *et al.*, 1974; Blumenthal *et al.*, 1981) even though the immunological mechanisms involved or the structural features of allergens that distinguish them from other tolerated food antigens are not fully understood.

Other adverse reactions to foods are food intolerance, an abnormal physiological response to ingested food or food additive; food poisoning, which is basically a toxic reaction; and pharmacological food reactions, due to

Nutrition and Chemical Toxicity. Edited by Costas Ioannides. © John Wiley & Sons Ltd. ISBN 0 471 97453 6

Table 4.1 Classification of adverse reactions to foods

Type of adverse reaction		Mechanism
Immunologically mediated (food allergy)	IgE-mediated	Cross-linking (bridging) of cell-bound allergen-specific IgE by allergen
	Not IgE-mediated	Diseases such as gastroenteropathy and coeliac disease; role of food in immunological mechanism is unknown
Not immunologically mediated (food intolerance)	Toxic	Caused by naturally occurring toxins, food-processing-induced compounds, or contaminants
	Enzymic	Lactose intolerance
	Pharmacological	Individuals with high reactivity to substances such as vasoactive amines (histamine)
	Undefined	Mechanism unknown, e.g. some reactions to food additives

Adapted from Anderson (1996).

substances such as biogenic amines (e.g. histamine) that produce a drug-like effect and mimic symptoms of food allergy.

Diagnosis of food allergy

The diagnosis of food allergy is still considered difficult. A major problem is that many extracts used for *in vivo* and *in vitro* diagnosis are neither well-characterised and most are not well-standardised; the allergenic potency of some of these extracts is at best questionable. Even the value of the 'gold standard' of food allergy diagnosis, the double-blind, placebo-controlled food challenge (DBPCFC) may be impaired by low-quality extracts since DBPCFC is only as accurate as the activity of the food material used in an oral challenge test (Atkins *et al.*, 1985; Sampson and Metcalfe, 1991).

EXTRACTS FOR DIAGNOSTIC USE

In contrast to extracts of many inhalant and stinging insect allergens such as grass pollen, house dust mite and bee venom extract, extracts of allergenic foods are only used in food allergy diagnosis but not for therapy (immunotherapy of food allergy is not considered to be safe and advantageous). The most important requirement of a well-prepared extract is that it contains relevant allergens in an immunologically active form in sufficient amounts. An extract containing immunologically inactive allergens or only a small amount of active allergen may yield false negative results. For example, apple extracts and extracts of other fruits are frequently inactive, and fresh fruits rather than extracts are often recommended for use in skin prick testing. Other extracts such as peanut or shrimp, that contain more stable food allergens are more reliable, but can also vary in their allergen content (Jeoung et al., 1997). In general, the quality of food extracts has to be improved to obtain reliable, standardised reagents since the reliability of in vitro and in vivo diagnostic tests and procedures depends on high-quality extracts.

IN VIVO DIAGNOSIS

A skin test is the most common in vivo method to demonstrate sensitisation to an allergen. Allergen is pricked (skin prick test) or injected intracutaneously (intracutaneous test) into the skin. If the subject is sensitised, a localised allergic reaction (wheal-and-flare reaction) occurs. The skin prick test is the preferred method over intracutaneous testing since it does not result in as many false positive reactions and the risk of systemic reactions is diminished.

As mentioned earlier, the DBPCFC is considered the gold standard for the diagnosis of adverse reactions to foods (Bock et al., 1988). The subject ingests masked allergen or placebo, and any reactions and symptoms are noted. Neither subject nor physician have prior knowledge whether the oral provocation is performed with allergen or with placebo. It is important that the allergen is carefully masked, so that the subject cannot identify the allergen-containing sample by smell, taste or texture.

IN VITRO DIAGNOSIS

In vitro tests measure allergen-specific IgE. The detection of specific IgE in and of itself is not sufficient to diagnose an allergy since the presence of specific IgE does not always correlate with clinical symptoms. RAST (radio allergosorbent test) is the most commonly used assay to measure allergen-specific IgE. CAP and ELISA are performed according the same principle, using solid-phase-bound allergen which is probed with patient's serum and a labelled, IgE-specific antibody or antiserum. Immunoblotting is useful as a research and diagnostic tool to identify IgE antibody reactivity to individual allergenic molecules in crude, multi-allergen extracts.

Radio allergosorbent test (RAST)

In the RAST, the allergen extract is covalently bound to a suitable solid phase, frequently a paper disc. The disc is incubated with serum from an allergic subject, allowing the allergen-specific IgE antibodies to bind to the allergen. The bound IgE antibodies are then detected with ^{125}L-labelled anti-human IgE.

Histamine release test

This test measures the amount of histamine released from blood basophils. Allergen is added to peripheral blood cells from allergic subjects, basophils carrying allergen-specific IgE antibodies degranulate, and released histamine is measured by fluorescence or radioimmuno assay (RIA). This test is not routinely used in allergy *in vitro* diagnosis as the test requires viable blood cells and must be performed within a short time after the blood is drawn.

Allergen characterisation

Identifying and characterising individual allergens in allergenic foods is a step to improve extract quality and to study and understand the interactions between the immune system and allergen on a molecular level. Allergen characterisation encompasses the detection of individual allergens in a given allergenic source, allergen identification, and analysis of immunological properties of its structural features. This encompasses the characterisation of their primary structures and the identification of portions of the allergen molecule (epitopes) which interact with antibodies or cells of the immune system. Epitopes that bind to peptide-specific receptors on T cells are called T-cell epitopes, whereas epitopes that bind to B cell-produced antibodies are called B-cell epitopes. In general, it is thought that T-cell epitopes do not depend on protein conformation (linear epitopes) whereas B-cell epitopes do (conformational epitopes). However, there may be exceptions to this rule (King, 1994).

ALLERGEN CLASSIFICATION AND NOMENCLATURE

The most general classification of allergenic proteins used is the division into major and minor allergens. According to this definition, major allergens are defined as allergens to which >50% of specifically sensitised allergic subjects react; minor allergens are detected by < 50% of allergic subjects. For example, Pen a 1 is a major shrimp allergen because >80% of all shrimp-allergic subjects have Pen a 1-specific IgE antibodies. This classification does not include the percentage of specific IgE bound by a particular allergen molecule and may not necessarily reflect the clinical importance of a particular allergen.

According to nomenclature rules (King *et al.*, 1995), allergens are designated according to the accepted taxonomic name of their source. The first three letters of the genus, followed by a space, the first letter of the species' name, another space, and an arabic number. Numbers are assigned in chronological order of characterisation and homologous allergens from related species are generally assigned the same number. For example, the first allergen described in brown shrimp, *Penaeus aztecus*, was designated Pen a 1 and the homologous allergens in Indian shrimp, *P. indicus*, and greasyback shrimp (*Metapenaeus ensis*) are named Pen i 1 and Met e 1, respectively. However, these nomenclature rules are not strictly applied to all major allergens, some well-known proteins that were studied for other purposes than their later discovered allergenicity are not named according to these roles. For example, the well-characterised milk allergen β-lactalbumin is not named according to the nomenclature rules.

METHODS TO DETECT INDIVIDUAL ALLERGENS

The first step of allergen characterisation is to analyse the IgE antibody response to individual proteins. This is usually achieved by separating proteins according to their biophysical properties and probing the separated proteins with sera of allergic subjects who are allergic to a particular allergen.

Crossed radio-immuno electrophoresis (CRIE) was one of the first methods to identify individual allergens (Weeke, 1973; Løwenstein et al., 1976; Aukrust and Aas, 1997). CRIE provides qualitative and semiquantitative information concerning the IgE reactivity and the amount of allergen present in the extract; however, it is not widely used anymore, since this method is not suitable for general extract standardisation and allergen identification because polyclonal antisera from different immunisations or laboratories used to precipitate the allergens may vary, and allergens may be missed if the antiserum does not precipitate a particular allergen or binds to IgE-binding sites.

Immunoblotting

Immunoblotting is now the most frequently used methodology to identify and characterisation allergens. It consists basically of four steps: electrophoretic separation of proteins; transfer of separated proteins onto a carrier membrane; incubation with the subject's serum; and detection of IgE antibodies which bind to individual bands (allergens).

Allergens can be separated according to molecular size (sodium dodecylsulphate polyacrylamide gel electrophoresis, SDS–PAGE), isoelectric point (pI.) (isoelectric focusing, IEF), or two-dimensionally (2D) using IEF for the first dimension and SDS–PAGE for the second dimension. SDS–PAGE is the most frequently used separation technique even though treatment with SDS and reducing agents such as β-mercaptoethanol, dithiothreitol (DTT) or dithioerythriol (DTE) may destroy allergenic epitopes with a loss of IgE binding. Separated proteins are transferred from the gel onto carrier membranes electrophoretically (semi-dry blotting) (Kyhse-Andersen, 1984), tank blotting or if an agarose gel is used, by capillary force (Peltre et al., 1982). Nitrocellulose, CNBr-activated nitrocellulose (Demeulemester et al., 1987) and polyvinylidine difluoride (PVDF) membranes are the most frequently used carrier membranes. 2D immunoblotting can be a valuable tool to purify small amounts of allergen sufficient for N-terminal sequencing (Petersen et al., 1993, 1994).

RAST inhibition

RAST inhibition is a modified version of the standard RAST. Serum is incubated in the presence of different concentrations of allergen extract in the fluid phase. If IgE antibodies bind to either solid phase and fluid phase allergens, IgE binding to solid phase allergens decreases with increasing inhibitor concentration. This assay format is used to trace allergens contaminating other foods (Yunginger et al., 1983; Keating et al., 1990; Gern et al., 1991; Jones et al., 1992; Nordlee et al., 1993) to assess the effect of processing on the allergenicity of various products made from peanuts and soybeans (Nordlee et al., 1981; Herian et al., 1993), and to study cross-reactivities among allergens. RAST inhibition test was also used to identify Brazil nut allergen in transgenic soybeans (Nordlee et al., 1994, 1996).

ALLERGEN IDENTIFICATION AND MOLECULAR CHARACTERISATION

The characterisation of allergen structure is a prerequisite to study the interaction of immune system and allergen on a molecular level. Without the knowledge of the amino acid sequence of an allergen, it is impossible to identify IgE binding sites (B-cell epitopes) and T-cell-binding peptides (T-cell epitopes). Different strategies have been employed; peptides, obtained from enzymatically digested, purified allergens were sequenced, and expression cDNA expression libraries were screened with IgE antibodies. Food allergens that have been characterised are summarised in Table 4.2. Since many food proteins have been studied for reasons other than their allergenicity (i.e. because they are important storage, structural and functional proteins), it is often possible to identify a food allergen by searching protein databases using only a small part of its entire amino acid sequence. In this context, electrophoretically purified and blotted allergens may provide a simple approach to obtain sufficient amounts of purified proteins for N-terminal sequencing. For example, the major shrimp allergen Pen a 1 was isolated by preparative SDS–PAGE, eluted from the gel, digested with proteinase Lys-C, and a 21 amino acid residue-long peptide was sequenced. This sequence identified Pen a 1 as the muscle protein tropomyosin (Daul et al., 1994).

Common properties of food allergens

Most foods contain a large number of different proteins, though only a few of these elicit allergic reactions. This prompts the question whether allergens share common properties that distinguish them from other, non-allergenic food proteins. In our view, there is no convincing answer to this question today. However, some very broad characteristics common to several food allergens have been identified. These include abundance of a given protein in a particular food, and physicochemical properties, such as a molecular

Table 4.2 Identified and characterised major food allergens

Allergen source	Allergens (systematic and original names)	Molecular weight (kDa)	Sequence data	References[a]
Gadus calarias (cod)	Gad c 1; allergen M	12	C	Elsayed and Bennich, 1975
Gallus domesticus	Gal d 1; ovomucoid	28	C	Hoffman, 1983
(chicken)	Gal d 2; ovalbumin	44	C	Langeland, 1983b
	Gal d 3; conalbumin (Ag22)	78	C	Williams *et al.*, 1982
	Gal d 4; lysozyme	14	C	Blake *et al.*, 1965
Penaeus aztecus (brown shrimp)	Pen a 1; tropomyosin	36	P	Daul *et al.*, 1993, 1994
Penaeus indicus (Indian shrimp)	Pen i 1; tropomyosin	34	P	Shanti *et al.*, 1993
Metapenaeus enis (greasyback shrimp)	Met e 1; tropomyosin	34	C	Leung *et al.*, 1994
Brassica juncea (oriental mustard)	Bra j 1; 25 albumin	14	C	Monsalve *et al.*, 1993
Hordeum vulgare (barley)	Hor v 1; BMAI-1	15	C	Mena *et al.*, 1992
Sinapis alba (yellow mustard)	Sin a 1; 25 albumin	14	C	Menendez-Arias *et al.*, 1988
Arachis hypogea (peanut)	Ara h 1	63.5	C	Burks *et al.*, 1995a,b,c
	Ara h 2	17.5	C	Stanley *et al.*, 1997
Malus domestica (apple)	Mal d 1	17.7	C	Vanek-Krebitz *et al.*, 1995
Apium graveolens (celery)	Api g 1	16.2	C	Breiteneder *et al.*, 1995

Modified from Lehrer *et al.* (1997).
[a]References for partial (P) or complete (C) sequence data.

weight (10–70 kDa), acidic isoelectric point, glycosylation and resistance to heat and digestion (Taylor *et al.*, 1987). These characteristics have been associated with protein allergenicity; many of these properties, however, characterise a vast number of non-allergenic proteins as well and thus are not unique to food allergens.

Abundance

Food allergens frequently account for a major fraction of the total protein content within a given food. For example, in peanuts and soybeans (Herian *et al.*, 1990; Burks *et al.*, 1991, 1992) important allergens were identified as major storage proteins. Similarly, the muscle protein tropomyosin, the major allergen in shrimp, accounts for about 25–30% of the total shrimp tail muscle protein (Daul *et al.*, 1991, 1992). An exception to this rule is the major allergen of codfish parvalbumin (Gad c 1) that is not a dominant protein in codfish muscle (Elsayed and Bennich, 1975).

Molecular size

Three reasons make molecular size relevant for protein allergenicity. First, the protein must be large enough to elicit an immune response. Second, it must be of sufficient size for at least two IgE binding sites to bridge mast cell-bound IgE; and third, the protein must be small enough to cross the gut mucosal membrane barrier. Most known food allergens have molecular weights between 10 and 70 kDa, thus fulfilling these requirements. The molecular weight of 10 kDa probably represents a lower limit of immunogenicity; the upper limit of 70 kDa probably reflects restricted mucosal absorption of large molecules (Taylor *et al.*, 1987). However, there are exceptions to these size restrictions. For example, native peanut allergens Ara h 1 and Ara h 2 are large polymers with molecular weights between 200–300 kDa (Burks *et al.*, 1991, 1992). It is not known whether the polymer itself or the subunits cleaved during digestion act as allergens. In contrast, mellitin, a 21-amino acid residue peptide from bee venom, induces histamine release from basophils and mast cells (King *et al.*, 1993). Even though this 3-kDa peptide is not a food allergen, it demonstrates that a protein smaller than 10 kDa can act as an allergen; it induces an immune response, binds specific IgE and causes mast cell and basophil degranulation.

Acidic isoelectric point and glycosylation

Most allergens are glycoproteins with an acidic isoelectric point (pI). However, these characteristics are not unique to allergens and many other non-allergenic proteins also exhibit them.

Heat resistance

Heat-resistance is probably the most common feature of potent food allergens. The fact that heat denaturation may cause loss of the native protein's conformation, yet patients' IgE antibodies still react with these denatured food proteins, indicates that the native conformation may not always be crucial for IgE binding. Thus, food allergens may contain a large number of non-conformational, sequential epitopes. Cow's milk caseins and whey proteins, for example, retain their allergenicity after heating (Kilshaw *et al.*, 1982, Ford *et al.*, 1983; Host and Samuelsson, 1988; Lee, 1992).

Resistance to digestion

The ability of food allergens to cross the mucosal membrane of the intestinal tract is most likely an important feature. As mentioned earlier, size is one parameter in this context. Another property may be resistance to digestion. Studies that used a gastric model for mammalian digestion to study the digestibility of food allergens point in this direction (Fuchs and Astwood, 1996; Metcalfe *et al.*, 1996). In this study, the digestibility of allergens from egg, milk, peanut, soybean and mustard were evaluated. Food allergens tested resisted digestion for up to an hour whereas the few non-allergens that were tested were digested within a minute. However, not all allergens are resistant to digestion and many non-allergenic proteins may be resistant so that there is still insufficient information to conclude that the resistance to digestion is the most important property that characterises a food allergen.

Important food allergens

A number of plant- and animal-derived foods have been identified as major sources of food allergens. Important plant-derived food allergens have been identified in legumes, particularly peanuts and soybeans; seeds and nuts; fruit; vegetables; grains; and spices. A number of foods from animal sources have been implicated to cause allergic reactions; however, only a few have been well studied. Major sources of allergens in this group are milk, eggs, fish and shellfish, particularly crustaceans.

PEANUT ALLERGENS

Peanut (*Arachis hypogaea*) ranks first as the cause of severe and lethal, anaphylactic reactions to foods; very small amounts may trigger an allergic reaction. Several children die every year from allergic reactions to peanut. Peanut allergens are subject to intense analysis due to their high allergenic potential and the economic importance of peanuts as a protein source for the food processing industry. Peanuts contain a large number of allergens; up to 37 allergenic peanut components have been identified (Barnett *et al.*, 1983; Bush *et al.*, 1983). Four peanut allergens have been described as major allergens. Peanut 1, Concanavalin A-reactive protein, Ara h 1 and Ara h 2.

Burks and coworkers (Burks *et al.*, 1991, 1995a,b) recently identified Ara h 1 and Ara h 2; their ongoing studies are some of the most advanced with regard to understanding the interaction of molecular structure of food allergens and the immune system. Ara h 1, a 63.5-kDa glycoprotein (Burks *et al.*, 1991, 1995a) is vicilin, a peanut storage protein, a major protein from the globulin fraction (Burks *et al.*, 1995b). Ara h 2, a second major peanut allergen (Burks *et al.*, 1992), is smaller than Ara h 1 with a molecular weight of 17.5 kDa and an isoelectric point of 5.2 (Burks *et al.*, 1992); it showed homology to the conglutinin family of seed storage proteins. Experiments with Ara h 1- and Ara h 2-specific monoclonal antibodies and human IgE identified three (Burks *et al.*, 1994; Stanley *et al.*, 1995) and two antigenic sites on Ara h 1 and Ara h 2 (Burks *et al.*, 1995c), respectively.

In recent studies, the major linear IgE-binding epitopes of Ara h 1 and Ara h 2 were systematically mapped using overlapping peptides synthesised on an activated cellulose membrane and pooled serum IgE from peanut-sensitive patients (Burks *et al.*, 1997; Stanley *et al.*, 1997). Twenty-three Ara h 1 and ten different linear Ara h 2 IgE-binding epitopes, located throughout the lengths of the molecules, were identified; no obvious sequence motif was shared by all peptides. Four Ara h 1 and three Ara h 2 peptides were immunodominant epitopes as they were recognised by more than 80% of the patients tested. Mutational analysis of the immunodominant epitopes revealed that single amino acid changes within these peptides could have dramatic effects on IgE-binding characteristics: single amino acid substitutions resulted in loss or increase of IgE binding.

SOYBEAN ALLERGENS

Similar to peanuts, soybeans (*Glycine max*) contain multiple allergens. A small study with four subjects suggested the 2S-globulin fraction as a major source of allergens (Shibasaki *et al.*, 1980); further, significant IgE binding to proteins with molecular weights between 14 and 70 kDa was demonstrated in the 7S fraction with major binding to a 30-kDa band (Ogawa *et al.*, 1991). This band was designated as Gly m 1. The 15-amino acid N-terminal sequence of Gly m 1 has been determined and is identical with the 34-kDa oil body-associated protein from soybean. This soybean protein also reacts with human IgE and Gly m 1-specific monoclonal antibodies. Some 65% of soybean-reactive subjects had specific Gly m 1-specific IgE antibodies; however, none of these individuals experienced severe or anaphylactic reactions to soybeans.

Other proteins were also identified as soybean allergens. The Kunitz soybean trypsin inhibitor was identified as a soybean allergen by skin test, RAST and RAST inhibition in a soybean-allergic subject (Moroz and Yang, 1980); the IgE reactivity to soybean was inhibited completely by the Kunitz soybean trypsin inhibitor. However, the RAST reactivity of two other sera from soy-allergic individuals indicate that the Kunitz soybean trypsin inhibitor is a relatively minor allergen.

A 68-kDa allergen was identified as a minor soy allergen (Ogawa *et al.*, 1995). It reacted with sera from approximately 25% of soy-allergic subjects and was identified as the α-subunit of β-conglycinin. IgE only bound to the α subunit but not to the α_1 and β-subunits, even though these structures are highly homologous.

Allergenic activity of other legumes was reported. For example, albumins in pea (*Pisum sativum*) were described as allergens (Grant *et al.*, 1976). The allergens appeared to be stable as they retained their allergenic activity when heated or boiled. A 1.8-kDa allergen from green peas with a carbohydrate content of 30% was purified from pea dialysate (Malley *et al.*, 1975, 1976), but was not further characterised.

RICE

The major allergens from rice (*Oryza sativa*) are encoded by a multigene family (Adachi *et al.*, 1993). Rice allergens range from 14 to 60 kDa (Matsuda *et al.*, 1993) and are resistant to heat and proteolysis. The cDNA sequence coding for the major rice allergen Ory s 1 has been determined (Izumi *et al.*, 1992; Adachi *et al.*, 1993). The mature protein has a molecular weight of approximately 14 kDa and has an amino acid sequence homology of 20% and 40% with the barley trypsin inhibitor and the wheat α-amylase inhibitor, respectively. Attempts have been made to select hypoallergenic strains (Izumi *et al.*, 1992; Adachi *et al.*, 1993; Matsuda *et al.*, 1993; Watanabe, 1993). Protease treatment was used to reduce the allergenicity of the rice (Watanabe, 1993) though this process requires large amounts of enzyme. To reduce the allergenicity of rice, synthesis of rice allergen was suppressed (Matsuda and Nakamura, 1993). Matsuda and colleagues have cloned and sequenced a 16-kDa rice seed protein that was identified as the major rice allergen. Based on its nucleotide sequence, an antisense RNA strategy was applied to repress expression of this allergen in maturing rice seeds. Seeds from transgenic rice plants with the antisense gene have substantially reduced amounts of the allergen (Adachi *et al.*, 1993; Matsuda and Nakamura, 1993; Matsuda *et al.*, 1993; Watanabe, 1993).

CORN

Corn (*Zea mays*) is generally not considered as an important food allergen. In a recent study, however, the IgE-binding proteins in corn were identified (Lehrer *et al.*, 1997b). As with most cereals, corn contains mostly alcohol-soluble proteins. These proteins have not been considered in terms of their allergenicity. In order to assess IgE-reactive corn proteins, aqueous and alcohol extracts were prepared of corn seeds according to established biochemical procedures and analysed by immunoblotting. Forty-seven sera of corn-reactive individuals were tested. Individuals were considered corn-reactive if they met two out of three criteria: a history of food allergy consistent with corn allergy, positive skin test to corn, or positive IgE response to corn. Two-thirds of these subjects had significant IgE antibodies to proteins present in aqueous extracts and, more interestingly, approximately 60% of the corn-reactive subjects also showed significant reactivity to proteins in the alcohol extracts. The allergenic reactivity to alcohol-soluble proteins did not necessarily correlate with that to proteins present in the aqueous extract. Twenty water-soluble and eight alcohol-soluble IgE-reactive bands were identified in corn. Two proteins of the aqueous corn fraction with molecular weights of 28 kDa and 10 kDa reacted with more than 50% of the subjects' sera, whereas one 28-kDa band of the alcohol fraction can be considered a major allergen. These results demonstrate the need for proper extraction methods for preparing food allergen extracts that are based on properties of the proteins present, rather than merely employing historically used standard extraction procedures. However, to establish the clinical relevance of corn IgE reactivities, double-blind, placebo-controlled food challenges must be performed.

NUTS

Brazil nuts (*Bertholletia excelsa*) can cause systemic anaphylaxis in some individuals. Several allergenic fractions were identified by immunoblotting using sera from Brazil nut-allergic subjects (Arshad *et al.*, 1991). The major allergen from Brazil nut Ber e 1 is a high-methionine, 2S protein (Nordlee *et al.*, 1994, 1996) with a molecular weight of 12 kDa. Ber e 1 is a dimer that consists of 9-kDa and 3-kDa subunits. The cDNA sequence of Ber e 1 was determined (Altenbach *et al.*, 1987) and its amino acid sequence deduced. Ber e 1 is homologous to high-methionine proteins from castor bean and rapeseed.

Other nuts are also a source of allergens. Bargman *et al.* (1992) used immunoblotting techniques to detect IgE binding proteins in almond extracts. A number of IgE-binding proteins ranging from 38 to 70 kDa were detected. A 70-kDa heat-labile and a 40–50-kDa heat-stable allergen were identified. Furthermore, chestnuts and pistachio were implicated as potential allergens. Reactivity to chestnuts was demonstrated in latex-allergic subjects (Anibarro *et al.*, 1993; Fernandez de Corres *et al.*, 1993).

EGG ALLERGENS

Food allergy to proteins from egg of the domestic chicken (*Gallus domesticus*) is one of the most frequently implicated causes of immediate food allergic reactions in children in the United States and Europe (Crespo *et al.*, 1994).

Egg sensitivity frequently disappears by the fourth or fifth year of life; however, one-third of individuals have clinical sensitivity that lasts over 6 years (Crespo *et al.*, 1994). Egg white (albumin) appears to be more allergenic than yolk, and egg white proteins have been extensively studied and sequenced (Yunginger, 1990).

Four proteins, ovomucoid, ovalbumin, ovotransferrin (conalbumin) and lysozyme, have been identified as major egg white allergens. Ovomucoid (Gal d 1) is a glycoprotein with a molecular weight of 28 kDa, and an isoelectric point of 4.1. Its primary structure (Kato *et al.*, 1987) is a polypeptide chain of 186 amino acids. The tertiary structure consists of three tandem domains each homologous to the pancreatic secretory trypsin inhibitor. Ovalbumin (Gal d 2) (Langeland, 1983a,b) is a monomeric phosphoglycoprotein with a molecular weight between 43 and 45 kDa and an isoelectric point of 4.5. Gal d 2 contains 385 amino acid residues (McReynolds *et al.*, 1978; Nisbet *et al.*, 1981). Ovotransferrin (Conalbumin, Gal d 3) has a molecular weight of 77 kDa, an isoelectric point of 6.0 and is 686 amino acid residues long (Jeltsch and Chambon, 1982; Williams *et al.*, 1982). Lysozyme (Gal d 4) has a molecular weight of 14.3 kDa and an isoelectric point of 10.7. Gal d 4 contains 129 amino acid residues in a single polypeptide chain cross-linked by four disulphide bounds (Canfield, 1963). The importance of Gal d 4 as an allergen is still not well established. In one study (Miller and Campbell, 1950), lysozyme was found to be a major allergen by skin testing whereas in another study (Langeland, 1983a) no sera from egg-allergic patients had positive IgE reactivity to Gal d 4. In contrast, a third study (Anet *et al.*, 1985) showed that about half of the egg-sensitive patients reacted to lysozyme by RAST.

Only minimal information is available concerning epitopes of egg allergens; ovalbumin has been the best egg allergen studied so far. IgE was found to bind the two CNBr-fragments of ovalbumin (residues 41–172 and 301–385) (Kahlert *et al.*, 1992), and in another study (Honma *et al.*, 1996) a ten-amino acid residue peptide (OVA357-366) inhibited histamine release from basophils. Two T-cell reactive ovalbumin peptides (OVA 105-122 and OVA 323-339) were reported (Shimojo *et al.*, 1994; Holen and Elsayed, 1996) which did not bind IgE.

In addition to ovomucoid, ovalbumin, ovotransferrin and lysozyme, a variety of other egg proteins have been described as minor allergens. These include ovomucin, ovoinhibitor, ovaflavoprotein, apovitellenin and phosvitin (Anet *et al.*, 1985; Scott *et al.*, 1987; Taylor *et al.*, 1987; Walsh *et al.*, 1987, 1988), but these proteins were not studied in more detail.

COW'S MILK ALLERGENS

Cow's milk is one of the most common food allergens. It is estimated that between 0.3 and 7.5% of infants and young children suffer from cow's milk allergy (Wershil and Walker, 1988; Amonette *et al.*, 1993). Cow's milk is a very complex mixture of proteins; two major groups of cow's milk proteins, caseins and β-lactoglobulin, have been identified as major allergens (Savilathi, 1981; Alexander et al., 1989; Amonette et al., 1992; Savilathi and Kuitonen, 1992). Caseins are phosphoproteins that precipitate from raw skim milk upon acidification to pH 4.6 at 20°C. They comprise 80% of the total milk protein. Whey proteins are those proteins remaining in the fluid ('serum') after casein precipitation (Whitney, 1988).

The biochemistry of milk proteins has been extensively studied; many cow's milk proteins have been sequenced (Swaisgood, 1985; Whitney, 1988), and computer-based molecular modelling of the three-dimensional structure of several milk proteins has also been reported (Kumosinski et al., 1991a,b, 1993). Surprisingly, even though cow's milk is a major food allergen and the structures of cow's milk allergens are well studied, the major IgE binding sites and T-cell epitopes of milk allergens have not been determined in humans.

Caseins and β-lactoglobulin appear to be the major allergens in cow's milk (Savilathi, 1981; Amonette et al., 1992; Savilathi and Kuitonen, 1992). The caseins are a family of chemically related proteins. The frequency of reactivity to different casein variants has not been systematically studied. α-S1 casein has at least five genetic variants, with varying degrees of post-translational phosphorylation, and four α-S2 casein variants have been identified. β-Caseins are a group of proteins which have one major component with seven genetic variants and eight minor components which are proteolytic fragments of the major component. The molecular weight of the major component is 24 kDa. β-Lactoglobulin is a whey protein that comprises approximately 20% of total milk proteins. It has a molecular weight of 18 kDa and at least six genetic variants have been identified. The primary structure has been determined (Swaisgood, 1985; Whitney, 1988) and the protein has a 91% sequence homology with egg β-lactoglobulin (Alexander et al., 1989).

The whey proteins α-lactalbumin and bovine serum albumin (BSA) have been identified as minor cow's milk allergens (Goldman et al., 1963). α-Lactalbumin has a molecular weight of 14 kDa and its amino acid sequence has been determined (Swaisgood, 1985; Hurley and Schuler, 1987; Whitney, 1988). BSA has a molecular weight of 67 kDa and comprises 1% of total milk protein.

FISH ALLERGENS

The consumption of fish (Elsayed et al., 1972) is a frequent cause of IgE-mediated reactions. Fish is one among the most commonly implicated allergenic foods, and have been incriminated in fatal anaphylactic reactions (Yunginger et al., 1988). Species-specific analysis of IgE reactivities have not been performed since most studies were either performed with cod, or information about the species tested are not provided.

One of the first and most comprehensive analyses of a food allergen was the purification and characterisation of the major codfish allergen, Gad c 1. This was originally designated allergen M from Baltic cod, *Gadus callarius*. It belongs to a group of muscle proteins called parvalbumins (Elsayed and Bennich, 1975) and constitutes approximately 0.05–0.1% of the white cod muscle tissue. Gad c 1 has a molecular weight of 12.3 kDa and an isoelectric point of 4.75. Its amino acid sequence has been established; it contains 113 amino acid residues (Elsayed and Aas, 1970; Elsayed and Bennich, 1975; Elsayed *et al.*, 1976). Gad c 1 contains at least five IgE binding sides (Elsayed and Apold, 1983). Studies using synthetic peptides established that region 49 to 64 encircled two repetitive sequences. These two tetrapeptides appear to be mutually important for IgE binding as region 49–64 showed relatively high RAST inhibition compared with Gad c 1 and could produce a Praunitz–Küstner reaction.

Minor cod fish allergens distinct from Gad c 1 (Aukrust *et al.*, 1978) were identified but were not further characterised. Some 25% of fish-allergic subjects bound to an allergen designated as Ag-17-cod (Aukrust *et al.*, 1978) and approximately 10% of cod-allergic individuals reacted to a cod blood serum protein (Aas and Elsayed, 1975). Protamine sulphate, a low-molecular-weight sperm protein of fish species belonging to the families Salmonidae and Clueidea, has been implicated as a fish allergen. However, based on the results of several studies, (Caplan and Beckman, 1976; Knape *et al.*, 1981; Greenberger *et al.*, 1989; Levy *et al.*, 1989), it can be concluded that protamine sulphate is rarely allergenic for fish-allergic subjects.

CRUSTACEA ALLERGENS

Crustacea such as prawns, crabs, lobster and crawfish are a common cause of food hypersensitivity. Like fish, a higher incidence of crustacea allergy can be expected in geographical areas where more shellfish are consumed on a regular basis, such as the Gulf coast region of the United States.

Several studies (Hoffman *et al.*, 1981; Nagpal *et al.*, 1989; Daul *et al.*, 1994; Leung *et al.*, 1994) described the identification of shrimp allergens. As with all other allergenic foods, several allergens were found in shrimp; it is now known that the muscle protein tropomyosin is the most important major allergen. The results of our studies indicate that the structural features responsible for the allergenicity of Pen a 1 are located in the phylogenetically diverse parts of tropomyosin rather than the conserved parts. This was confirmed for different shrimp species; Pen a 1 from brown shrimp (*Penaeus aztecus*) (Daul *et al.*, 1994), Pen i 1 from Indian shrimp (*Penaeus indicus*) (Shanti *et al.*, 1993) and Met e 1 from greasyback shrimp (*Metapenaeus ensis*) (Leung *et al.*, 1994). There is very good evidence that clinically relevant cross-reactivity is due to virtually identical primary structures: the cDNA of Pen a 1 showed 26 base pair substitutions when compared with the sequence of Met e 1; these base pair substitutions, however, resulted in only one amino acid substitution (Figure 4.1). Furthermore, Pen a 1 and tail muscle tropomyosin of American lobster (*Homarus americanus*) differ only in three amino acid positions. Slow tropomyosin from the claws of American lobster differ from Pen a 1 in 18 positions mainly clustered around position 57 (Mykles *et al.*, 1998); the differences in the allergenicity have not been studied but based on epitope studies on Pen i 1 and Pen a 1, its allergenicity is probably not critically affected.

In Pen i 1 (Shanti *et al.*, 1993) two peptides, of 17 and 9 amino acid residues each, were identified as important IgE-binding epitopes, since they inhibited more than 50% of specific IgE reactivity to Pen i 1. Four IgE-binding Pen a 1 epitopes were identified recently (Reese *et al.*, 1997). One of two IgE-reactive peptides, previously identified in the Indian shrimp, *P. indicus* as peptide 153–161 (Daul *et al.*, 1994), partially overlaps with IgE-reactive peptide from *P. aztecus* 157–166 (Reese *et al.*, 1997), indicating that this part of shrimp tropomyosin is a major IgE binding site (Figure 4.1).

In our view, the shrimp allergen tropomyosin provides a unique opportunity to study the contribution of protein structure to a protein's allergenicity since sequences of non-allergenic tropomyosins from pork, beef and poultry are known and shrimp-allergic subjects usually do not suffer from allergies to vertebrate meats (Ayuso *et al.*, 1998). Comparison of allergenic Pen a 1 epitopes with homologous sequences of vertebrate tropomyosins and sequential amino acid substitution experiments may help to understand and predict the allergenicity of proteins.

Food cross-reactivities

Cross-reactivities are found among foods of related phylogenetic origin and foods of seemingly unrelated non-food allergens. Allergens from legumes, fishes, crustaceans, fruits, tree nuts are examples for phylogenetically related, cross-reacting allergens. In addition to cross-reactivity of foods within the same group, cross-reactivity has been described between foods that are unrelated or only distantly related. For example, it has been reported that ragweed pollen cross-reacts with melons and bananas (Anderson *et al.*, 1970; Enberg *et al.*, 1987); grass and mugwort pollens cross-react with celery and a variety of vegetables (Wütrich and Dietschi, 1985; Calkhoven *et al.*, 1987, 1991); and birch pollen cross-reacts with a number of fruits (Halmepuro *et al.*, 1984; Calkhoven *et al.*, 1991). Studies from our laboratory have shown that marine animals belonging to different phyla such as oysters and crustacea (Lehrer and McCants, 1988), or clams and shrimp (Desjardins *et al.*, 1995), cross-react.

The origin of food allergen cross-reactivity is still unknown; it is thought to be due to similar protein structure or multiple sensitisation to similar proteins in cross-reacting foods. The clinical relevance of food allergen cross-reactivity depends on the food in question. For example, the *in vitro* cross-reactivities among crustacea are thought to be clinically relevant – shrimp-allergic subjects

```
                 10        20        30        40        50        60        70        80        90        100
Pen i 1                                      AEKSEEAVHELQRMIQTUEDELDVTQESLLKANIQLVEKDKALSNAEGEVAALNRRIQLLEEDLE
Pen a 1                     DRADTLEQQNKEANNRAEKSEEVHNLQKRMQQLENDLDQVQESLLKANIQLVEKDKALSNAEGEVAALNRRIQLLEEDLE
Met e 1            MKLEKDNAMDRADTLEQQNKEANNRAEKSEEVHNLQKRMQQLENDLDQVQESLLKANNQLVEKDKALSNAEGEVAALNRRIQLLEEDLE
HomaTMf  MDAIKKKMQAMKLEKDNAMDRADTLEQQNKEANNRAEKSEEVHNLQKRMQQLENDLDQVQESLLKANNQLVEKDKALSNAEGEVAALNRRIQLLEEDLE
HomaTMs  MDAIKKKMQAMKLEKDNAMDRADTLEQQNKEANIRAEKTEEEIRITHKKMQQLENELDQVEQLSLANTKLEEKKALQNAEGEVAALNRRIQLLEEDLE
                                                        |——————|
                                                       50  Pen i 1  66

                 110       120       130       140       150       160       170       180       190       300
Pen i 1  R          LAEASQAADESER                              FLAEEADRKYDEVAR               ERAEQGESKIVELEEELRVV
Pen a 1  RSEERLNTATTKLAEASQAADSERMRKVLENRSLSDEERMDALENQLKEARFLAEEADRKYDEVARKLAMVEADLERAEBRAETGESKIVELEEELRVV
Met e 1  RSEERLNTATTKLAEASQAADSERMRKVLENRSLSDEERMDALENQLKEARFLAEEADRKYDEVARKLAMVEADLERAEBRAETGESKIVELEEELRVV
HomaTMf  RSEERLNTATTKLAEASQAADSERMRKVLENRSLSDEERMDALENQLKEARFLAEEADRKYDEVARKLAMVEADLERAEBRAETGESKIVELEEELRVV
HomaTMs  RSEERLNTATTKLAEASQAADSERMRKVLENRSLSDEERMDALENQLKEARFLAEEADRKYDEVARKLAMVEADLERAEBRAETGESKIVELEEELRVV
                         |———————|        |—Pen i 1—|     |—Pen a 1—|
                        136 Pen a 1 148  153       161   167       179
                                          157       169

                 210       220       230       240       250       260       270       280 284
Peni1    GNNLK        NKREEYKNQIK        AEFAER        DELVNEKEKYKQ
Pena1    GNNLKSLEVSEEKANQREEAYKEQIKTLTNKLKAAARAEFAERSVQKLQKEVDRLEDELVNEKEKYKSITDELDQTFSELSGY
Mete1    GNNLKSLEVSEEKANQREEAYKEQIKTLTNKLKAAARAEFAERSVQKLQKEVDRLEDELVNEKEKYKSITDELDQTFSELSGY
HomaTMf  GNNLKSLEVSEEKANQREEAYKEQIKTLTNKLKAAEARAEFAERSVQKLQKEVDRLEDELVNEKEKYKSITDELDQTFSELSGY
HomaTMs  GNNLKSLEVSEEKANQREEAYKEQIKTLANKLKAAARAEFAERSVQKLQKEVDRLEDELVNEKEKYKSITDELDQTFSELSGY
                                                        |——————|
                                                       262 Pen a 1 282
```

Figure 4.1 Sequence comparison of shrimp allergens Pen i 1, Pen a 1, Met e 1 and slow (HomaTMs; GenBank# AF034953) and fast muscle (HomaTMf; GenBank# AF034954) of American lobster (*Homarus americanus*). Pen i 1 and Pen a 1 epitopes are marked. (From Shanti *et al.*, 1993 and Reese *et al.*, 1997.)

can have clinical symptoms after ingesting lobster and crab (Lehrer, 1986; Daul *et al.*, 1987; Halmepuro *et al.*, 1987) whereas cross-reactivities among legumes seem to be of less clinical importance; peanut-allergic subjects who show *in vitro* IgE antibody reactivity to beans or peas usually do not show clinical symptoms after ingestion of beans or peas (Barnett *et al.*, 1987; Taylor *et al.*, 1987; Bernhisel-Broadbent and Sampson, 1989).

EXAMPLES OF CROSS-REACTING, PHYLOGENETICALLY RELATED FOODS

Legumes

Positive skin reactions and RASTs are frequently observed in peanut-allergic subjects to other leguminosae such as soybean, peas and beans (Barnett *et al.*, 1987; Bernhisel-Broadbent and Sampson, 1989; Bernhisel-Broadbent *et al.*, 1989; Bock and Atkins, 1990; Bernhisel-Broadbent, 1995). However, multiple positive skin tests to different leguminosae did not necessarily correlate with positive oral provocation (Bernhisel-Broadbent and Sampson, 1989) and the IgE reactivities to different leguminosae, analysed by Western blotting, did not correlate with clinically relevant symptoms either (Bernhisel-Broadbent *et al.*, 1989). An example of a seemingly clinically relevant cross-reactivity among legumes was reported by Hefle and Bush (1994) when a peanut-allergic child reacted to a lupin-fortified pasta product. The IgE-binding proteins of the lupin have an approximate molecular weight of 21 kDa (range from 35 to 55 kDa), and are heat-stable.

Fishes

The majority of consumed fishes belong to one of five taxonomic orders (Moody *et al.*, 1993): Perciformes (e.g. mackerel, tuna fish), Gadiformes (e.g. codfish), Pleuronectiformes (e.g. flounder), Cypriniformes (e.g. carp, catfish) and Clupeiformes (e.g. trout, salmon, herring). The reactivity to different fishes by RAST and skin test suggest cross-reactivity; however, the majority of fish-allergic subjects could eat other fish species or did not react during food challenge (Aas, 1996; Bernhisel-Broadbent *et al.*, 1992) indicating that the *in vitro* cross-reactivity may be of limited clinical relevance.

Crustacea

The substantial cross-reactivity among crustacea appears to be clinically important (Waring *et al.*, 1985; Daul *et al.*, 1987); for example shrimp-allergic subjects may react to other crustaceans without prior exposure. The cause for this cross-reactivity is probably the major allergen tropomyosin, a highly conserved muscle protein. Tropomyosin has been identified in three shrimp species: brown shrimp (*P. aztecus*) (Daul *et al.*, 1993, 1994), Indian shrimp (*P. indicus*)

(Shanti *et al.*, 1993) and greasyback shrimp (*M. ensis*) (Leung *et al.*, 1994). Pen a 1-like proteins were detected in crab, crawfish and lobster using sera of shrimp-allergic subjects and Pen a 1-specific monoclonal antibodies (Daul *et al.*, 1993, 1994). The amino acid sequence similarity among these different shrimp tropomyosin is very high; for example, Met e 1 and Pen a 1 only differ in one position (Leung *et al.*, 1994; Reese *et al.*, 1997).

EXAMPLES OF CROSS-REACTING, NON-RELATED FOODS

Cross-reactivity between foods and pollens

Birch, mugwort and ragweed pollen have been associated with various food allergies. For example, ragweed pollen cross-reacts with melons and bananas (Anderson *et al.*, 1970; Enberg *et al.*, 1987); grass and mugwort pollens cross-react with celery and a variety of vegetables (Wütrich and Dietschi, 1985; Calkhoven *et al.*, 1987, 1991); and birch pollen cross-reacts with a number of fruits (Halmepuro *et al.*, 1984; Calkhoven *et al.*, 1991). As the interest in cross-reactivity between foods and non-food allergens has increased, more and more information about the structural basis of cross-reactivity has become available, and these cross-reactivities are now the best studied examples of the cross-reactions between food and non-food allergens.

The association of allergic reactions to pollen allergens and apple, hazelnut, potatoes, celery and carrots has been attributed to cross-reactivities among pathogenesis-related plant proteins and profilin, an ubiquitous cyctoskeleton protein. The structural relationship of birch pathogenesis-related plant protein (Bet v 1), profilin (Bet v 2) and the reactivity to fruits has been studied in more detail (Vieths *et al.*, 1994, 1995; Ebner *et al.*, 1995; Fahlbusch *et al.*, 1995; Vanek-Krebitz *et al.*, 1995). The structural and immunological homology of the major apple allergen Mal d 1 and Bet v 1 has been demonstrated (Vieths *et al.*, 1994, 1995; Fahlbusch *et al.*, 1995; Vanek-Krebitz *et al.*, 1995). The immunological properties of recombinant Mal d 1 were tested and cross-reactivity with Bet v 1 was shown (Vanek-Krebitz *et al.*, 1995). The association between celery, apple, peanut and kiwi fruit, and mugwort pollen was ascribed to the homologous mugwort allergen Art v 1 (Valenta and Kraft, 1995) and pollen profilins (Vallier *et al.*, 1992; Valenta *et al.*, 1992; Breiteneder *et al.*, 1995).

Cross-reactivity between foods and latex

Over the past decade, latex allergy has increased and studies have shown that some allergic reactions to fruits such as avocado, chestnut and banana are due to cross-reacting allergens (Anibarro *et al.*, 1993; Fernandez de Corres *et al.*, 1993; Fisher, 1993; Blanco *et al.*, 1994a,b; Makinen-Kiljunen, 1994; Lavaud *et al.*, 1995). Papaya, fig, celery, passion fruit and peach have been suggested as sources for cross-reacting allergens.

Transgenic foods

Recombinant DNA technology has been used to introduce traits such as resistance to disease, herbicides, insects or environmental stress; delayed ripening; male sterility; synthesis of modified starch and oils; or increased synthesis of major components into a variety of plants. To date, more than 60 different plant species have been successfully genetically engineered. This field is rapidly expanding and more than 20 new plant products are expected to be introduced into the marketplace within the next 5 years (Table 4.3). Since the introduced traits result from the expression of proteins that are not necessarily part of the species' original genome, there is concern about the safety of transgenic foods as they enter the marketplace. A major aspect in this regard is the potential allergenicity of new products (Harlander, 1991; Kessler et al., 1992; Olempska-Beer et al., 1993; Fuchs and Astwood, 1996; Lehrer et al., 1996; Metcalfe et al., 1996; O'Neil et al., 1998).

It is relatively straightforward to evaluate the allergenicity of genetically engineered foods derived from plants known to be allergenic as information about the allergen and allergen-specific human sera or monoclonal antibodies is available. Using the parental variety as a control, in vitro immunological assays can be employed to assess the IgE reactivity of transgenic foods. RAST and RAST inhibition and/or ELISA are the tests of choice to quantify possible differences in total allergen content and allergen composition. Immunoblotting, although less quantitative than other solid phase assays, can also be used to identify allergens and compare IgE reactivity to individual allergens. If results from the in vitro testing are negative or equivocal, more definitive in vivo testing such as skin prick tests and DBPCFC can be performed. For example, a storage protein from Brazil nut was expressed in soybean to improve the nutritional quality of soy as animal feed. In vitro tests, using sera from Brazil nut-sensitive subjects, confirmed that an immunologically functional Brazil nut allergen was produced by the transgenic soybeans (Nordlee et al., 1994, 1996). Another example was the evaluation of two sulphur-rich corn proteins (Lehrer and Reese, 1997). Sera from 42 individuals, demonstrated by skin test, RAST or clinical history and immunoblot to be corn-reactive, were tested for IgE antibody reactivity to the two zein corn proteins using SDS–PAGE/immunoblotting. None of the sera from corn-reactive subjects demonstrated IgE reactivity against either zein proteins, suggesting that products encoding these genes do not pose an increased risk of allergy to consumers.

Another study investigated transgenic soybeans with elevated oleic acid levels (McCants et al., 1997) for differences in their allergenic potency and levels of endogenous allergens. Transgenic and wild-type soybeans were extracted and sera from 31 subjects with histories of soy allergy, positive soy skin test and/or IgE antibody response were tested for reactivity to soy allergens by RAST and immunoblotting. Both wild-type and transgenic soy

Table 4.3 Foods obtained from plant varieties derived through recombinant DNA technology

Plant	Product	Company	Year of FDA evaluation
Corn	Glufosinate-tolerant corn	Pioneer Hi-Bred	Ongoing
	Glyphosate-tolerant corn	Monsanto Co.	Ongoing
	Glufosinate-tolerant corn	AgrEvo Inc.	Ongoing
	Glufosinate-tolerant corn	Dekalb Genetics Corp.	1996
	Glufosinate-tolerant corn	AgrEvo Inc.	1995
	Glyphosate-tolerant/ insect-protected corn	Monsanto Co.	1996
	Insect-protected corn	Dekalb Genetics Corp.	1997
	Insect-protected corn	Monsanto Co.	1996
	Insect-protected corn	Northrup King	1996
	Insect-protected corn	Ciba-Geigy Corp.	1995
	Lepidopteran-resistant corn	Plant Genetics System	Ongoing
	High-oleic oil corn	Dupont	Ongoing
	Male sterile corn	Pioneer Hi-Bred	Ongoing
	Male sterile corn	Plant Genetic Systems	1996
Tomato	Cherry tomato with lowered ethylene content	DNA Plant Technology	Ongoing
	Tomato with lowered ethylene content	DNA Plant Technology	Ongoing
	Modified fruit ripening tomato	Agritope Inc.	1996
	Flavr Savr tomato	Calgene Inc.	1994
	Improved ripening tomato	DNA Plant Technology	1994
	Delayed softening tomato	Zeneca Plant Science	1994
	Improved ripening tomato	Monsanto Co.	1994
Cotton	Bromoxynil-tolerant cotton	Calgene Inc.	Ongoing
	Bromoxynil-tolerant cotton	Calgene Inc.	1994
	Sulfonylurea-tolerant cotton	Dupont	1996
	Glyphosate-tolerant cotton	Monsanto Co.	1995
	Insect-protected cotton	Monsanto Co.	1996
Canola	Canola with altered phytase activity	BASF	Ongoing
	Glufosinate-tolerant canola	AgrEvo Inc.	1997
	Glufosinate-tolerant canola	AgrEvo Inc.	1995
	Glyphosate-tolerant canola	Monsanto Co.	1995
	Laurate canola	Calgene Inc.	1995
Potato	Disease-resistant, increased potato	Frito Lay	Ongoing
	Colorado potato beetle-resistant potato	Monsanto Co.	Ongoing
	Insect-protected potato	Monsanto Co.	1996
	Insect-protected potato	Monsanto Co.	1994
Soybean	Glyphosate-tolerant soybean	Monsanto Co.	1994
	High-oleic, low-linoleic oil soybean	Dupont	Ongoing
	High oleic acid soybean	Dupont	1997

Table 4.3 (continued)

Plant	Product	Company	Year of FDA evaluation
Pepper	Sweet pepper with improved texture	DNA Plant Technology	Ongoing
	Pepper with increased sweetness	DNA Plant Technology	Ongoing
Squash	Virus-resistant squash	Seminis Vegetable Seeds	1997
	Virus-resistant squash	Asgro Seed Co.	1994
Miscellaneous	High-protein lupin	Resource Seeds Inc.	Ongoing
	Pea with increased sweetness	DNA Plant Technology	Ongoing
	Glufosinate-tolerant sugar beet	AgrEvo Inc.	Ongoing
	Phosphinothricin-tolerant rice	AgrEvo Inc.	Ongoing
	Sulfonylurea-tolerant flax	Univ. of Saskatchewan	1997
	Male sterile radicchio rosso	Bejo Zaden BV	1997
	Virus-resistant papaya	Univ. Hawaii & Cornell Univ.	1997
	Male sterile/fertility restorer oilseed rape	Plant Genetic Systems	1996

Modified from Astwood *et al.* (1997).

extracts yielded substantial inhibition of the wild-type RAST. Both inhibition curves, analysed by logit-log transformation and linear regression were identical. Immunoblot analysis showed no significant differences in the number of bands or the intensity of the IgE antibody reactivities. These studies indicate that increased oleic acid content did not substantially affect soy allergens either quantitatively or qualitatively and that such transgenic soy-beans do not pose increased risk of allergy to consumers.

A much more difficult problem is evaluation of the allergenic potential of foods engineered using proteins from sources of undetermined allergenicity. Predicting potential allergenicity is a major challenge since there is no single predictive assay to assess the potential allergenicity of any proteins. An initial step, evaluation of amino acid sequence homology with known allergens, may be useful in predicting allergenicity of a transgenic protein. If sequence homo-logies are observed, particularly with regions containing IgE-binding epitopes, it is essential that *in vitro* testing with RAST or ELISA should be performed to assess IgE reactivity. If no IgE antibody reactivity is detected, the second step should be to compare the physicochemical and biological characteristics, including molecular size, stability, solubility and isoelectric point of these proteins with major food allergens.

Contamination and hidden allergens

As of today, avoidance is the only accepted form of food allergen therapy (Taylor *et al.*, 1986; Taylor, 1989) as even minute amounts of allergen-containing foods can cause anaphylactic reactions. Avoidance is therefore the primary means to prevent actual incidence of acute episodes. However, hidden allergens and contaminations can pose a serious risk for highly allergic individuals. Food preparation at home, restaurants and commercial food processing plants can result in prepared or processed foods that contain allergens. This may be due to shared utensils or equipment used to prepare and process foods, or equipment that was not adequately cleaned between runs. Another source of hidden allergens is undeclared or insufficiently declared ingredients in processed food products when certain ingredients make up only a small percentage and do not have to be indexed separately on the ingredient list. For example, small amounts of peanut do not have to be declared and spices used do not have to be identified individually. Another possibility for unexpected exposure is ingredients that are sometimes, but not always, contaminated. For example, an anaphylactic reaction to beignets, a form of doughnuts, was traced to a contamination of the beignet mix with house dust mites, a potent inhalent allergen (Erben *et al.*, 1993).

Conclusion and future directions

In comparison with inhalant allergens such as grass pollen, house dust mite allergens and hymenoptera allergens such as bee venom allergens, food allergens are not well characterised. Of the hundreds of foods which can cause allergy, only a small number have been characterised; the primary structure of only a few food allergens is known, and very little information about allergenic epitopes is available even though some of the most advanced epitope studies on allergens have been performed on codfish and peanut allergens. The route of exposure to food allergens is different from other allergens: food allergens are normally ingested; the gut-associated lymphoid tissue (GALT) may respond differently compared with peripheral lymphoid tissue in spleen and lymph nodes from which most of our information concerning the immune response has been obtained. Food antigens, in such an environment, may therefore have different properties as compared with other non-food allergens.

Features that make proteins resistant to digestion, heat and acid denaturation and preserve the immunological integrity must be studied since these properties have been linked to protein allergenicity. The clinical relevance of *in vitro* cross-reactivity must be further explored. Is it the structure of cross-reacting proteins that reduces the IgE antibody affinity and thus prevents the mediator release from mast cells, or is the number of epitopes reduced? These questions concerning the structural features responsible for the allergenicity of a protein need to be studied in detail.

Even though the characterisation of food allergens lags behind that of inhalant allergens, studying food allergens may provide a unique opportunity to understand the contribution of structure to the allergenicity of proteins. The studies of peanut allergens Ara h 1 and Ara h 2 show that a single amino substitution may render a given IgE-binding epitope non-reactive, although it remains to be seen whether it is possible to reduce or abolish the IgE reactivity of the entire allergen molecule. Another interesting food allergen is tropomyosin, the major shrimp allergen. Since tropomyosin is ubiquitous and structurally a well-characterised muscle protein, and tropomyosins of meats including poultry, pork and beef are not allergenic, sequence comparison, systematic amino acid substitutions and IgE binding and T-cell activation assays of modified epitopes may help to understand protein allergenicity. Using genetically modified allergens that do not bind IgE, but are still able to interact with T cells inducing T-cell tolerance/anergy may be developed into new concepts of allergen-specific and safer immunotherapy. If the basis of allergenicity is better defined, genetically modified plants may be developed with reduced allergenic potential. Furthermore, it is important to develop better methods to assess genetically engineered varieties as the introduced traits may result from the expression of proteins that are not necessarily part of the species' original genome.

In conclusion, more information is needed about the primary and tertiary structures of food allergens and allergenic epitopes in order to understand the relationship between protein structure and allergenicity, to provide insights into the basic mechanisms of food allergy, to develop an approach to the immunotherapy of food allergy, to use this knowledge to address the immunological safety of transgenic crops and to develop new, less-allergenic varieties.

Acknowledgements

The writing of this chapter was partially supported by funds from the Department of Medicine, Tulane University School of Medicine, Dupont, and the National Fisheries Institute (NFI).

References

Aas K (1966) Studies of hypersensitivity to fish. A clinical study. *International Archives of Allergy and Immunology*, **29**, 346–363.

Aas K and Elsayed S (1975) Physicochemical properties and specific activity of a purified allergen (codfish). *Developments in Biological Standardization*, **29**, 90–98.

Adachi, T. Izumi H, Yamada, T, Tanaka K, Takeuchi S, Nakamura R and Masuda T (1993) Gene structure and expression of rice seed allergenic proteins belonging to the α-amylase/trypsin inhibitor family. *Plant Molecular Biology*, **21**, 239–248.

Alexander, LJ, Hayes G, Pearse MJ, Beattie CW, Stewart AF, Willis IM and Mackinlay AG (1989) Complete sequence of the bovine beta-lactoglobulin cDNA. *Nucleic Acids Research*, **17**, 6739–6745.

Altenbach SB, Pearson KW, Leung FW and Sun SSM (1987) Cloning and sequence analysis of a cDNA encoding a Brazil nut protein exceptionally rich in methionine. *Plant Molecular Biology*, **8**, 239–259.

Amonette MS, Rosenfeld SI and Schwartz RH (1993) Serum IgE antibodies to cow's milk proteins in children with differing degrees of IgE-mediated cow's milk allergy: analysis by immunoblotting. *Pediatric Asthma Allergy and Immunology*, **7**, 99–109.

Anderson JA (1996) Allergic reactions to foods. *Critical Reviews in Food Science and Nutrition*, **36**, S19–S38.

Anderson LB, Dreyfuss EM, Logan J and Johnston DE (1970) Melon and banana sensitivity coincident with ragweed pollinosis. *Journal of Allergy and Clinical Immunology*, **45**, 310–319.

Anet J, Back JF, Baker, RS, Barnett D, Burley RW and Howden MEH (1985) Allergens in the white and yolk of hen's eggs: a study of IgE binding by egg proteins. *International Archives of Allergy and Applied Immunology*, **77**, 364–371.

Anibarro B, Garcia-Ara C and Pascual C (1993) Associated sensitization to latex and chestnut. *Allergy*, **48**, 130–131.

Arshad SH, Malmberg E, Krapt K and Hide DW (1991) Clinical and immunological characteristics of Brazil nut allergy. *Clinical and Experimental Allergy*, **21**, 373–376.

Astwood JD, Fuchs RL and Lavrik PB (1997) Food biotechnology and genetic engineering. In *Food Allergy: Adverse Reactions to Foods and Food Additives*, Metcalfe DD, Sampson HA, Simon RA (eds), Blackwell Scientific Publications, Cambridge, pp. 65–92.

Atkins, FM, Steinberg SS and Metcalfe DD (1985) Evaluation of immediate adverse reactions to foods in adults. I. Correlation of demographic, laboratory, and prick skin test data with response to controlled oral food challenge. *Journal of Allergy and Clinical Immunology*, **75**, 348–353.

Aukrust A and Aas K (1977) The reference in crossed radioimmunoelectrophoresis. *Scandinavian Journal of Immunology*, **6**, 1093–1099.

Aukrust L, Apold J, Elsayed S and Aas K (1978) Crossed immunoelectro-phoretic and crossed radioimmunoelectrophoretic studies employing a model allergen from codfish. *International Archives of Allergy and Applied Immunology*, **57**, 253–262.

Ayuso R, Reese G, Tanaka L, Ibanez MD, Pascual C, Burks AW, Sussman GL, Dalton AC, Lahoud C, Lopez M and Lehrer SB (1998) IgE antibody response to raw and cooked vertebrate meats and tropomyosins (abstract). *Journal of Allergy and Clinical Immunology*, **101**, S239.

Bargman TJ, Rupnow JH and Taylor SL (1992) IgE-binding proteins in almonds (*Prunus amygdalus*): identification by immunoblotting with sera from almond-allergic adults. *Journal of Food Science*, **57**, 717–720.

Barnett D, Baldo BA and Howden MEH (1983) Multiplicity of allergens in peanuts. *Journal of Allergy and Clinical Immunology*, **72**, 61–68.

Barnett D, Bonhan B and Howden MEH (1987) Allergenic cross-reactions among legume foods – in vitro study. *Journal of Allergy and Clinical Immunology*, **79**, 433–438.

Bernhisel-Broadbent J (1995) Allergenic cross-reactivity of foods and characterization of food allergens and extracts. *Annals of Allergy, Asthma and Immunology*, **95**, 295–303.

Bernhisel-Broadbent J and Sampson HA (1989) Cross-allergenicity in the legume botanical family in children with food hypersensitivity. *Journal of Allergy and Clinical Immunology*, **83**, 435–440.

Bernhisel-Broadbent J, Taylor S and Sampson HA (1989) Cross-allergenicity in the legume botanical family in children with food hypersensitivity. II. Laboratory correlates. *Journal of Allergy and Clinical Immunology*, **84**, 701–709.

Bernhisel-Broadbent J, Scanlon SM and Sampson HA (1992) Fish hypersensitivity. I. In vitro and oral challenge results in fish-allergic patients. *Journal of Allergy and Clinical Immunology*, **89**, 730–737.

Blanco C, Carrillo T, Castillo R, Quiralte J and Cuevas M (1994a) Latex allergy: clinical features and cross-reactivity with fruits. *Annals of Allergy*, **73**, 309–314.

Blanco C, Carillo T, Castillo R, Quialte J and Cuevas M (1994b) Avocado hypersensitivity. *Allergy*, **49**, 454–459.

Blake CCF, Koenig DF, Mair FA, North ACT, Phillips DC and Sarma VR (1965) Structure of hen egg white lysozyme. *Nature*, **206**, 757–758.

Blumenthal MN, Namboodiri K, Mendell N, Gleich G, Elston RC and Yunis E (1981) Genetic transmission of serum IgE levels. *American Journal of Medical Genetics*, **10**, 219–222.

Bock SA and Atkins FM (1990) Patterns of food hypersensitivity during sixteen years of double-blind, placebo-controlled food challenges. *Journal of Pediatrics*, **117**, 561–567.

Bock SA, Sampson HA, Atkins FM, Zeiger RS, Lehrer SB, Sachs MR, Bush K and Metcalfe DD (1988) Double-blind, placebo-controlled food challenges (DBPCFC) as an office procedure: a manual. *Journal of Allergy and Clinical Immunology*, **82**, 986–997.

Breiteneder H, Hoffmann-Sommergruber K, O'Riordan G, Susani M, Ahorn H, Ebner C, Kraft D and Scheiner O (1995) Molecular characterization of Api g 1, the major allergen of celery (*Apium graveolens*), and its immunological and structural relationships to a group of 17 kDa tree pollen allergens. *European Journal of Biochemistry*, **233**, 484–489.

Burks, AW, Williams LW, Helm RM, Connaughton C, Cockrel G and O'Brien TJ (1991) Identification of a major peanut allergen, *Ara h 1*, in patients with atopic dermatitis and positive peanut challenges. *Journal of Allergy and Clinical Immunology*, **88**, 712–719.

Burks, AW, Williams LW, Connaughton C, Cockrell, O'Brien TJ and Helm RM (1992) Identification and characterization of a second major peanut allergen, *Ara h 2*, with use of the sera of patients with atopic dermatitis and positive peanut challenge. *Journal of Allergy and Clinical Immunology*, **90**, 962–969.

Burks AW, Cockrell G, Connaughton C and Helm RM (1994) Epitope specificity and immunoaffinity purification of the major peanut allergen, Ara h I. *Journal of Allergy and Clinical Immunology*, **93**, 743–750.

Burks AW, Cockrell G, Stanley JS, Helm RM and Bannon GA (1995a) Recombinant peanut allergen Ara h 1 expression and IgE binding in patients with peanut hypersensitivity. *Journal of Clinical Investigation*, **96**, 1715–1721.

Burks AW, Helm RM, Cockrell G, Stanley J and Bannon GA (1995b) The identification of a family of vicilin-like gene encoding allergens responsible for peanut hypersensitivity (abstract). *Journal of Allergy and Clinical Immunology*, **96**, 332.

Burks AW, Cockrell G, Connaughton C, Karpas A and Helm RM (1995c) Epitope specificity of the major peanut allergen, Ara h II. *Journal of Allergy and Clinical Immunology*, **95**, 607–611.

Burks AW, Shin D, Cockrell G, Stanley JS, Helm RM and Bannon GA (1997) Mapping and mutational analysis of the IgE-binding epitopes on Ara h 1, a legume vicilin protein and a major allergen in peanut hypersensitivity. *European Journal of Biochemistry*, **245**, 334–339.

Bush RK, Voss M, Taylor SL, Nordlee J, Busse W and Yunginger JW (1983) Detection of peanut allergens by crossed radioimmuno-electrophoresis (CRIE). *Journal of Allergy and Clinical Immunology*, **71**, 95.

Calkhoven PG, Aalbers M, Koshte VL, Pos O, Oei HD and Aalberse RC (1987) Cross-reactivity among birch pollen, vegetables and fruits as detected by IgE antibodies is due to at least three distinct cross-reactive structures. *Allergy*, **42**, 382–390.

Calkhoven PG, Aalbers M, Koshte VL, Schilte PP, Yntema JL, Griffioen RW, Van Nierop JC, Oranje AP and Aalberse RC (1991) Relationship between IgG1 and IgE4 antibodies to foods and the development of IgE antibodies to inhalant allergens. II. Increased levels of IgG antibodies to foods in children who subsequently develop IgE antibodies to inhalant allergens. *Clinical and Experimental Allergy*, **21**, 99–107.

Canfield RE (1963) The amino acid sequence of egg white lysozyme. *Journal of Biological Chemistry*, **238**, 2698–2707.

Caplan SN and Berkman EM (1976) Protamine sulfate and fish allergy. *New England Journal of Medicine*, **295**, 172.

Crespo JF, Pascual C, Ferrer A, Burks AW, Diaz Pena JM and Esteban MM (1994) Egg white-specific IgE level as a tolerance marker in the follow-up of egg allergy. *Allergy Proceedings*, **15**, 73–76.

Daul CB, Morgan JE, Waring NP, McCants ML, Hughes J and Lehrer SB (1987) Immunological evaluation of shrimp-allergic individuals. *Journal of Allergy and Clinical Immunology*, **80**, 716–722.

Daul CB, Slattery M, Morgan JE and Lehrer SB (1991) Isolation and characterization of an important 36 kD shrimp allergen. *Journal of Allergy and Clinical Immunology*, **87**, 192.

Daul CB, Slattery M, Morgan JE and Lehrer SB (1992) Identification of a common major crustacea allergen. *Journal of Allergy and Clinical Immunology*, **89**, 194.

Daul CB, Slattery M, Morgan JE and Lehrer SB (1993) Common crustacea allergens: identification of B cell epitopes with the shrimp specific monoclonal antibodies. In *Molecular Biology and Immunology of Allergens*, Kraft D and Sehon A (eds), CRC Press, Boca Raton, pp. 291–294.

Daul CB, Slattery M, Reese G and Lehrer SB (1994) Identification of the major brown shrimp (*Penaeus aztecus*) allergen as the muscle protein tropomyosin. *International Archives of Allergy and Immunology*, **105**, 49–55.

Demeulemester C, Peltre G, Laurent M, Pankeleux D and David B (1987) Cyanogen bromide-activated nitrocellulose membranes: a new tool for immunoprint techniques. *Electrophoresis*, **8**, 71–73.

Desjardins A, Malo JL, L'Archevêque J, Cartier A, McCants M and Lehrer SB (1995) Occupational IgE-mediated sensitization and asthmatic reactions to clam and shrimp. *Journal of Allergy and Clinical Immunology*, **96**, 608–617.

Ebner C, Hirschwehr R, Bauer L, Breiteneder H, Valenta R, Ebner H, Kraft D and Scheiner O (1995) Identification of allergens in fruits and vegetables. IgE cross-reactivities with the important birch pollen allergens Bet v 1 and Bet v 2 (birch profilin). *Journal of Allergy and Clinical Immunology*, **95**, 962–969.

Elsayed S and Aas K (1970) Characterization of a major allergen (cod): chemical composition and immunological properties. *International Archives of Allergy and Applied Immunology*, **38**, 536–548.

Elsayed S and Apold J (1983) Immunological analysis of cod fish allergen M: locations of the immunoglobulin binding sites as demonstrated by native and synthetic peptides. *Allergy*, **38**, 449–459.

Elsayed S and Bennich H (1975) The primary structure of allergen M from cod. *Scandinavian Journal of Immunology*, **4**, 203–208.

Elsayed S, Aas K, Slette K and Johansson SGO (1972) Tryptic cleavage of a homogeneous cod fish allergen and isolation of two active polypeptide fragments. *Immunochemistry*, **9**, 647–661.

Elsayed SM, Apold S, Aas K and Bennich H (1976) The allergenic structure of allergen M from cod. Tryptic peptides of fragment TM1. *International Archives of Allergy and Applied Immunology*, **52**, 59–63.

Enberg RN, Leickley FE, McCoullough J, Bailey J and Ownby DR (1987) Watermelon and ragweed share allergens. *Journal of Allergy and Clinical Immunology*, **79**, 867–875.

Erben EM, Rodriguez JL, McCullough J and Ownby DR (1993) Anaphylaxis after ingestion of beignets contaminated with Dermatophahoides farinae. *Journal of Allergy and Clinical Immunology*, **993**, 846–891.

Fahlbusch B, Rudeschko O, Müller WD, Schlenvoigt G, Vettermann S and Jäger L (1995) Purification and characterization of the major allergen from apple and its allergenic cross-reactivity with Bet v 1. *International Archives of Allergy and Immunology*, **108**, 119–126.

Fernandez de Corres L, Moneo L, Munoz D, Bernaola G, Fernandez E, Audicana M and Urrutia I (1993) Sensitization from chestnuts and bananas in patients with urticaria and anaphylaxis from contact with latex. *Annals of Allergy*, **70**, 35–39.

Fisher AA (1993) Association of latex and food allergy. *Cutis*, **52**, 70–71.

Ford JE, Heppell LMJ and Kilshaw PJ (1983) Effects of heat treatment of milk on its nutritional value and antigenic properties. *Kieler Milchwirtschaftlicher Forschungsbericht*, **35**, 321–322.

Fuchs RL and Astwood JD (1996) Allergenicity assessment of foods derived from genetically modified foods. *Food Technology*, **50**, 83–88.

Geha RS (1984) Human IgE. *Journal of Allergy and Clinical Immunology*, **74**, 109–120.

Gern JE, Yang E, Evrard HM and Sampson HA (1991) Allergic reactions to milk-contaminated 'nondairy' products. *New England Journal of Medicine*, **324**, 976–979.

Goldman AS, Sellars WA, Halpern SR, Anderson DW, Furlow TE and Johnson CH (1963) Milk allergy II. Skin testing of allergic and normal children with purified milk proteins. *Pediatrics*, **32**, 572–579.

Grant DR, Sumner AK and Johnson J (1976) An investigation of pea seed albumins. *Journal of the Canadian Institute of Food Technology*, **9**, 84–91.

Greenberger PA, Patterson R, Tobin MC, Liota JL and Roberts M (1989) Lack of cross-reactivity between IgE to salmon and protamine sulfate. *American Journal of Medical Science*, **298**, 104–108.

Halmepuro L, Vuontela K, Kalimo K and Björlstén (1984) Cross-reactivity of IgE antibodies with allergens in birch pollen, fruits and vegetables. *International Archives of Allergy and Applied Immunology*, **74**, 235–240.

Halmepuro L, Salvaggio J and Lehrer SB (1987) Crawfish and lobster allergens: identification and structural similarities with other crustacea. *International Archives of Allergy and Applied Immunology*, **82**, 213–220.

Harlander SK (1991) Biotechnology – A means for improving our food supply. *Food Technology*, **45**, 84, 86, 91–92, 95.

Hefle SL and Bush RK (1994) Adverse reaction to lupin. *Journal of Allergy and Clinical Immunology*, **94**, 167–172.

Herian AM, Taylor SL and Bush RK (1990) Identification of soybean allergens by immunoblotting with sera from soy-allergic adults. *International Archives of Allergy and Applied Immunology*, **92**, 193–198.

Herian AM, Taylor SL and Bush RK (1993) Allergenicity of various soybean products as determined by RAST inhibition. *Journal of Food Science*, **58**, 385–388.

Hoffman DR (1983) Immunochemical identification of the allergens in egg white. *Journal of Allergy and Clinical Immunology*, **71**, 481–486.

Hoffman DR, Day ED and Miller JS (1981) The major heat stable allergen of shrimp. *Annals of Allergy*, **47**, 17–22.

Holen E and Elsayed S (1996) Specific T cell lines for ovalbumin, ovomucoid, lysozyme and two OA synthetic epitopes, generated from egg allergic patients' PBMC. *Clinical and Experimental Allergy*, **26**, 1080–1088.

Honma K, Kohno Y, Saito K, Shimojo N, Horiuchi T, Hayashi H, Suzuki N, Hosoya T, Tsunoo H and Niimi H (1996) Allergenic epitopes of ovalbumin (OVA) in patients with hen's egg allergy: inhibition of basophil histamine release by haptenic ovalbumin peptide. *Clinical and Experimental Immunology*, **103**, 446–453.

Host A and Samuelsson EG (1988) Allergic reactions to raw, pasteurized and homogenized/pasteurized cow milk: a comparison. *Allergy*, **43**, 113–118.

Hurley WL and Schuler LA (1987) Molecular cloning and nucleotide sequence of bovine α-lactalbumin. *Gene*, **61**, 119–122.

Izumi H, Adachi T, Fujii N, Matsuda T, Nakamura R, Tanaka K, Urisu A and Kurosawa Y (1992) Nucleotide sequence of a cDNA clone encoding a major allergenic protein in rice seeds. Homology of the deduced amino acid sequence with a member of α-amylase/trypsin inhibitor family. *FEBS Letters*, **302**, 213–216.

Jeltsch JM and Chambon P (1982) The complete sequence of the chicken ovotransferrin mRNA. *European Journal of Biochemistry*, **122**, 291–295.

Jeoung BJ, Reese G, Hauck P, Oliver JB, Daul CB and Lehrer SB (1997) Quantification of the major brown shrimp allergen Pen a 1 (tropomyosin) by a monoclonal antibody-based sandwich ELISA. *Journal of Allergy and Clinical Immunology*, **100**, 229–234.

Jones RT, Squillace DL and Yunginger JW (1992) Anaphylaxis in a milk-allergic child after ingestion of milk-contaminated kosher-pareve-labeled 'dairy-free' dessert. *Annals of Allergy*, **68**, 223–227.

Kahlert H, Petersen A, Becker WM and Schlaak M (1992) Epitope analysis of the allergen ovalbumin (Gal d II) with monoclonal antibodies and patients' IgE. *Molecular Immunology*, **29**, 1191–1201.

Kato I, Schrode J, Kohr WJ and Laskowski M (1987) Chicken ovomucoid: determination of its amino acid sequence, determination of the trypsin reactive site, and preparation of all three of its domains. *Biochemistry*, **26**, 193–201.

Kessler OA, Taylor MR, Maryanski JH, Flamm EL and Kahl LS (1992) The safety of foods developed by biotechnology. *Science*, **256**, 1747–1749, 1832.

Keating MU, Jones RT, Worley NJ, Shively CA and Yunginger JW (1990) Immunoassay of peanut allergens in food-processing materials and finished foods. *Journal of Allergy and Clinical Immunology*, **86**, 41–44.

Kilshaw PJ, Heppel LMJ and Ford JE (1982) Effect of heat treatment of cow's milk on the nutritional quality and antigenic properties. *Archives of Disease in Childhood*, **57**, 842–847.

King TP (1994) Antigenic Determinants: B cells. Conference on Scientific Issues Related to Potential Allergenicity in Transgenic Food Crops, Sponsored by FDA, EPA and USDA, Annapolis, MD.

King TP, Coscia MR and Kochoumian L (1993) Structure-immunogenicity relationship of a peptide allergen, mellitin. In *Molecular Biology and Immunology of Allergens*, Kraft D and Sehon (eds), CRC Press, Boca Raton, pp. 11–20.

King TP, Hoffmann D, Lowenstein H, Marsh DG, Platts-Mills TA and Thomas W (1994) Allergen nomenclature. WHO/IUIS Allergen Nomenclature Subcommittee. *International Archives of Allergy and Immunology*, **105**, 224–233.

King TP, Hoffman D, Lowenstein H, Marsh DG, Platts-Mills TA and Thomas W (1995) Allergen nomenclature. *Allergy*, **50**, 765–774.

Knape JTA, Schuller JL, De Haan P, de Jong AP and Bovill JG (1981) An anaphylactic reaction to protamine in a patient allergic to fish. *Anaethesiology*, **55**, 324–325.

Kumosinski TF, Brown EM and Farrell HM (1991a) Three-dimensional molecular modelling of bovine caseins: kappa-caseins. *Journal of Dairy Science*, **74**, 2879–2887.

Kumosinski RF, Brown EM and Farell HM (1991b) Three-dimensional molecular modelling of bovine caseins. α_{s1}-casein. *Journal of Dairy Science*, **74**, 2889–2895.

Kumosinski TF, Brown EM and Farrell HM (1993) Three-dimensional molecular modelling of bovine caseins. An energy-minimizing β-casein structure. *Journal of Dairy Science*, **76**, 931–945.

Kyhse-Andersen J (1984) Electroblotting of multiple gels: a simple apparatus without buffer tank for rapid transfer of proteins from polyacrylamide to nitrocellulose. *Journal of Biochemical and Biophysical Methods*, **10**, 203–209.

Langeland T (1983a) A clinical and immunological study of allergy to hen's egg white. III. Allergens in hens' egg white studied by cross radio immunoelectrophoresis. *Allergy*, **38**, 500–521.

Langeland T (1983b) A clinical and immunological study of allergy to hen's egg white. IV. Specific IgE antibodies to individual allergens in hen's egg white related to clinical and immunological parameters in egg-allergic patients. *Allergy*, **38**, 493–500.

Lavaud F, Prevost A, Cossart C, Guerin L, Bernard J and Kochman S (1995) Allergy to latex, avocado pear, and banana: evidence for a 30 kd antigen in immunoblotting. *Journal of Allergy and Clinical Immunology*, **95**, 557–564.

Lee YH (1992) Food processing approaches to altering allergenic potential of milk-based formula. *Journal of Pediatrics*, **121**, S47–S50.

Lehrer SB (1986) The complex nature of food antigens: studies of cross-reacting crustacea allergens. *Annals of Allergy*, **57**, 267–272.

Lehrer SB and McCants ML (1988) Reactivity of IgE antibodies with crustacea and oyster allergens: evidence for common antigenic structures. *Journal of Allergy and Clinical Immunology*, **76**, 803–809.

Lehrer SB and Reese G (1997) Recombinant proteins in newly developed foods: identification of allergenic activity. *International Archives of Allergy and Immunology*, **113**, 122–124.

Lehrer SB, Horner WE and Reese G (1996) Why are some proteins allergenic? Implications for Biotechnology. *Critical Reviews in Food Science and Nutrition*, **36**, 553–564.

Lehrer SB, Taylor SL, Hefle SL and Bush RK (1997a) Food Allergens. In *Allergy and Allergic Diseases*, Kay AB (ed), Blackwell Scientific Publications, Oxford, pp. 961–980.

Lehrer SB, Reese G, Ortega H, El-Dahr JM, Goldberg B and Malo JL (1997b) IgE antibody reactivity to aqueous-soluble, alcohol-soluble and transgenic corn proteins. *Journal of Allergy and Clinical Immunology*, **99**, S147.

Leung PSC, Chu KH, Chow WK, Aftab A, Bandea CI, Kwan HS, Nagy SM and Gershwin ME (1994) Cloning, expression, and primary structure of *Metapenaeus ensis* tropomyosin, the major heat-stable shrimp allergen. *Journal of Allergy and Clinical Immunology*, **92**, 837–845.

Levy JH, Schwieger IM, Zaidan JR, Faraj BA and Weintraub WS (1989) Evaluation of patients at risk for protamine reactions. *Journal of Thoracic and Cardiovascular Surgery*, **98**, 200–204.

Løwenstein H, Markussen B and Weeke B (1976) Identification of allergens in extracts of horsehair and dander by means of crossed radioimmunoelectrophoresis. *International Archives of Allergy and Applied Immunology*, **51**, 39.

Makinen-Kiljunen S (1994) Banana allergy in patients with immediate-type hypersensitivity to natural rubber latex: characterization of cross-reacting antibodies and allergens. *Journal of Allergy and Clinical Immunology*, **93**, 990–996.

Malley A, Baecher L, Mackler B and Perlman F (1975) The isolation of allergens from the green pea. *Journal of Allergy and Clinical Immunology*, **56**, 282–290.

Malley A, Baecher L, Mackler B and Perlman F (1976) Further characterization of a low molecular weight allergen fragment isolate from green pea. *Clinical and Experimental Immunology*, **25**, 159–164.

Marsh DG, Bias WB and Ishizaka K (1974) Genetic control of basal serum immunoglobulin E level and its effect on specific reaginic sensitivity. *Proceedings of the National Academy of Science of the USA*, **71**, 3588–3592.

Matsuda T and Nakamura R (1993) Molecular structure and immunological properties of food allergens. *Trends in Food Science and Technology*, **4**, 289–293.

Matsuda T, Alvarez AM, Tada Y, Adachi T and Nakamura R (1993) Gene engineering for hypo-allergenic rice: repression of allergenic protein synthesis in seeds of transgenic rice plant by antisense RNA. In: *Proceedings, International Workshop on Life Science in Production and Food-Consumption of Agricultural Products*, Tsukuba, Japan.

McCants M, Lehrer SB, Reese G and Tracey D (1997) Allergy assessment of high oleic acid transgenic soy beans (G94-1) (abstract). *Journal of Allergy and Clinical Immunology*, **99**, S479.

McReynolds L, O'Malley BW, Nisbet AD, Fothergill JE, Givol D, Fields S, Roberson M and Bownlee GG (1978) Sequence of chicken ovalbumin mRNA. *Nature*, **273**, 723–728.

Mena M, Sanchez-Monge R, Gomez L, Salcedo G and Carbonero P (1992) A major barley allergen associated with baker's asthma disease is a glycosylated monomeric inhibitor of insect α-amylase: cDNA cloning and chromosomal location of the gene. *Plant Molecular Biology*, **20**, 451–458.

Menendez-Arias L, Moneo I, Dominguez J and Rodriguez R (1988) Primary structure of the major allergen of yellow mustard (*Sinapis alba* L.) sed, Sin a I. *European Journal of Biochemistry*, **177**, 159–166.

Metcalfe DD, Astwood JD, Townsend R, Sampson HA, Taylor SL and Fuchs RL (1996) Assessment of the allergenic potential of foods derived from genetically engineered crop plants. *Critical Reviews in Food Science and Nutrition*, **36** (suppl.), S165–S186.

Miller H and Campbell DH (1950) Skin test reactions to various chemical fractions of egg white and their possible clinical significance. *Journal of Allergy*, **21**, 522–524.

Monsalve RE, Gonzalez de la Pena MA, Menendez-Arias L, Lopez-Otin C, Villalba M and Rodriguez R (1993) Characterization of a new mustard allergen, Bra j IE. Detection of an allergenic epitope. *Biochemical Journal*, **294**, 625–632.

Moody MW, Roberts KJ and Huner JV (1993) Phylogeny of commercially important seafood and description of the seafood industry. *Clinical Reviews in Allergy*, **11**, 159–181.

Moroz LA and Yang WH (1980) Kunitz soybean trypsin inhibitor, a specific allergen in food anaphylaxis. *New England Journal of Medicine*, **302**, 1126–1128.

Mykles D, Cotton JLS, Taniguchi H, Sano K-I and Maeda Y (1998) Cloning of tropomysins from lobster (*Homarus americanus*) striated muscle: fast and slow isoforms may be generated from the same transcript. *Journal of Muscle Research and Cell Motility*, **19**, 105–116.

Nagpal S, Rajappa L, Metcalfe DD and Rao PV (1989) Isolation and characterization of heat-stable allergens from shrimp (*Penaeus indicus*). *Journal of Allergy and Clinical Immunology*, **83**, 26–36.

Nisbet AD, Saundry RH, Moire AJG, Fothergill LA and Fothergill JE (1981) The complete amino acid sequence of hen ovalbumin. *European Journal of Biochemistry*, **115**, 335–345.

Nordlee JA, Taylor SL, Jones RT and Yunginger JW (1981) Allergenicity of various peanut products as determined by RAST inhibition. *Journal of Allergy and Clinical Immunology*, **68**, 376–382.

Nordlee JA, Atkins FM, Bush RK and Taylor SL (1993) Anaphylaxis from undeclared walnut in commercially processed cookies (abstract). *Journal of Allergy and Clinical Immunology*, **91**, 154.

Nordlee JA, Taylor SL, Townsend JA and Thomas LA (1994) High methionine Brazil nut protein binds human IgE. *Journal of Allergy and Clinical Immunology*, **93**, 209.

Nordlee JA, Taylor SL, Townsend JA and Thomas LA (1996) Identification of a Brazil nut allergen in transgenic soybeans. *New England Journal of Medicine*, **334**, 688–692.

Ogawa T, Bando N, Tsuji H, Okajima H, Nishikawa K and Sasoka K (1991) Investigation of the IgE-binding proteins in soybeans by immunoblotting with the sera of soybean-sensitive patients with atopic dermatitis. *Journal of Nutritional Science and Vitaminology*, **37**, 555–565.

Ogawa T, Bando N, Tsuji H, Nishikawa K and Kitamura K (1995) Alpha-subunit of beta-conglycinin, an allergenic protein recognized by IgE of soybean-sensitive patients with atopic dermatitis. *Bioscience, Biotechnology and Biochemistry*, **59**, 831–833.

Olempska-Beer ZS, Kuznesof PM, DiNovi M and Smith MJ (1993) Plant biotechnology and food safety. *Food Technology*, **47**, 64–72.

O'Neil C, Reese G and Lehrer SB (1998) Allergenic potential of recombinant food proteins. *ACI Clinical Trends*, **101**, 5–9.

Peltre G, Lapeyre J and David B (1982) Heterogeneity of grass pollen allergens (*Dactylus glomerata*) recognized by IgE antibodies in human patient sera by a new nitrocellulose immunoprint technique. *Immunology Letters* **5**, 127–131.

Petersen A, Schramm G, Becker WM and Schlaak M (1993) Comparison of four grass pollen species concerning their allergens of grass group V by 2D immunoblotting and microsequencing. *Biological Chemistry Hoppe-Seyler* **374**, 855–861.

Petersen A, Becker WM and Schlaak M (1994) Epitope analysis of isoforms of the major allergen Phl p V by fingerprinting and microsequencing. *Clinical and Experimental Allergy* **24**, 250–256.

Reese G, Jeoung BJ, Daul CB and Lehrer SB (1997) Characterization of recombinant shrimp allergen Pen a 1 (tropomyosin). *International Archives of Allergy and Immunology*, **113**, 240–242.

Roitt IM, Brostoff J and Male DK (1985) *Immunology*, Gower Medical Publishing, London, New York.

Sampson HA and Metcalfe DD (1991) Immediate reactions to foods. In *Food Allergy: Adverse Reactions to Foods and Food Additives*, Metcalfe DD, Sampson HA and Simon RA (eds), Blackwell Scientific Publications, Oxford, pp. 99–112.

Savilathi E (1981) Cow's milk allergy. *Allergy*, **36**, 73–88.

Savilathi E and Kuitonen M (1992) Allergenicity of cow's milk proteins. *Journal of Pediatrics*, **121**, S12–S20.

Scott MJ, Huckaby CS, Kato I, Kohr WJ, Laskowski M, Tsai MJ and O'Malley BW (1987) Ovoinhibitor introns specify functional domains as in the related and linked ovomucoid gene. *Journal of Biological Chemistry*, **262**, 5899–5907.

Shanti KN, Martin BM, Nagpal S, Metcalfe DD and Sabba-Rao PV (1993) Identification of tropomyosin as the major shrimp allergen and characterization of its IgE binding epitopes. *Journal of Immunology*, **151**, 5354–5363.

Shibasaki M, Suzuki S, Tajima S, Nemoto H and Kuroume T (1980) Allergenicity of major component proteins of soybeans. *International Archives of Allergy and Applied Immunology*, **61**, 441–448.

Shimojo N, Katsuki T, Coligan JE, Nishimura Y, Sasazuki T, Tsunoo H, Sakamaki T, Kohno Y and Niimi H (1994) Identification of the disease-related T cell epitope of ovalbumin and epitope-targeted T cell inactivation in egg allergy. *International Archives of Allergy and Immunology*, **105**, 155–161.

Stanley JS, Burks AW, Helm RM, Cockrell G and Bannon GA (1995) Ara h I, a major allergen involved in peanut hypersensitivity, has multiple IgE binding sites. *Journal of Allergy and Clinical Immunology*, **95**, 333.

Stanley JS, King N, Burks AW, Huang SK, Sampson H, Cockrell G, Helm RM, West CM and Bannon GA (1997) Identification and mutational analysis of the immunodominant IgE binding epitopes of the major peanut allergen Ara h 2. *Archives of Biochemistry and Biophysics*, **342**, 244–253.

Swaisgood HE (1985) Characterization of edible fluids of animal origin: milk. In *Food Chemistry*, Fennema OR (ed), Marcel Dekker, New York, pp. 791–827.

Taylor SL (1989) Elimination diets in the diagnosis of atopic dermatitis. *Allergy*, **44**, 97–102.

Taylor SL, Bush RK and Busse WE (1986) Avoidance diets – how selective should we be? *New England Allergy Proceedings*, **7**, 527–532.

Taylor SL, Lemanski RF, Bush RK and Busse WW (1987) Food allergens: structure and immunologic properties. *Annals of Allergy*, **59**, 93–99.

Valenta R and Kraft D (1995) Type I allergic reactions to plant-derived food: a consequence of primary sensitization to pollen allergens. *Journal of Allergy and Clinical Immunology*, **95**, 893–895.

Valenta R, Duchene M, Ebner C, Valent P, Sillaber C, Deviller P, Ferreira F, Tejkl M, Edelmann H, Kraft D and Scheiner O (1992) Profilins constitute a novel family of functional plant pan-allergens. *Journal of Experimental Medicine*, **175**, 377–385.

Vallier P, DeChamp C, Valenta R, Vial O and Deviller P (1992) Purification and characterization of an allergen from celery immunochemically related to an allergen present in several other plant species. Identification as a profilin. *Clinical and Experimental Allergy*, **22**, 774–782.

Vanek-Krebitz M, Hoffmann-Sommerguber K, Laimer da Camara Machado M, Susani M, Ebner C, Kraft D, Scheiner O and Breiteneder H (1995) Cloning and sequencing of Mal d 1, the major allergen from apple (*Malus domestica*), and its immunological relationship to Bet v 1, the major birch pollen allergen. *Biochemical and Biophysical Research Communications*, **214**, 538–551.

Vieths S, Schoning B and Petersen A (1994) Characterization of the 18-kDa apple allergen by two-dimensional immunoblotting and microsequencing. *International Archives of Allergy and Immunology*, **104**, 399–404.

Vieths S, Janek K, Aulepp H and Petersen A (1995) Isolation and characterization of the 18-kDa major apple allergen and comparison with the major birch pollen allergen (Bet v I). *Allergy*, **50**, 421–430.

Walsh BJ, Elliott C, Baker RS, Barnett D, Burley RW, Hill DJ and Howden MEH (1987) Allergenic cross-reactivity of egg-white and egg-yolk proteins. *International Archives of Allergy and Applied Immunology*, **84**, 228–232.

Walsh BJ, Barnett D, Burley RW, Elliott C, Hill DJ and Howden MEH (1988) New allergens from hen's egg white and egg yolk: *in vitro* studies of ovomucin, apovitellin I and VI, and phosvitin. *International Archives of Allergy and Applied Immunology*, **87**, 81–86.

Waring NP, deShazo RD, Daul CB, McCants M and Lehrer SB (1985) Hypersensitivity reactions to ingested crustaceans: clinical evaluation and diagnostic studies in shrimp sensitive individuals. *Journal of Allergy and Clinical Immunology*, **76**, 440–445.

Watanabe M (1993) Hypoallergenic rice as a physiologically functional food. *Trends in Food Science and Technology*, **4**, 125–128.

Weeke B (1973) Crossed immunoelectrophoresis. *Scandinavian Journal of Immunology*, **1**, 47.

Wershil BK and Walker WA (1988) Milk allergens and other food allergies in children. *Immunology and Allergy Clinics of North America*, **8**, 485–504.

Whitney RM (1988). Proteins of milk. In: *Fundamentals of Dairy Chemistry*, 3rd edn, Wong NP, Jernes R, Keeney M, Marth EH (eds), Van Nostrand Reinhold, New York, pp. 81–169.

Williams J, Elleman TC, Kingston IB, Wilkens AG and Kuhn KA (1982) The primary structure of hen ovotransferrin. *European Journal of Biochemistry*, **122**, 297–303.

Wütrich B and Dietschi R (1985) The celery-carrot-mugwort-condiment syndrome: skin test and RAST results. *Schweizerische Medizinische Wochenschrift*, **115**, 258–264.

Yunginger JW (1990) Classical food allergens. *Allergy Proceedings*, **11**, 7–9.

Yunginger JW, Gauerke MB, Jones RT, Dahlberg MJE and Ackerman SJ (1983) Use of radioimmunoassay to determine the nature, quantity and source of allergenic contamination of sunflower butter. *Journal of Food Protection*, **46**, 625–628.

Yunginger JW, Sweeney KG, Sturner WQ, Giannandrea LA, Teigland JD, Bray M, Benson PA, York JA, Biedrzycki L, Squillace DL and Helm RM (1988) Fatal food-induced anaphylaxis. *Journal of the American Medical Association*, **260**, 1450–1452.

5 Nutritional Modulation of Cytochromes P450

Costas Ioannides

Molecular Toxicology Group, School of Biological Sciences, University of Surrey, Guildford, Surrey, GU2 5XH, UK

Introduction

A plethora of epidemiological studies have highlighted the importance of dietary habits in the aetiology of many major degenerative diseases including cancer and cardiovascular disease. It is, for example, well established that high intake of fat increases the tumour incidence at a number of sites whereas large intake of fruit and vegetables is associated with a low tumour incidence. Moreover, chemicals having the potential to induce cancer are inherent to some types of food, are present as contaminants, or are generated during the cooking process. Humans, through their diet, are exposed daily to major groups of chemical carcinogens such as nitrosamines, polycyclic aromatic hydrocarbons and heterocyclic amines. Although the precise underlying mechanisms through which diet influences the appearance of tumours are not completely understood, it is widely recognised that a change in our dietary habits may be the most promising avenue to exploit if we are successfully to combat fatal diseases such as cancer.

It has become increasingly evident during the past two decades that dietary components, other than macronutrients such as fat, or micronutrients such as minerals and vitamins, could also modulate the carcinogenic response of chemicals in animal models of the disease. These components, having no biological value, are often referred to as anutrients and are primarily of plant origin. Plant products such as green tea and brassica vegetables have been shown to effectively antagonise the carcinogenicity induced in animals by structurally diverse chemical carcinogens (Yang and Wang, 1993; Verhoeven *et al.*, 1997). The isolation and identification of the constituents of these plant products

Nutrition and Chemical Toxicity. Edited by Costas Ioannides. © John Wiley & Sons Ltd. ISBN 0 471 97453 6

responsible for their anticarcinogenic effect are currently of major research interest.

The anticarcinogenic effects of these naturally occurring plant products most likely involve a number of distinct mechanisms. One such mechanism is modulation of the metabolism of the chemical carcinogen so as to minimise the generation of the reactive intermediates which, as a result of their electrophilicity, readily interact covalently with DNA to initiate the process of carcinogenesis. Metabolism of a carcinogen may be perturbed in such a way so as to: (i) decrease the enzymic generation of the reactive intermediates; (ii) direct metabolism of the carcinogen towards the production of innocuous metabolites; and (iii) detoxicate reactive intermediates by facilitating their interaction with endogenous nucleophiles, e.g. glutathione, to generate inactive, readily excretable products. Thus, diet can influence the toxicological fate of a chemical by modulating the enzyme systems that catalyse the pathways of its metabolism. Since the same enzyme systems that metabolise chemical carcinogens are also responsible for the metabolism of drugs, it is logical to expect that dietary habits can also interfere with the clinical efficacy of drugs. It is feasible that the nature of the diet can alter the pharmacokinetic characteristics, and consequently, the pharmacological effect of a drug, by influencing its metabolic deactivation leading to changes in its intensity and duration of action. Inhibition of the drug-metabolising enzymes may increase plasma levels and, in the case of chronically administered drugs, give rise to accumulation and the appearance of adverse effects associated with overdosage. Alternatively, an increase in the activity of the drug-metabolising enzymes will result in low plasma levels, attenuating or even totally abolishing the pharmacological effect. Clearly, diet and nutrition can play a major role in determining how the body deals with the numerous xenobiotics which find their way into the body, and an understanding of how the enzyme systems that metabolise chemicals are influenced by dietary habits is of paramount importance.

Although a number of enzymes systems contribute to the metabolism of xenobiotics, undoubtedly the most important are the cytochromes P450, a ubiquitous family of haemoproteins endowed with unprecedented versatility, being capable of metabolising structurally very diverse substrates. This enzyme is sensitive to various external stimuli, including changes in nutritional and dietary habits, with toxicologically significant consequences in the metabolism of chemicals. The effects of nutrition on chemical toxicity have been periodically reviewed (Parke and Ioannides, 1981, 1994; Guengerich, 1984; Parke, 1991) and will not be addressed in the present chapter, which will deal exclusively with the nutritional modulation of cytochrome P450 proteins.

Nutrition and cytochromes P450

Almost every lipophilic chemical that finds its way into the human body is metabolised, at least partly, by the cytochrome P450 superfamily of proteins. This enzyme system owes its broad substrate specificity to the fact that it exists as a number of individual proteins, or isoforms, which based on their structural similarity are grouped into families that are further subdivided into subfamilies and which may comprise one or more isoforms. The families which are active in the metabolism of xenobiotics are CYP1, CYP2, CYP3 and, to a much lesser extent, CYP4 (Ioannides, 1996). Table 5.1 shows the cytochrome P450 proteins participating in xenobiotic metabolism in humans and laboratory animals. The most frequent outcome of cytochrome P450-mediated metabolism is loss of biological activity (deactivation). However, in many cases a chemical may be metabolically converted by the same enzyme system to reactive intermediates (activation) which, having escaped the defensive detoxicating mechanisms that protect the living organism, readily interact covalently with cellular macro-molecules, such as DNA and proteins, giving rise to mutations, malignancy, immunotoxicity and cytotoxicity. Thus, cytochromes P450 can catalyse both, the activation and the deactivation of chemicals. Of the cytochrome P450 subfamilies, CYP1A appears to be the most important in the activation of

Table 5.1 Species distribution of xenobiotic-metabolising cytochrome P450 proteins

CYP subfamily	Human	Rabbit	Rat	Hamster	Mouse
CYP1A	1A1, 1A2	1A1, 1A2	1A1, 1A2	1A1, 1A2	1A1, 1A2
CYP2A	2A6, 2A7 2A13	2A10, 2A11	2A1, 2A2 2A3	2A8, 2A9	2A4, 2A5 2A12
CYP2B	2B6	2B4, 2B5	2B1, 2B2 2B3, 2B12 2B15, 2B16		2B9, 2B10 2B13
CYP2C	2C8, 2C9, 2C18, 2C19	2C1, 2C2, 2C3, 2C4 2C5, 2C14 2C15, 2C16 2C30	2C6, 2C7, 2C11, 2C12 2C13, 2C22 2C23, 2C24	2C25, 2C26 2C27, 2C28	2C29
CYP2D	2D6		2D1, 2D2 2D3, 2D4 2D5, 2D18	2D20	2D9, 2D10 2D11, 2D12, 2D13
CYP2E	2E1	2E1, 2E2	2E1	2E1	2E1
CYP3A	3A4, 3A5 3A7	3A6	3A1, 3A2 3A9, 3A18 3A23	3A10	3A11, 3A13 3A16
CYP4A	4A9, 4A11	4A4, 4A5 4A6, 4A7	4A1, 4A2 4A3, 4A8		4A10, 4A12 4A14

chemicals (Ioannides and Parke, 1990; Gonzalez and Gelboin, 1994), although other xenobiotic-metabolising subfamilies, such as CYP2E in the case of small molecular weight compounds (Raucy, 1995), may make the predominant contribution in the activation of some chemicals.

The levels of individual cytochrome P450 isoforms are most frequently determined by a combination of approaches. The first involves the use of substrates whose metabolism through a defined pathway is selectively catalysed by the isoform in question. However, as there is considerable overlap in the substrate specificity of individual cytochrome P450 proteins, it is prudent to support such studies using a different approach, namely immunological determination of the apoprotein levels. Antibodies to cytochrome P450 isoforms are rapidly becoming commercially available. Table 5.2 shows the substrates most commonly employed to assess the activity of individual isoforms.

Table 5.2 Chemical probes commonly used to monitor individual cytochrome P450 isoforms[a]

Cytochrome P450 protein	Chemical probe
CYP1A1	Ethoxyresorufin O-deethylase
CYP1A2	Methoxyresorufin O-demethylase
	Caffeine N-demethylase
	Acetanilide hydroxylase
CYP2A	Testosterone 7α-hydroxylase
	Coumarin 7-hydroxylase
CYP2B	Pentoxyresorufin O-depentylase
	Testosterone 16β-hydroxylase
	Testosterone 16α-hydroxylase
CYP2C6	Progesterone 21-hydroxylase
CYP2C11	Androstenedione 16α-hydroxylase
	Testosterone 16α-hydroxylase
	Testosterone 2α-hydroxylase
	Benzphetamine N-demethylase
CYP2D1	Debrisoquine 4-hydroxylase
CYP2D6	Debrisoquine 4-hydroxylase
CYP2E1	p-Nitrophenol hydroxylase
	Dimethylnitrosamine N-demethylase
	Aniline p-hydroxylase
	Chlorzoxazone 6-hydroxylase
CYP3A	Testosterone 6β-hydroxylase
	Progesterone 6β-hydroxylase
	Androstenedione 6β-hydroxylase
	Erythromycin N-demethylase
	Cortisol 6β-hydroxylase
CYP4A	Lauric acid ω-hydroxylase

[a]Certain probes can only be used in some animal species.

Nutrition and xenobiotic metabolism

During the 1970s, numerous studies showed that nutritional changes could influence the response to chemicals, and that this was due to modifications in their rate of metabolism (Parke and Ioannides, 1981). At the time, the understanding of the cytochrome P450 system was still in its infancy, and it was believed that it comprised at most two proteins. Consequently, the effect of nutrition on cytochrome P450 expression was monitored using substrates that, as we now appreciate, were not selective for a particular isoform. The past decade, however, has witnessed a re-emergence of the interest in the effects of nutrition on the cytochrome P450 system, with emphasis now having been placed on the modulation of individual isoforms. The importance of nutrition on cytochrome P450 expression was emphasised in elegant studies in which the cytochrome P450 profile in the liver of rabbits was determined during and following weaning. The expression of CYP3A6 was monitored using the N-demethylation of erythromycin, and apoprotein and mRNA levels. A sharp rise in all these parameters was observed between the 2nd and 4th week of age, the period of weaning. In order to confirm that this change was due to the change in diet, weaning was commenced earlier or delayed. The change in CYP3A6 expression paralleled the time of weaning (Pineau et al., 1991). A similar picture was obtained when the CYP1A1 and A2 isoforms were monitored by determining apoprotein and mRNA levels as well as the O-deethylation of ethoxyresorufin and acetanilide hydroxylase, probes for CYP1A1 and A2 respectively. In order to exclude the possibility that contaminating chemicals were responsible for this change in cytochrome P450 expression, the animals were fed diets containing alfalfa, the main component of the solid chow diet. The same changes in the cytochrome P450 composition were noted, indicating that these can be ascribed to the intake of solid food. The effects of weaning on cytochrome P450 expression were selective in that CYP2B4, 2C3, 2C5 and 2E1 isoforms were not modulated (Pineau et al., 1991).

Changes in cytochrome P450 activity may be brought about by:

1. Changes in the levels of macronutrients.
2. Changes in the levels of micronutrients.
3. Starvation and changes in caloric intake.
4. Anutrients present in the diet.

Effect of macronutrients on cytochrome P450 expression

Dietary macronutrients can influence xenobiotic metabolism directly by altering the enzyme levels or indirectly by modulating the availability of essential cofactors (Parke and Ioannides, 1981; Guengerich, 1984).

PROTEIN

Using various substrates, a number of investigators demonstrated that both the quantity and quality of protein present in the diet can perturb cytochrome P450 activity, a decrease in activity being observed in many animal studies following the consumption of protein-deficient diets (Campbell and Hayes, 1976). For example, when rats were fed diets having different protein content, namely inadequate (8%), adequate (12%) and excessive (22%), total cytochrome P450 levels in the liver and to a lesser extent the O-deethylation of ethoxycoumarin increased with increasing protein levels (Butler and Dauterman, 1989). Especially important is the presence of protein rich in sulphur amino acids, which are required for the synthesis of glutathione, whose conjugation with reactive chemical intermediates is the principal defence mechanism against chemical injury, and to provide inorganic sulphate for conjugation in the Phase II metabolism of many chemicals and of their metabolites.

The plasma half-life in human volunteers of the drug theophylline, whose metabolism is catalysed by the CYP1 family, diminished by about 30% when the protein content of the diet was increased, the diets being isocaloric, and the volunteers were fed the diet for two weeks (Alvarez et al., 1976; Kappas et al., 1976; Fagan et al., 1987). It is worth noting that in these studies a marked difference in the response of the volunteers to the new diets was observed, with no change seen in some subjects. Interestingly, the plasma half-life of theophylline decreased when the volunteers were shifted from their customary diet to the high-protein, low-carbohydrate diet. Moreover, in a subsequent study involving 12 volunteers, changing from a high-protein, low-carbohydrate diet to an isocaloric low-protein, high-carbohydrate prolonged the clearance of the same drug by about 30% (Anderson et al., 1991). A comprehensive study of the effects of dietary protein levels on cytochrome P450 isoforms has not been undertaken, but the fact that drugs such as antipyrine and propranolol generally respond to changes in the protein content of the diet in the same fashion as theophylline (Kappas et al., 1976; Fagan et al., 1987) suggests that isoform-specific changes may not occur.

CARBOHYDRATES

The consequences of altering the carbohydrate content of diets on the metabolism of xenobiotics in general and on the cytochrome P450 system in particular have not been adequately studied. In early studies (Strother et al., 1971), it was reported that fructose, glucose or sucrose administration to mice at high concentrations in the drinking water reduced the metabolism of xenobiotics in vitro and prolonged barbiturate-induced sleeping times. However, no studies have been performed where individual cytochrome P450 proteins were studied. Although conditions characterised with hyperglycaemia, such as insulin-dependent diabetes, are associated with pronounced and sustained changes in the hepatic cytochrome P450 profile of rats, these effects appear to be independent of the high glucose levels and are mediated by the changes in hormone levels and the pronounced hyperketonaemia that accompany this disease (Ioannides et al., 1996). However, intraperitoneal administration to animals of high doses of glucose or fructose modulated the metabolism of cytochrome P450 substrates, lowering cytochrome P450 content and associated activities such as the p-hydroxylation of aniline, preferentially but not exclusively catalysed by CYP2E1, and N-demethylation of ethylmorphine which has been linked to the CYP3A subfamily (Hartshorn et al., 1979). Glucose administration to mice prolonged the analgesia of a number of narcotics, and this effect was associated with reduced metabolism (Strother and Chau, 1980); not all narcotics were influenced by the glucose administration, suggesting that the effects of glucose on drug metabolism are selective.

LIPIDS AND LIPOTROPES

The realisation that consumption of high-fat diets promotes the spontaneous incidence of cancer and potentiates the carcinogenicity of chemicals has led to studies of the possible underlying mechanisms, including the cytochrome P450-mediated metabolism of chemical carcinogens. The lipid content of diets, both the level as well as nature, can alter the expression of cytochrome P450 isoforms in animals. Early studies revealed that maintaining rats on fat-free diets for three weeks reduced cytochrome P450 activity, compared with that in animals kept on 3% corn oil diets (Norred and Wade, 1972), whereas activity rose when diets were supplemented with 5–10% of olive oil (Hietanen et al., 1975).

Exposure of rats to diets containing 20% corn oil for only four days resulted in an increase in CYP2E1 levels in the liver, as determined using the N-demethylation of dimethylnitrosamine and immunologically in Western blots, when compared with animals fed fat-free diets (Yoo et al., 1990a, 1992). The same treatment did not influence CYP2B activity but elevated CYP2B2 apoprotein levels. The hydroxylation of testosterone at the 6β-position, the demethylation of erythromycin and CYP3A apoprotein levels were also higher in the corn oil-treated animals. The hydroxylation of the steroid at the 7α- and 2α-positions and benzphetamine N-demethylation were unaffected, showing that CYP2A1 and 2C11 expression is resistant to corn oil intake. Finally, the hepatic CYP1A2 apoprotein levels doubled following consumption of the corn oil diets. In studies where animals were fed high-fat, energy-dense diets for a year, a selective increase in CYP2E1 activity and apoprotein levels was observed (Raucy et al., 1991).

When the animals were maintained on diets containing different amounts of corn oil, the increase in CYP2E1 activity correlated with the plasma ketone concentrations, consistent with a role of ketone bodies in the induction of this isoform (Yang et al., 1992). Hyperketonaemia was also implicated in the effects of medium-chain triglycerides on the cytochrome P450 system. In these studies, rats were given daily intragastric doses of 8 g/kg for 22 days and the hepatic cytochrome P450 profile was monitored using diagnostic substrates and confirmed by immunological analysis (Barnett et al., 1988, 1990a,b). This treatment, which results in marked hyperketonaemia, increased the expression of the CYP1A, specifically CYP1A2, 2B, 2E and 4A subfamilies, but had no effect on 3A. Treatment of rats with acetone enhanced the levels and activities of CYP1A2, 2B and 2E, showing that, in the case of these cytochrome P450 proteins, acetone and possibly other ketone bodies are at least partly responsible for the increases following the administration of medium-chain triglycerides (Barnett et al., 1992). Similarly, maintaining animals on high-fat diets, containing 70% lard, which also induce hyperketonaemia stimulated CYP2E1 activity in both rat and kidney, as exemplified by an increase in the p-hydroxylation of aniline, apoprotein and mRNA levels (Yun et al., 1992). The increase in CYP2E1 mRNA exhibited a positive correlation with the plasma acetoacetate and β-hydroxybutyrate levels. However, no correlation was seen with the plasma levels of acetone but this is not surprising since the induction of CYP2E1 by acetone involves post-translational mechanisms and does not involve increase in mRNA levels (Song et al., 1989). The same treatment did not modify the hepatic levels of CYP2C and, in contrast, to previous studies where hyperketonaemia was induced by medium-chain triglycerides (Barnett et al., 1988) or where acetone was administered directly to the animals (Barnett et al., 1992), CYP1A levels were also unchanged (Yun et al., 1992).

The extent of modulation of cytochrome P450 proteins by lipids is also dependent on the nature of oil employed, indicating that other factors are important, such as degree of unsaturation. For example, corn oil and menhaden oil, when present in the diet at concentrations of 5 and 20%, were more efficient in inducing CYP2E activity compared with lard and olive oil (Yoo et al., 1991). Corn oil and menhaden oil are high in polyunsaturated fatty acids whereas lard and olive oil are high in saturated and monounsaturated fatty acids. Linolenic acid appears to be largely responsible for the corn oil-induced increase in CYP2E1 since feeding it to rats, at concentrations equivalent to that present in corn oil, induced the levels of this isoform. The induction of CYP2B1 was the same whether the fat is tallow, which is devoid of linolenic acid, or corn oil (Takahashi et al., 1992).

The effect of cholesterol-rich diets on xenobiotic metabolism appear to be species-specific, in that induction was noted in the rat (Hietanen et al., 1987), mouse (Mantyla et al., 1982) and guinea pig (Deliconstantinos et al., 1983), but in contrast activities in the rabbit were inhibited (Nakahama et al., 1992). In a recent study (Irizar and Ioannides, 1998), rabbits were maintained on a 1% cholesterol-supplemented diet for eight weeks. Activities associated with various cytochrome P450 proteins were measured in the liver and a marked inhibition was observed in all cases. However, when cytochrome P450 proteins were measured immunologically, no differences could be discerned between control and cholesterol-treated animals. As cholesterol failed to influence cytochrome P450 activities *in vitro* it was concluded that a metabolite(s) of cholesterol was bound avidly to the cytochrome, impairing its metabolic activity.

Lipid content of the diet not only influences the basal levels of cytochrome P450 proteins but can also modulate their induction by administration of potent inducing agents. The presence of unsaturated fat in the diet appears to potentiate the ethanol-induced increase in CYP2E1. For example, the induction of CYP2E1 in the liver of rats, measured using *p*-nitrophenol as a probe and immunologically, following the intragastric administration of alcohol was much higher when the animals were maintained on diets containing corn oil compared with tallow. Under the same conditions, the apoprotein levels of CYP2B1 were not perturbed (Takahashi *et al.*, 1992). Induction of CYP2B activity, determined using pentoxyresorufin, and apoprotein levels by phenobarbitone was more pronounced in animals fed a 20% corn oil diet compared with a fat-free diet, and the same difference was observed when mRNA levels were measured (Wade *et al.*, 1985; Yoo *et al.*, 1990a). When acetone served as the inducing agent, CYP2E1 induction was not influenced by the presence of fat in the diet (Yoo *et al.*, 1990a).

Dietary deficiencies in the lipotropes methionine and choline potentiated the carcinogenicity of many metabolically activated chemical carcinogens (Parke and Ioannides, 1994), and this may be, at least partly, related to the modulation of cytochrome P450 isoforms (Murray *et al.*, 1987). When male rats were made cirrhotic by the administration of choline-deficient diets for 30 weeks, total levels of the haemoprotein in the liver were halved but the effect was isoform-specific (Murray *et al.*, 1987). A marked drop was observed in the CYP2C11-mediated 16α-hydroxylation of androstenedione. Hydroxylation in the 6β-position and CYP3A2 apoprotein levels were lower, but hydroxylation at the 16β-position was unaffected. Finally, the apoprotein levels of CYP1A2, 2C6 and 2C12 were also unaffected. Similar results were obtained when female rats received the same treatment. The activity of the CYP2A1-catalysed steroid 7α-hydroxylase was halved, and the hydroxylation of aniline and hydroxylation of androstenedione at the 6β-position were decreased; the hydroxylation of the steroid at the 16α- and 16β-positions was not affected (Murray *et al.*, 1988).

FIBRE

Fibre appears to have no direct effect on cytochrome P450 expression but may influence the induction potential of other agents presumably by impeding their absorption. For example, the extent of induction of CYP1A1 in the proximal and distal portions of the colonic mucosa of rats following administration of 3-methylcholanthrene was lower when the animals were maintained for two weeks on high-fibre diets, containing 5% wheat bran, compared with control diets (Kawata *et al.*, 1992). When the inducing agent was injected intraperitoneally the extent of induction was not influenced by the nature of the diet.

The response of cytochromes P450 to changes in the dietary macronutrient composition is summarised in Table 5.3.

Effects of micronutrients on cytochrome P450 expression

Deficiency of minerals and vitamins in animals has long been known to modulate significantly the metabolism of xenobiotics such as drugs and influence the incidence of chemical toxicity and carcinogenesis, the effects being usually reversed on replenishing the depleted stores (Parke and Ioannides, 1981, 1994; Parke, 1991).

VITAMINS

Vitamin A

Vitamin A and retinoids have been shown to protect against chemical carcinogens in animal models and, moreover, epidemiological studies revealed an inverse relationship between plasma levels of the vitamin and cancer incidence, especially of the lung. Consequently, the effects of vitamin A deficiency and supplementation on xenobiotic metabolism have received considerable attention. It is relevant to point out that all-*trans*-retinoic acid, which mediates most biological properties of vitamin A, is one of the many endogenous compounds metabolised by cytochrome P450. The CYP1A1 protein appears to be involved in the catabolism of vitamin A (Li *et al.*, 1995), and this may explain why the potent inducer of CYP1A1 benzo(a)pyrene, a carcinogenic polycyclic aromatic hydrocarbon, depletes tissue vitamin A (Edes *et al.*, 1991). Moreover, the CYP1A1-inducing agents 3-methylcholanthrene and 3,3′, 4,4′, 5,5′-

Table 5.3 Modulation of cytochrome P450 proteins by macronutrients

Macronutrient	Supplementation/ deficiency	Changes in cytochrome P450 expression
Protein	Supplementation	CYP1A↑
Lipids and lipotropes		
Corn oil	Supplementation	CYP1A2↑ CYP2B2↑ CYP2E1↑
Medium-chain triglycerides	Supplementation	CYP1A2↑ CYP2B↑ CYP2E1↑ CYP4A1↑
Lard	Supplementation	CYP2E1↑
Linolenic acid	Supplementation	CYP2E1↑
Choline	Deficiency	CYP2A1↓ CYP2C11↓ CYP3A2↓

hexabromobiphenyl enhanced the 4-hydroxylation of all-*trans*-retinoic acid, that leads to its deactivation (Roberts *et al.*, 1979; Spear *et al.* 1988). In more recent studies, however, the CYP1A1 inducer β-naphthoflavone failed to stimulate the 4-hydroxylation of all-*trans*-retinoic acid, whereas the inducers of CYP2B and CYP3A phenobarbitone and dexamethasone induced this activity in rat hepatic microsomes (Roberts *et al.*, 1979; Martini and Murray, 1994a). In studies using eight purified rabbit cytochrome P450 isoforms in reconstituted systems, it was observed that CYP2B4, the major phenobarbitone-inducible form in the rabbit, as well as CYP1A2 were the forms most active in the 4-hydroxylation of retinoic acid, retinol and retinal (Roberts *et al.*, 1992). It has also been reported that rabbit CYP2C7 is also able to catalyse this reaction (Leo *et al.*, 1984) and, moreover, a human member of the CYP2C subfamily is also capable of doing so (Leo *et al.*, 1989). Evidence has also been presented that in the rat a member of the CYP3A subfamily participates in retinoic acid 4-hydroxylation, but is neither CYP3A1 nor CYP3A2 (Martini and Murray, 1993). Clearly, a number of cytochrome P450 proteins contribute to the metabolism of retinoic acid through 4-hydroxylation.

Vitamin A deficiency has been reported by many groups to depress cytochrome P450 activity (Colby *et al.*, 1975; Miranda *et al.*, 1979; Periquet *et al.*, 1986). In subsequent studies, however, in which rats were maintained for eight weeks on diets that were deficient in or supplemented with vitamin A, no major change was seen in the total cytochrome P450 levels or in the metabolism of substrates including aniline and ethoxyresorufin (Ayalogu *et al.*, 1988), diagnostic substrates for CYP2E1 and 1A1 respectively (Table 5.2). However, other members of the cytochrome P450 superfamily active in xenobiotic metabolism appear to be sensitive to vitamin A deficiency. CYP2C11-mediated hepatic 2α- and 16α-hydroxylation of testosterone, CYP2C11 apoprotein levels and mRNA levels in the liver of rats were decreased (Martini *et al.*, 1995). All these effects were prevented by the addition of all-*trans*-retinoic acid to the diet. No changes in the 7α- and 6β-hydroxylation of testosterone, catalysed predominantly by CYP2A1 and 3A respectively, were noted indicating that vitamin A deficiency perturbed the cytochrome P450 system in an isoform-specific manner. Androgen plays a major role in sustaining CYP2C11 levels in the male rat (Morgan *et al.*, 1985; Janeczko *et al.*, 1990). Vitamin A deficiency reduced the circulating levels of testosterone, the effect being prevented by addition of all-*trans*-retinoic to the diet, indicating that the down-regulation of CYP2C11 levels in vitamin A deficiency may be mediated, at least partly, by the lower testosterone levels (Martini *et al.*, 1995). Indeed, administration of the androgen methyltrienolone restored the 16α-hydroxylation of androstenedione, CYP2C11 apoprotein and mRNA levels (Murray *et al.*, 1996). Furthermore, administration of all-*trans*-retinoic acid to gonadectomised rats did not restore CYP2C11 expression, indicating that the decline in CYP2C11 levels encountered in the liver of vitamin A-deficient rats is the consequence of androgen deficiency. In the hamster, vitamin deficiency caused a marked inhibition in the metabolism of all activities studied, including the microsomal hydroxylation of testosterone at all sites, alluding to a species difference when compared with the rat (Ushio *et al.*, 1996).

In studies aimed at investigating the expression of cytochrome P450 enzymes in animals kept on diets containing different amounts of vitamin A, supplementation of the diet with the vitamin (25 IU/g) for 15 weeks led to higher total cytochrome P450 levels and to a selective increase in the hepatic levels of CYP3A2 in the rat, as denoted by an increase in the 6β-hydroxylation of androstenedione and progesterone and a parallel rise in the CYP3A2 apoprotein levels (Murray *et al.*, 1991). The 16α-hydroxylation of androstenedione, catalysed by CYP2C11, and the 21-hydroxylation of progesterone, catalysed by CYP2C6 were modestly decreased. In contrast, the CYP2A-mediated 7α-hydroxylation of androstenedione and the CYP1A1-mediated O-deethylation of ethoxyresorufin were slightly elevated (Murray *et al.*, 1991). Intraperitoneal administration of high, supraphysiological doses of all-*trans*-retinoic to rats for three days gave rise to a marked decrease in the hepatic 2α- and 16α-hydroxylation of testosterone with a concomitant decrease in CYP2C11 apoprotein levels (Martini *et al.*, 1995). However, feeding of a diet containing excess vitamin A (500 IU/g) to weanling rats for 10 weeks did not influence the expression of this cytochrome P450 enzyme in the liver (Martini and Murray, 1994b). Studies carried out in hamsters showed that supplementation of the diet with vitamin A (250 IU/g) for six weeks gave rise to a marked increase in the hepatic 7α-hydroxylation of testosterone, with hydroxylation at other positions being unaffected, paralleled by an increase in CYP2A1 apoprotein levels (Ushio *et al.*, 1996). The same workers noted a modest, but statistically significant, rise in the CYP2B-mediated dealkylation of pentoxyresorufin but not in the dealkylation of ethoxyresorufin. In *in vitro* studies, retinol, 9-*cis*-retinoic acid and all-*trans*-retinoic appear to induce the mRNA levels of CYP2C7 in primary hepatocytes isolated from female rats (Westin *et al.*, 1993).

When the carotenoids canthaxanthin, a naturally occurring carotenoid also used extensively as a food colouring, β-carotene and vitamin A were fed to rats through the diet, and the metabolism of various cytochrome P450 diagnostic substrates examined, the latter two carotenoids had no effect (Astorg *et al.*, 1994). Canthaxanthin, in contrast, gave rise to a very marked increase in the O-dealkylations of methoxy- and ethoxy-resorufin, indicative of enhanced expression of the CYP1A1 and 1A2 enzymes. Subsequent studies by the same workers established that canthaxanthin, astaxanthin and β-apo-8'-carotenal, but not β-carotene, lutein or lycopene, are potent inducers of CYP1A1 and A2 in the liver of rats (Gradelet *et al.*, 1996a,b).

When retinoic acid was applied to the skin of human volunteers, the levels of epidermal CYP1A1 mRNA were suppressed. Similarly, the levels of CYP1A2 were down-regulated as determined using reverse transcription–polymerase chain reaction (Li *et al.*, 1995). Furthermore, co-application of retinoic acid with coal tar attenuated the increase in CYP1A1 mRNA caused by coal tar applied alone.

Vitamin B

Thiamine deficiency, in contrast to other vitamin deficiencies, appears to enhance cytochrome P450 activity in the liver of rats whereas dietary administration of the vitamin leads to suppression (Grosse and Wade, 1971; Wade and Evans, 1977). It appears that thiamine deficiency induces selectively the CYP2E1 protein (Yoo *et al.*, 1990b). When weanling rats were fed a thiamine-deficient diet for three weeks, an increase was observed in the hepatic N-demethylation of dimethylnitrosamine and CYP2E1 apoprotein levels, with no change in CYP2C11 levels. The increased expression of CYP2E1 was antagonised by intraperitoneal administration of thiamine to the deficient animals. No hyperketonaemia was evident in the thiamine-deficient rats, indicating that the induction of CYP2E1 is mediated through a ketone-independent mechanism.

Deficiency in riboflavin, an essential component of NADPH-cytochrome P450 reductase, leads to reduced cytochrome P450 activity (Yang, 1974).

Vitamin C

Ascorbic acid deficiency in guinea pigs is associated with reduced cytochrome P450 function in the liver and lung, which, at least in the liver, could be reversed by the administration of the vitamin (Zannoni *et al.*, 1972; Kuenzig *et al.*, 1977; Peterson *et al.*, 1983); subsequent studies revealed that the various isoforms are differentially modulated in that only the CYP1A1, 1A2 and 2E1 proteins were decreased by the induction of deficiency (Kanazawa *et al.*, 1991; Mori *et al.*, 1992; Roomi *et al.*, 1997). Although the hydroxylation of testosterone and progesterone at the 6β-position was elevated in the vitamin C-deficient guinea pigs, this was not accompanied with changes in either CYP2B1 or 3A levels (Kanazawa *et al.*, 1991).

Vitamin C levels may also influence the response of animals to cytochrome P450-inducing agents. In ODS-od/od rats, a mutant strain with a hereditary osteogenic receptor lacking L-gulono-γ-lactone – the terminal enzyme system in the synthesis of ascorbic acid – induction of CYP1A2 and 2B mRNA levels by polyhalogenated biphenyls was higher in animals fed an ascorbic acid-supplemented diet (Suzuki *et al.*, 1993).

Vitamin E

Rats in which vitamin E deficiency has been induced are characterised by reduced cytochrome P450 activity (Carpenter and Howard, 1974; Yang and

Yoo, 1988). The response of individual isoforms to vitamin E deficiency has not been addressed.

Supplementation of diets with vitamin E (0.06%) elevated modestly the levels of CYP2C11 and of the associated androstenedione 16α-hydroxylase activity, but hydroxylation at other positions was unaffected highlighting the sensitivity of CYP2C11 to vitamin E (Murray, 1991).

The changes in cytochrome P450 expression mediated by vitamin deficiency and supplementation are summarised in Table 5.4.

MINERALS

Iron

As cytochrome P450 is a haemoprotein, it would be reasonable to assume that iron deficiency would lead to loss of metabolic activity. Initial studies indicated that feeding to rats and mice iron-deficient diets did not impair hepatic drug-metabolising activity and even increased activity was noted with some substrates (Catz et al., 1970; Becking, 1972). These observations suggest that the liver pool of iron is not readily depleted. In contrast, intestinal total cytochrome P450 levels and activity declined in rats fed iron-deficient diets (Hoensch et al., 1975; Pascoe et al., 1983; Dhur et al., 1989). Iron overload suppressed cytochrome P450 in the liver of rats (Bacon et al., 1989).

Selenium

Selenium is an essential component of gluatathione peroxidase, an enzyme that protects the cell from peroxides and the reactive oxygen species derived from these. It is well documented that deficiency in selenium is associated with increased risk of cancer. Induction of selenium deficiency is characterised by loss of cytochrome P450 in the intestine, but not the liver, of rats (Correia and Burk, 1978; Pascoe et al., 1983; Wrighton and Elswick, 1989; Olsson et al., 1993). In the intestine, deprivation of selenium for just a single day resulted in dramatic loss of cytochrome P450 and suppression of ethoxyresorufin O-de-ethylase, both effects being reversed by supplementation of the diet with

Table 5.4 Modulation of cytochrome P450 proteins by vitamins

Vitamin	Supplementation/ deficiency	Changes in cytochrome P450 expression
Vitamin A	Deficiency	CYP2C11↓
	Supplementation	CYP2A1↑ CYP2C6↓ CYP3A2↑
Thiamine	Deficiency	CYP2E1↑
Vitamin C	Deficiency	CYP1A1↓ CYP1A2↓ CYP2E1↓
Vitamin E	Supplementation	CYP2C11↑

selenium for one day (Pascoe *et al.*, 1983). This marked and rapid decline that occurs specifically in the intestine, is believed to be due to decreased ferro-chelatase activity leading to unavailability of haem. It has been suggested (Pascoe *et al.*, 1983) that the intestinal cell relies on the diet for its selenium requirements whereas the liver derives its needs from body stores which are very difficult to deplete.

Selenium deficiency also perturbs the induction of cytochromes P450. The induction of the CYP2B2 and 3A isoforms by phenobarbitone was impaired in rats maintained on selenium-deficient diets for four months (Wrighton and Elswick, 1989). However, mRNA levels were unaffected by the deficiency, suggesting that the underlying mechanism responsible for this effect is reduced translational efficiency or an accelerated degradation of these proteins. Moreover, when dexamethasone and troleandomycin served as inducers of CYP3A, or 3-methylcholanthrene was the inducing agent of CYP1A (Burk and Masters, 1975), selenium deficiency had no effect, indicating that such effect is specific to phenobarbitone (Wrighton and Elswick, 1989). It is conceivable that selenium deficiency alters the pharmacokinetics of the barbiturate inducer, facilitating its elimination. Cytochrome P450 induction by barbiturates is directly related to their plasma half-life (Ioannides and Parke, 1975).

Zinc

In rats fed zinc-deficient diets for three weeks hepatic cytochrome P450 levels and related activities declined through a free radical-mediated mechanism (Xu and Bray, 1992).

Copper

Induction of copper deficiency by feeding diets devoid in this mineral to rats led to increase in the metabolism of some cytochrome P450 substrates whereas in other cases metabolism was attenuated, suggesting differential regulation of the various isoforms (Hammermueller *et al.*, 1987; Arce and Keen, 1992).

Effects of starvation and caloric restriction on cytochrome P450 expression

STARVATION

Early studies revealed that fasting modulates differentially the metabolism of classic cytochrome P450 substrates, suggesting that the various isoforms display different sensitivity to food withdrawal (Kato and Gillette, 1965). The most sensitive cytochrome P450 protein to starvation is CYP2E1 whose expression is enhanced in both the liver and kidney of rats (Hong *et al.*, 1987a; Imaoka *et al.*, 1990a,b). Starvation of rats led to enhanced N-demethylation of dimethylnitrosamine, hydroxylation of p-nitrophenol and p-hydroxylation of aniline resulting from an increase in CYP2E1 expression (Miller and Yang, 1984; Hong et al., 1987a; Johansson et al., 1988; Brown et al., 1995). Following short-term starvation of rats, in addition to the increased expression of CYP2E1, a rise in the O-dealkylation of pentoxyresorufin and in CYP2B apoprotein levels were observed (Brown et al., 1995). When rats were starved for three days, total cytochrome P450 content in the kidney doubled, accompanied by an increase in the p-hydroxylation of aniline, lauric acid hydroxylation and in the CYP2E1 apoprotein levels. A kidney-specific isoform, catalytically active in the hydroxylation of lauric acid, was also induced (Imaoka et al., 1990b). In the hamster, starvation lasting four days stimulated the p-hydroxylation of aniline, O-de-ethylation of ethoxycoumarin and N-demethylation of dimethylnitrosamine in the liver, lung and kidney, and the N-demethylation of benzphetamine in the lung and, to a much lesser extent, in the liver (Ueng et al., 1993b). Immunoblotting revealed increases in the apoprotein levels of CYP2E1 and 1A1 in all three tissues, and in CYP2B1 in the lung. In contrast to these effects, in the liver of rats the male-specific form CYP2C11 was down-regulated by starvation as observed by a decrease in apoprotein levels and in the associated 2α- and 16α-hydroxylation of testosterone and N-demethylation of benzphetamine (Ma et al., 1989; Imaoka et al., 1990a). Similarly, CYP2C13, 1A2, and 2B2 were also down-regulated by starvation but, in contrast, the 6β-hydroxylation of testosterone, N-demethylation of erythromycin and CYP3A2 apoprotein levels as well as CYP2A1 levels and testosterone 6β-hydroxylase and CYP2B1 levels were increased (Ma et al., 1989; Imaoka et al., 1990a). In this study CYP1A1 was not modulated by starvation. The changes in cytochrome P450 expression induced by starvation are summarised in Table 5.5

The changes in cytochrome P450 expression consequent to starvation may be partially mediated by the increased circulating levels of ketones or the decreased levels of growth hormone that occur during starvation

Table 5.5 Modulation of cytochrome P450 proteins by starvation and calorie restriction

Factor	Tissue	Changes in cytochrome P450 expression
Starvation	Liver	CYP1A1↑ CYP1A2↓
		CYP2A1↑ CYP2B1↑
		CYP2B2↓ CYP2C11↓
		CYP2C13↓ CYP2E1↑
		CYP3A2↑
	Kidney	CYP1A1↑ CYP2E1↑
	Lung	CYP1A1↑ CYP2B1↑
		CYP2E1↑
Calorie restriction	Liver	CYP2C11↓ CYP2E1↑
	Testicular Leydig cells	CYP2A1↓

(Tannenbaum *et al.*, 1979; Miller and Yang, 1984). However, hyperketonaemia cannot fully account for the starvation-induced changes in cytochrome P450. In the case of CYP2E1 induction, fasting elevates the level of mRNA as a result of transcriptional activation (Hong *et al.*, 1987b; Johansson *et al.*, 1990) whereas acetone induction of this isoform appears to involve protein stabilisation (Song *et al.*, 1989). Studies in humans do not concord with observations made in laboratory animals. Prolonged starvation in humans, associated with a rise in the circulating levels of ketone bodies, led to a decrease in the metabolism of the CYP2E1 substrate chlorzoxazone (O'Shea *et al.*, 1994). It was suggested that, on prolonged fasting, reactive oxygen species generated from this protein result in its destruction. A synergistic effect has been reported in the increase of CYP2B apoprotein and mRNA levels by acetone treatment and fasting (Johansson *et al.*, 1988).

It is now standard procedure to starve animals overnight prior to conducting studies on the metabolism and pharmacokinetics of chemicals. The intention is to reduce liver glycogen that may interfere in the preparation of microsomal fractions, to prevent lipid-associated turbidity of serum, and to prevent food from influencing the absorption process. Even in elective surgery, patients are fasted overnight to prevent regurgitation of fluids. What is not appreciated is that such procedure, as a result of increased CYP2E1 expression, may result in enhanced metabolism of small molecular weight compounds and the generation of reactive oxygen species (Ronis *et al.*, 1996). CYP2E1 activity and apoprotein levels were elevated in rats following starvation for only 8 hours (Brown *et al.*, 1995). It must be emphasised that many gaseous anaesthetics are substrates of the CYP2E1 protein (Raucy, 1995). Moreover, glutathione levels decline as a result of starvation (Pessayre *et al.*, 1979) so that this critical protective system is compromised. Thus, the combination of increased CYP2E1 activity and low glutathione levels may result in increased production of chemical reactive intermediates and reactive oxygen species at a time that the body defences that normally deal with these are compromised.

CALORIC RESTRICTION

One of the most effective means of attenuating cancer incidence in animals is through restriction of caloric intake. Rodents maintained on calorie-restricted diets exhibited a much lower incidence of spontaneous and chemically induced tumours than animals fed *ad libitum* diets. These observations prompted further work to clarify the underlying mechanisms and, consequently, the effects of calorie restriction on energy metabolism and on the enzymes that catalyse the metabolism of chemicals have been the subject of many studies (Manjgaladze *et al.*, 1993).

Early studies established that restriction in the intake of energy influences the levels of the drug-metabolising enzymes as well as their inducibility (Sachan, 1982; Hashmi *et al.*, 1986). Rats receiving calorie-restricted diets displayed modest changes in metabolising substrates associated with cytochrome P450 enzymes (Leakey *et al.*, 1989; Chou *et al.*, 1993). Maintaining rats on diets of 60% of the *ad libitum* intake for 22 months resulted in an increase in the *p*-hydroxylation of nitrophenol, a CYP2E1 probe. The same food restriction for only six weeks stimulated the hydroxylation of testosterone in the 6β-, 16α- and 16β-positions (Sohn *et al.*, 1994). In contrast, one of the initial effects of food restriction is down-regulation of the expression of the male-specific form CYP2C11 in the liver of rats, with the increase in CYP2E1 being evident after more prolonged treatment (Manjgaladze *et al.*, 1993). In a study designed to established what level of caloric restriction can modify drug metabolism, diets equivalent to 85, 70 and 55% of the *ad libitum* intake were fed to rats for four weeks. An increase in total cytochrome P450 levels and aniline *p*-hydroxylation was evident only at the 55% diet restriction (Sachan and Su, 1986). Extrahepatic cytochrome P450 expression appears also to be sensitive to food restriction. Caloric restriction to 60% of the *ad libitum* intake in rats led to a dramatic decrease in testosterone 7α-hydroxylase and CYP2A1 apoprotein levels in testicular Leydig cells (Seng *et al.*, 1996). Table 5.5 shows the effects of caloric restriction of cytochrome P450 expression. These are discussed more extensively in Chapter 8.

Effects of anutrients on cytochrome P450 expression

Diet is probably the most important route through which the body is exposed to chemical anutrients. Such chemicals are inherent to the diet, may be generated during storage, e.g. fungal mycotoxins and chemicals leaking into the food from storage material, may be added into the food in the form of food additives or, finally, may be generated during the cooking process. By far the largest group are those inherent to the food, a vast array of structurally very diverse chemicals. Interest in these chemicals grew when it was realised that these have biological activity that can be exploited for the benefit of mankind. It is now widely recognised that chemicals in food can antagonise the carcinogenicity of chemicals or, because of their antioxidant activity, can have a protective effect against conditions such as heart disease (Wattenberg, 1993). Moreover, it is now realised that such chemicals can influence the cytochrome P450 expression at the levels ingested by humans. In many instances the precise nature of the chemicals that mediate the modulation of the cytochrome P450 profile in a particular type of food have not been fully identified.

CRUCIFEROUS VEGETABLES

Rats fed diets containing cruciferous vegetables, such as cabbage and sprouts, displayed higher activity in metabolising a number of cytochrome P450 substrates in the intestine (Pantuck *et al.*, 1976). In what are now regarded as classical studies, the same workers showed that humans exposed to similar diets for seven days exhibited enhanced metabolism of the drug phenacetin, a CYP1A substrate (Tassaneeyakul *et al.*, 1993), indicating that the capacity of humans to metabolise xenobiotics is also influenced by the nature of the diet. They suggested that indoles, present at high concentrations in cruciferous vegetables, were responsible for these effects (Pantuck *et al.*, 1979). In one of the first studies aimed at investigating the effects of commonly consumed vegetables on xenobiotic-metabolising enzymes (Bradfield *et al.*, 1985), the O-deethylation of ethoxycoumarin in the liver of mice was induced by exposure for ten days to diets containing kidney beans, cauliflower, carrots, etc.

Both white and Savoy cabbage when added to the diet at a concentration of 25% dry weight, and fed to rats for only five days induced the CYP1A1-mediated O-deethylation of ethoxyresorufin in the small and large intestine; Savoy cabbage also induced this activity in the liver (McDanell *et al.*, 1987). Boiling the vegetables attenuated the extent of induction. When a 10% broccoli diet was fed to rats for a week, hepatic apoprotein levels of CYP1A1 and 1A2, as well as total CYP1A mRNA levels were elevated (Vang *et al.*, 1991). Similarly, the CYP2B1/B2 and 2E1 apoprotein levels increased but the CYP2B mRNA levels were unaffected; CYP2E1 mRNA levels were not determined. The same treatment increased the apoprotein levels of CYP1A1 and 2B1/B2 in the colon. The CYP1A1 mRNA levels also rose in this tissue but, in contrast, those of CYP2B1/B2 were reduced (Vang *et al.*, 1991). In rats fed cooked Brussels sprouts-supplemented diets, at concentrations of 2.5, 5.0 and 20%, for 2–28 days, the cytochrome P450 protein primarily induced in the liver was CYP1A2, and to a lesser degree 1A1 and 2B, all being determined by using chemical probes and immunoblotting; in contrast, the CYP2C11-mediated 2α-hydroxylation of testosterone was decreased. In the intestine the form primarily increased was CYP2B1 but, at the highest dose, an increase in the O-deethylation of ethoxyresorufin was observed, indicative of an increase in CYP1A1 levels (Wortelboer *et al.*, 1992a). Some of these effects were evident just two days after exposure to these diets. Indeed, a marked rise in intestinal O-deethylation of ethoxyresorufin was reported in rats some 4–6 hours after the intake of a single meal of 25% Brussels sprouts (McDanell *et al.*, 1990).

Indole-3-carbinol is a hydrolysis product of glucobrassicin, an indolymethyl glucosinolate, which is released by the action of the enzyme myrosinase (Figure 5.1). Another hydrolysis product is indole-3-carbonitrile. It appears that, at the physiological gastric acid pH, indole-3-carbinol condenses non-enzymatically to form dimers, including 3,3'-diindolymethane, probably the major product, and indolo[3,2-*b*]carbazole, linear and cyclic trimers and tetramers as well as some high-molecular weight oligomers (de Kruif *et al.*, 1991; Stresser *et al.*, 1995). When added to the diet, indole-3-carbinol caused a marked increase in the hepatic and intestinal O-deethylation of ethoxyresorufin whereas other glucobrassicin metabolites, namely diindolymethane and indole-3-carbonitrile also induced the hepatic activity, but to a much lesser degree, and had no effect on the intestinal activity (McDanell *et al.*, 1987).

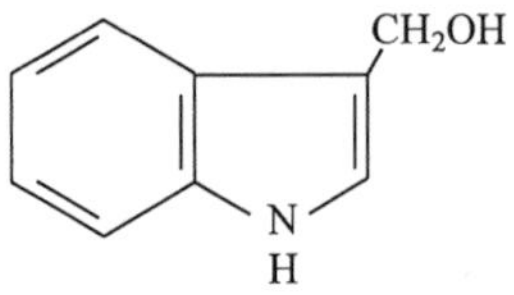

Indole-3-carbinol

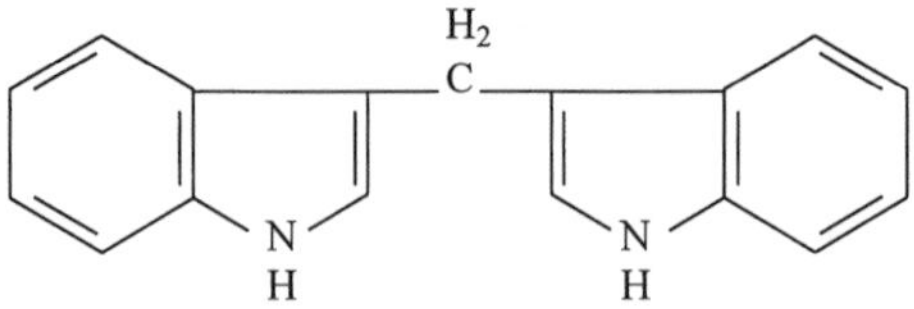

3,3'-Diindolylmethane

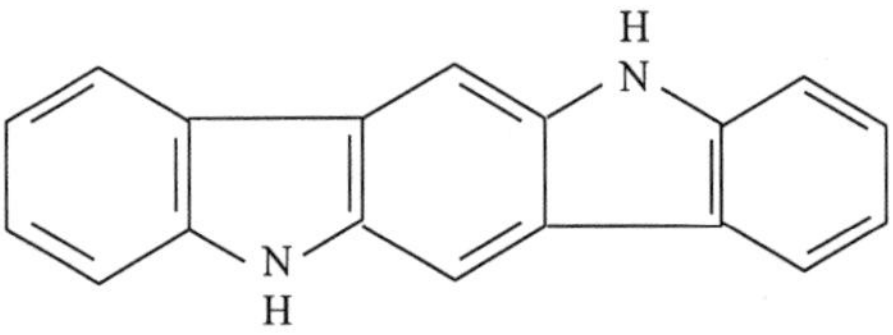

Indolo-[3,2-*b*]carbazole

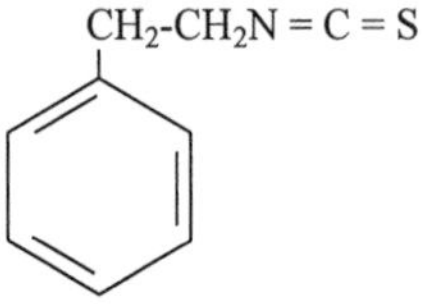

Phenethyl isothiocyanate

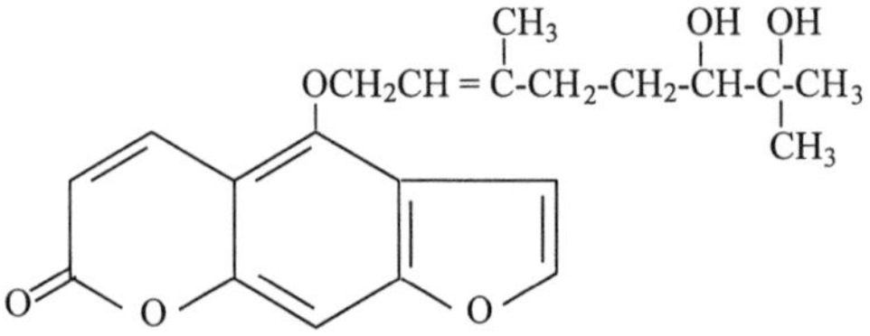

6',7'-Dihydroxybergamottin

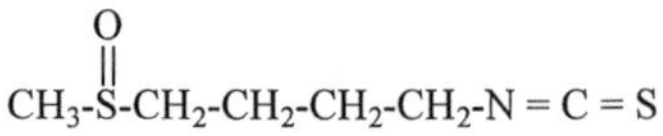

Sulphoraphane

$CH_2 = CH\text{-}CH_2\text{-}S\text{-}CH_2\text{-}CH = CH_2$

Diallyl sulphide

$CH_2 = CH\text{-}CH_2\text{-}S\text{-}S\text{-}CH_2\text{-}CH = CH_2$

Diallyl disulphide

Figure 5.1 Structure of dietary anutrients that modulate cytochrome P450 expression.

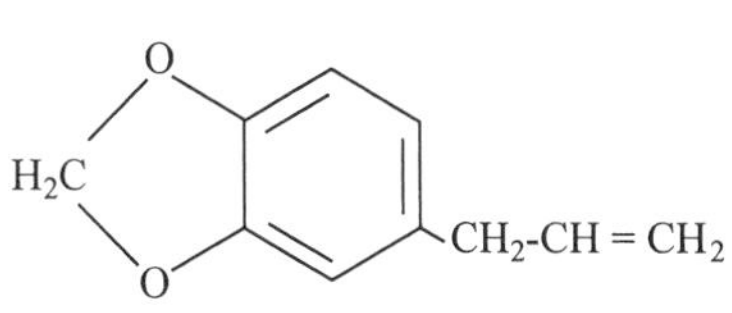

Safrole

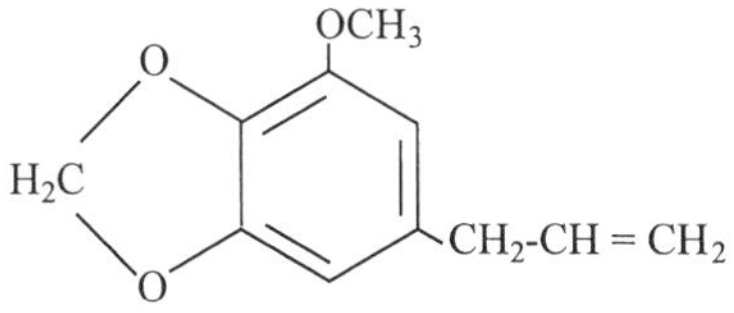

Myristicin

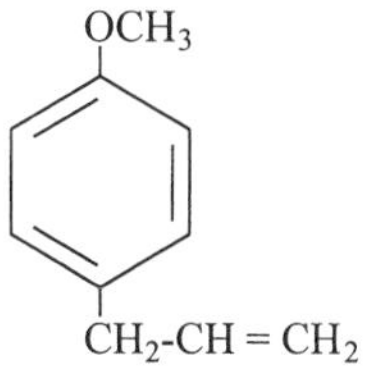

Estragole

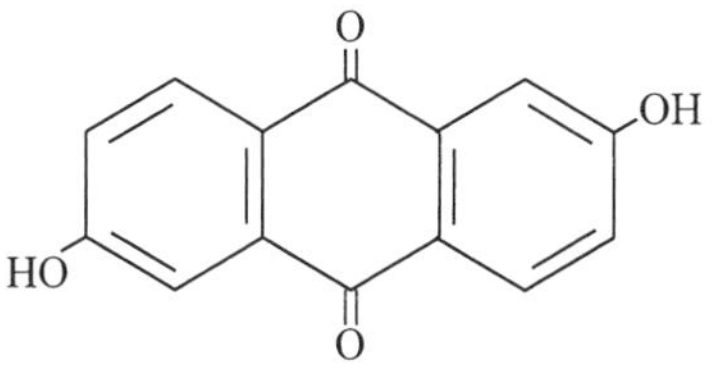

Anthraflavic acid

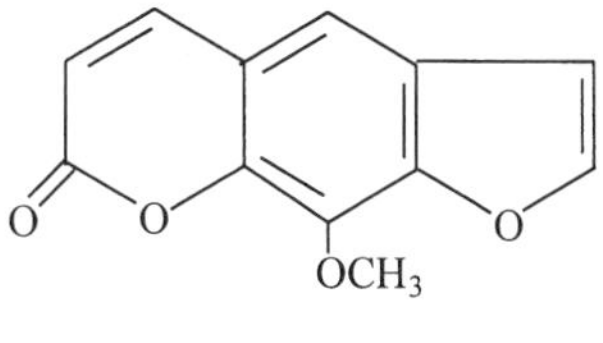

Methoxsalen

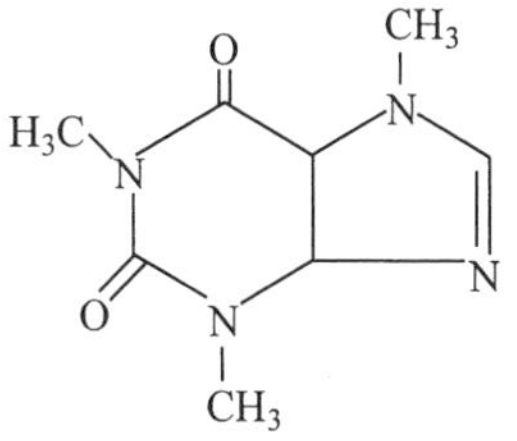

Caffeine

Figure 5.1 (*continued*)

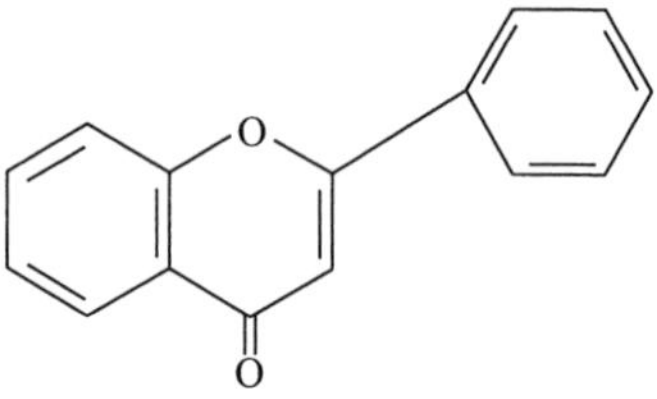

Flavone

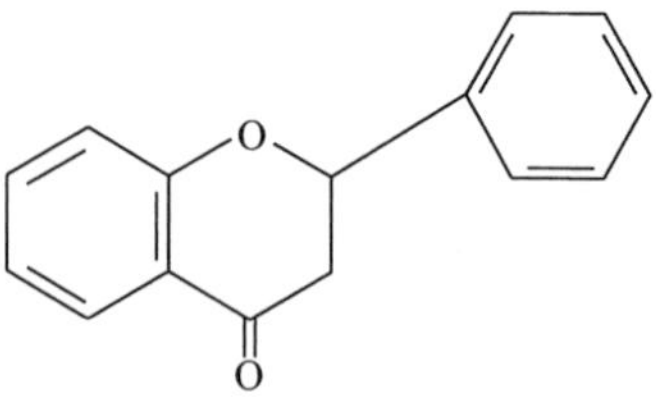

Flavanone

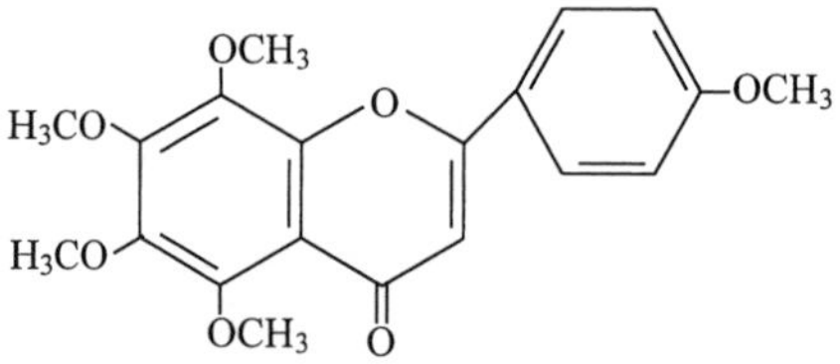

Tangeretin

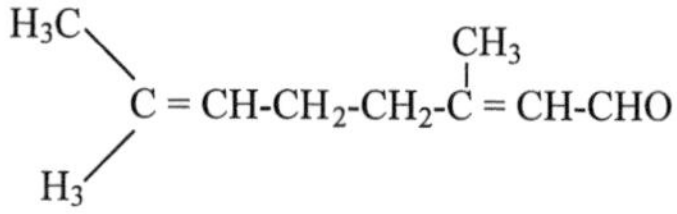

Citral

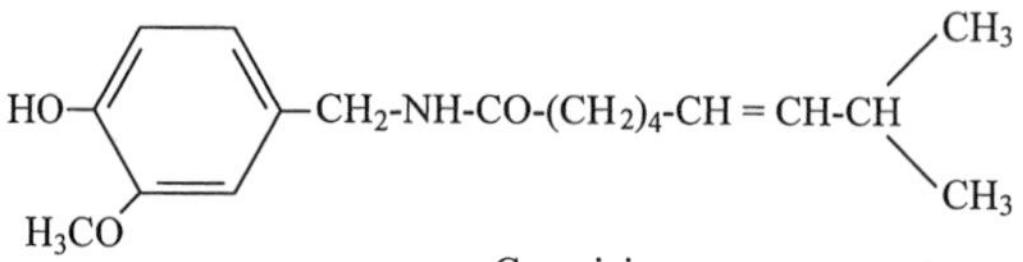

Capsaicin

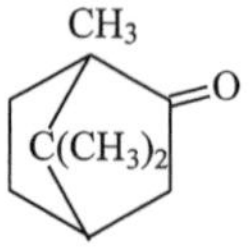

Camphor

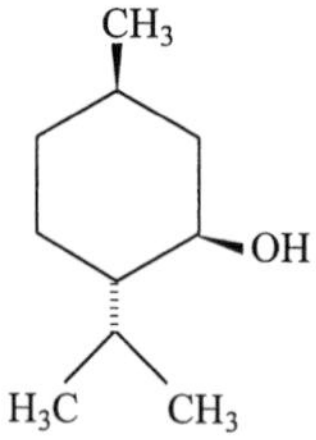

Menthol

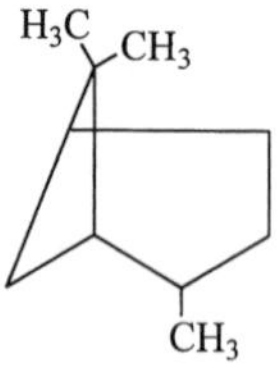

α-Pinene

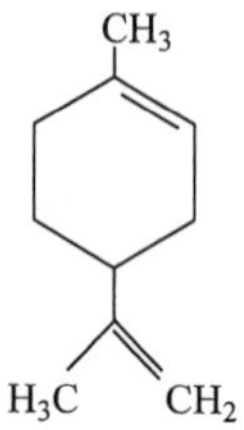

Limonene

Figure 5.1 (*continued*)

When indole-3-carbinol was administered to animals through the diet, at a concentration of 0.2% for three days, an increase in the hepatic apoprotein levels of CYP1A1, A2, 3A and to a lesser extent 2B was observed (Stresser *et al.*, 1994). In more extensive studies (Wortelboer *et al.*, 1992b), rat diets were supplemented with indole-3-carbinol at the dose levels of 200 and 500 mg/kg for various periods of time ranging from 2 to 28 days. The hepatic O-dealkylations of ethoxy- and pentoxy-resorufin were stimulated in a dose-dependent fashion, accompanied by increased apoprotein levels of CYP1A1, 1A2, 2B1. Both dealkylations were also induced in the intestine following the same treatment but in this case the apoprotein levels of only CYP1A1 and CYP2B1 were elevated. In the liver a modest transient rise in testosterone 6β-hydroxylation was also noted, suggesting an increase in the expression of CYP3A proteins. The increased expression of the CYP1A subfamily appears to be the result of increased transcription since a single dose of indole-3-carbinol increased CYP1A1 mRNA in the rat liver and colon, and CYP1A2 mRNA only in the liver (Vang *et al.*, 1990). However, when hepatocytes were exposed to indole-3-carbinol no increase in the CYP1A1-mediated O-dealkylation of ethoxyresorufin was observed whereas 3,3′-diindolymethane was a potent inducer; a more modest increase in activity was achieved by indole-3-acetonitrile (Wortelboer *et al.*, 1992b), suggesting that the *in vivo* effects of indole-3-carbinol may be mediated by condensation products such as 3,3′-diindolylmethane. In accordance with this hypothesis is the fact that hepatic CYP1A1 activity is induced when indole-3-carbinol is administered orally, but not intraperitoneally (Shertzer, 1982; Bradfield and Bjeldanes, 1987). Furthermore, acid treatment of indole-3-carbinol generated a mixture that induced this activity following both oral and intraperitoneal administration (Bradfield and Bjeldanes, 1987). Finally, 3,3′-diindoylmethane has higher affinity than indole-3-carbinol for the Ah receptor, a cytosolic receptor protein that regulates CYP1A induction (Jellinck *et al.*, 1993). Another condensate that may contribute to the induction characteristics of indole-3-carbinol is indolo[3,2-*b*]carbazole, which binds avidly to the Ah receptor, with an affinity orders of magnitude higher than that of indole-3-carbinol (Gillner *et al.*, 1985; Bjeldanes *et al.*, 1991).

Cruciferous vegetables also contain isothiocyanates, a class of compounds that have proved successful in antagonising the carcinogenicity of a number of chemicals. In *in vitro* studies these compounds functioned as inhibitors of CYP1A1 and other cytochrome P450 isoforms in hamsters (Hamilton *et al.*, 1994; Hamilton and Teel, 1996). The extent of inhibition was related to the length of the alkyl chain, phenethyl isothiocyanate being the most potent. Phenethyl isothiocyanate (Figure 5.1) is formed from the glucosinolate, gluconasturtiin by the action of the enzyme murosinase (Chung *et al.*, 1992). Subsequent studies have shown that the phenethyl derivative markedly inhibited human CYP1A2 activity in a reconstituted system (Smith *et al.*, 1996). In human liver microsomes it also inhibited the 4-hydroxylation of debrisoquine, but when watercress (50 g), a rich source of this isothiocyanate, was fed to human volunteers the activity was not modified, presumably because the concentrations achieved in the liver were not sufficiently high (Carporaso et al., 1994). Administration of this isothiocyanate to rats induced CYP2B1 apoprotein levels and induced the O-dealkylation of pentoxyresorufin, but it suppressed the CYP2E1-catalysed N-demethylation of dimethylnitrosamine and the CYP3A-catalysed N-demethylation of erythromycin (Guo et al., 1992; Huang et al., 1993). It appears to impair CYP2E1 activity by a suicide mechanism (Ishizaki et al., 1990). The related isothiocyanate, sulphoraphane (Figure 5.1), another constituent of cruciferous vegetables, is also a potent inhibitor of CYP2E1 activity (Barcelo et al., 1996).

The effects of cruciferous vegetables on cytochrome P450 expression have also been studied in humans. Individual proteins were investigated using established in vivo probes such as caffeine, for monitoring CYP1A2, and chlorzoxazone, for monitoring CYP2E1. Human volunteers received diets supplemented with broccoli so that the daily intake of this vegetable was 500 g/day. Following consumption of this diet for 10–12 days the metabolism of caffeine, but not of chlorzoxazone, was elevated (Vistisen et al., 1992; Kall et al., 1996). Similarly, just three meals containing cruciferous vegetables were sufficient to shorten the half-life of caffeine by about 20%, but large inter-individual variation was observed (McDanell et al., 1992). Finally, consumption of watercress (50 g twice daily for a week) by human volunteers reduced the metabolism and prolonged the half-life of chlorzoxazone, indicating inhibition of CYP2E1 activity (Kim and Wilkinson, 1996).

GARLIC

In epidemiological studies and in laboratory experiments the consumption of garlic (Allium sativum) has been associated with a reduced risk of cancer incidence. Organosulphur compounds, such as the lipophilic ethers allyl sulphides, formed from the oxidation of allicin, are believed to contribute to the anticarcinogenic properties of this vegetable. The most extensively studied component of garlic is diallyl sulphide (Figure 5.1) which is encountered in crushed garlic at concentrations of 0.03–0.1 g/kg (Yu et al., 1989).

Administration of diallyl sulphide and diallyl disulphide (Figure 5.1) to rats resulted in a time- and dose-dependent selective inhibition of hepatic CYP2E1 whereas 2B, 3A1/2 and to a lesser extent 1A were up-regulated (Brady et al., 1991a; Haber et al., 1994; Dragnev et al., 1995). Selective inhibition of CYP2E1 was also demonstrated for other organosulphur compounds such as allyl methyl sulphide and allyl mercaptan (Kwak et al., 1994; Reicks and Cranckshaw, 1996). Interestingly, inhibition of CYP2E1 activity was paralleled by a similar decline in the apoprotein levels (Reicks and Crankshaw, 1996), but no change in mRNA levels (Kwak et al., 1994) suggesting that possibly a metabolite of these compounds, such as an epoxide, may act as suicide inhibitor, and that no transcriptional inactivation is involved. Indeed, diallyl sulphide inhibits CYP2E1 activity by a dual mechanism involving competitive inhibition and irreversible suicide-inhibition caused by a sulphone metabolite rather than an epoxide (Brady *et al.*, 1991b; Jin and Baillie, 1997). Indeed, the decrease in CYP2E1 activity occurred more rapidly following administration of diallyl sulphone when compared with diallyl sulphide (Brady *et al.*, 1991a). However, these authors also emphasised the importance of the allyl group since the analogue dipropyl sulphide failed to suppress CYP2E1 activity. In recent studies, diallyl sulphide was shown to be readily oxidised by CYP2E1 to form the sulphoxide, which in turn is oxidised to form the sulphone. The sulphone is further metabolised by the same enzyme to form an active metabolite that inactivates the enzyme or generates an epoxide that is subject to detoxication through glutathione conjugation (Figure 5.2) (Jin and Baillie, 1997).

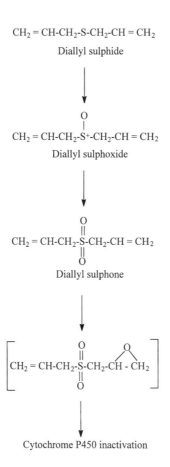

Figure 5.2 Bioactivation of diallyl sulphide. (Adapted from Jin and Baillie, 1997).

TEA

Following an increasing number of laboratory studies showing that tea, and in particular green tea, can prevent the carcinogenicity induced by chemicals and radiation, extensive effort is currently devoted into identifying the tea constituents responsible for its anticarcinogenic potential. Although flavanols, because of their antioxidant properties, are considered to play a predominant role experimental evidence is still lacking.

When aqueous infusions of green or black tea (2.0–2.5%, w/v) were given to rats as the sole drinking fluid for 4–6 weeks, selective increases were observed in the O-dealkylations of methoxy-, ethoxy- and pentoxy-resorufin and in the hydroxylation of lauric acid (Bu-Abbas *et al.*, 1994; Sohn *et al.*, 1994). Immunoblot analyses revealed elevated CYP1A2 and 4A1 apoprotein levels (Bu-Abbas *et al.*, 1994). Caffeine appears to be responsible for the tea-induced up-regulation of CYP1A2, since decaffeinated black tea failed to induce CYP1A2 (Bu-Abbas A, Clifford MN, Walker R and Ioannides C, unpublished observations; Chen *et al.*, 1996). Indeed, caffeine administration to rats in the drinking water at a concentration range of 0.1–1.0% (w/v) for two weeks caused a selective, dose-dependent rise in hepatic CYP1A2 and CYP2B expression, without influencing CYP2E1 and 3A activity or apoprotein levels (Ayalogu *et al.*, 1995). Similar findings have been reported following short-term intragastric administration to rats (50–150 mg/kg) and, in addition, a rise in the CYP1A1 mRNA levels and activity was seen in the kidney (Goasduff *et al.*, 1996). It is relevant to point out that heavy coffee drinkers may consume as much as 3 g of caffeine daily, and since the half-life in humans is five times longer compared with rats, thus achieving higher plasma levels (Barone and Roberts, 1996), it is possible that in such persons caffeine may play an important role in the regulation of CYP1A2 expression in the liver.

GRAPEFRUIT JUICE

Drug–drug interactions leading to a modest increase in drug levels are emphasised, whereas drug–nutrient interactions where drug levels rise dramatically do not receive the same attention (Spence, 1997). The extensively studied interactions involving grapefruit juice have helped to highlight the importance of drug–nutrient interactions and demonstrate that these are of clinical relevance when drugs of narrow therapeutic index are concerned. For example, the interaction of grapefruit with terfenadine is of concern since this drug can cause fatal arrhythmia related to torsade de pointes. The increase in felodipine plasma levels observed in patients with hypertension when they also consumed grapefruit juice was associated with an increase in the blood pressure, heart rates and adverse effects induced by the drug (Bailey *et al.*, 1991).

Ingestion of grapefruit juice increases markedly the plasma levels of drugs that are subject to extensive first-pass effect. Such drugs include the dihydropyridine calcium channel blockers felodipine, nisoldipine and nifedipine (Bailey *et al.*, 1991, 1993a), quinidine (Min *et al.*, 1996), midazolam (Kupferschmidt *et al.*, 1995), terfenadine (Benton *et al.*, 1996) and cyclosporine (Yee *et al.*, 1995). The mode of action involves the inhibition of the presystemic metabolism of these drugs. Human intestinal mucosa contains high levels of CYP3A4 (Kolars *et al.*, 1992), one of the most active isoforms in the metabolism of drugs. For example, the 3-hydroxylation of quinidine, catalysed by CYP3A4, is inhibited by grapefruit juice (Min *et al.*, 1996). Such interactions are not seen when the drugs are taken intravenously but only following oral intake (Ducharme *et al.*, 1995). Grapefruit juice is rich in flavonoids, the principal compound being naringin, constituting up to 10% of dry weight, and to a lesser extent quercetin. Naringin, one of the bitter components of grapefruit juice, is converted to the aglycone naringetin by the intestinal microflora. In studies conducted *in vitro*, naringetin, but not naringin, perturbed the metabolism of calcium channel blockers (Guengerich and Kim, 1990). However, when administered *in vivo* naringin failed to alter the pharmacokinetics of felodipine (Bailey *et al.*, 1993b). Similarly, quercetin, another flavonoid present in grapefruit juice, had no effect on nifedipine pharmacokinetics and is, thus, unlikely to contribute to the interactions with this juice (Rashid *et al.*, 1993). The compound responsible for the interactions of grapefruit juice with drugs appears to be the furanocoumarin (psoralen) 6′-,7′-dihydroxybergamottin (Figure 5.1), a potent CYP3A inhibitor (Edwards *et al.*, 1996). Grapefruit juice also inhibited CYP1A2 activity as exemplified by suppressed caffeine clearance, but surprisingly it had no effect on the pharmacokinetics of another CYP1A2 drug, theophylline (Fuhr *et al.*, 1993, 1995). Finally, it has been reported that simultaneous ingestion of grapefruit juice with coumarin resulted in inhibition of the 7-hydroxylation of the anticoagulant in humans, a pathway catalysed by CYP2A6 (Merkel *et al.*, 1994).

OTHER FLAVONOIDS

In addition to naringetin, many other flavonoids have been studied for their ability to interact with the cytochrome P450. Indeed, synthetic flavonoids such as β-naphthoflavone, are established potent inducers of CYP1A activity. It is widely believed that flavonoids, which are abundant in fruit and vegetables, as a result of their antioxidant characteristics can protect against diseases that may be caused by oxidative stress, such as cardiovascular disease and cancer. It is also conceivable that they may also act by preventing the bioactivation of chemical carcinogens or by inhibiting the cytochrome P450-catalysed generation of reactive oxygen species. The human daily consumption of flavonoids is estimated to be about 1 g.

When administered to rats through the diet (0.3%, w/w) for two weeks, flavone and, to a lesser extent, tangeretin (Figure 5.1) enhanced selectively the O-dealkylations of ethoxy- and pentoxy-resorufin with a concomitant rise in the apoprotein levels of CYP1A1, A2, B1 and B2 (Canivenc-Lavier *et al.*, 1996a). Under the same conditions, flavanone (Figure 5.1), a flavonoid present in citrus fruit, stimulated the O-dealkylation of pentoxyresorufin and CYP2B1 and B2 apoprotein levels whereas quercetin did not modify any of these activities. These differences reflect the fact that flavones and flavonols are fairly planar molecules (Glusker and Rossi, 1986), and consequently can induce CYP1A activity (Lewis *et al.*, 1986). In contrast, flavanones are buckled molecules where the exocyclic phenyl group lies almost perpendicular to the rest of the molecule. Northern blot analysis indicated that flavone and tangeretin increased the mRNA levels of CYP1A2 whereas the levels of the mRNAs coding for CYP1A1 and CYP2B1/2 were slightly or not affected (Canivenc-Lavier *et al.*, 1996b), indicating that these flavonoids may modulate cytochrome P450 expression also by post-transcriptional mechanisms.

OTHER PLANT CONSTITUENTS

Capsaicin (*trans*-8-methyl-*N*-vanillyl-6-nonenamide; Figure 5.1) is one of the major pungent components of chillies and hot peppers. In *in vivo* studies it has been shown to prolong the sleeping time induced by barbiturates, alluding to inhibition of their metabolism (Miller *et al.*, 1983). It is an inhibitor of CYP2E1 activity and this characteristic appears to be important in its anticarcinogenic activity against chemical carcinogens that rely on the CYP2E1 enzyme for their activation (Surh *et al.*, 1995). The mechanism of action is believed to involve cytochrome P450-mediated metabolism to form an electrophile that binds covalently to proteins, including CYP2E1 where it is generated (Miller *et al.*, 1983).

Consecutive daily intraperitoneal administrations for three days to rats of both sexes of the naturally occurring terpenoids (50 mg/kg) camphor, menthol or pinene (Figure 5.1), increased selectively the hepatic apoprotein and mRNA levels of the CYP2B subfamily, camphor being the most potent (Austin *et al.*, 1988). Under the same conditions myrcene had no effect and limonene caused a modest increase only in female animals. However, limonene, when added to the diet (5% w/w) and fed to rats for two weeks also elevated the hepatic apoprotein levels of CYP2B1 and B2 (Maltzman *et al.*, 1991). Finally, short-term intragastric administration of citral to rats resulted in an increase in the hepatic microsomal hydroxylation of lauric acid accompanied by a rise in CYP4A1 apoprotein levels (Roffey *et al.*, 1990). Under the same conditions linalool was ineffective. Related to terpenoids is another naturally occurring compound, picrotoxin, which comprises two components, picrotoxinin and picrotin. Both components selectively enhanced the expression of both proteins of the CYP2B subfamily as exemplified by an increase in the 16α- and 16β-hydroxylation of testosterone and a rise in the apoprotein levels (Yamada *et al.*, 1993).

Methylenedioxyphenyl compounds such as safrole (Figure 5.1) are encountered in many spices such as nutmeg, cinnamon, cloves and black pepper. Safrole was the first chemical identified as an inducer of CYP1A2 but is also capable of inducing 1A1 and 2B isoforms (Ioannides *et al.*, 1981). Similarly, estragole and myristicine (Figure 5.1) are inducers of the O-dealkylation of ethoxyresorufin (Ioannides *et al.*, 1985). At very high doses, eugenol administration induced the O-dealkylations of ethoxy- and pentoxy-resorufin (Rompelberg *et al.*, 1993).

Psoralens (furanocoumarins) are present in many plant species such as celery, grapefruit, parsnip and figs. Administration of methoxsalen (Figure 5.1) to rats stimulated the O-dealkylation of methoxy-, ethoxy- and pentoxy-resorufin in a dose-dependent manner, and these effects were paralleled by increases in the apoprotein and mRNA levels of CYP1A and 2B (Gwang, 1996).

The planar anthraquinone, anthraflavic acid (2,6-anthraquinone; Figure 5.1), when administered to rats intraperitoneally (100 mg/kg) for three days selectively induced in the liver both proteins comprising the CYP1A subfamily, as exemplified by increases in the O-de-ethylation of ethoxyresorufin and apoprotein levels (Ayrton *et al.*, 1988).

ALCOHOL

Alcohol, in the strictest sense of the definition, cannot be considered an anutrient but it is one of the most widely consumed drinks whose ability to induce the cytochrome P450 system was recognised three decades ago (Rubin *et al.*, 1968). The most sensitive metabolic pathway to alcohol intake is aniline *p*-hydroxylation, and subsequent studies have attributed this to an up-regulation of CYP2E1 expression. Indeed, alcohol is the first documented inducer of this isoform. Subsequent studies have shown that alcohol was also a modest inducer of the CYP1A subfamily as indicated by a rise in the O-de-ethylation of ethoxyresorufin (Steele and Ioannides, 1986). Induction of CYP2E1, determined immunologically, also occurs in extrahepatic tissues such as kidney, brain and intestine (Roberts *et al.*, 1994). As a result of the short half-life of this isoform, the effect disappears rapidly, in both hepatic and extrahepatic tissues, after withdrawal of the alcohol. Finally, alcohol has also been reported to enhance CYP2B1 and 4A1 expression (Johansson *et al.*, 1988; Ma *et al.*, 1993; Nanji *et al.*, 1994). Similar observations were made in the hamster where CYP1A and 2E1 activities and apoprotein levels were induced in the liver; in extrahepatic tissues, with the exception of the intestine, CYP2E1 was induced following alcohol ingestion (Ioannides and Steele, 1986; Ueng *et al.*, 1993a). Increase in CYP2E1 and 2B expression in the rat was not accompanied by concomitant increases in mRNA levels indicating that the induction of these proteins involves post-translational mechanisms (Nanji *et al.*, 1994; Roberts *et al.*, 1994). In contrast to the rat, in the hamster CYP2E1 mRNA levels were elevated in the liver (Kubota *et al.*, 1988). Induction of CYP2E1 by alcohol intake has also been established in human liver (Perrot *et al.*, 1989).

In more recent studies carried out in rats (Hakkak *et al.*, 1996), chronic ethanol intake, in addition to CYP2E1, increased the expression in the liver and colon of the constitutive cytochrome P450 protein CYP2C7 that catalyses the 4-hydroxylation of retinal and retinoic acid (Leo and Lieber, 1985). Increased metabolism of retinoic acid may contribute to the lower hepatic storage vitamin A seen frequently in alcoholics (Leo and Lieber, 1982).

Table 5.6 summarises the effects of dietary anutrients on cytochrome P450 expression in the liver and other tissues.

Table 5.6 Modulation of cytochrome P450 expression by naturally occurring dietary anutrients

Anutrient	Tissue	Changes in cytochrome P450 expression
Indole-3-carbinol	Liver	CYP1A1↑ CYP1A2↑ CYP2B1↑ CYP3A↑
	Intestine	CYP1A1↑ CYP2B1↑
Phenethyl isothiocyanate	Liver	CYP2B1↑ CYP2E1↓ CYP3A↓
Sulphoraphane	Liver	CYP2E1↓
Diallyl sulphide	Liver	CYP1A↑ CYP2B↑ CYP2E1↓ CYP3A↑
Diallyl disulphide	Liver	CYP1A↑ CYP2B↑ CYP2E1↓ CYP3A↑
Caffeine	Liver	CYP1A2↑ CYP2B↑
6′,7′ -Dihydroxybergamottin	Intestine	CYP3A↓
Flavone	Liver	CYP1A1↑ CYP1A2↑ CYP2B1↑ CYP2B2↑
Flavanone	Liver	CYP2B1↑ CYP2B2↑
Tangeretin	Liver	CYP1A1↑ CYP1A2↑ CYP2B1↑ CYP2B2↑
Capsaicin	Liver	CYP2E1↓
Camphor	Liver	CYP2B↑
Menthol	Liver	CYP2B↑
Pinene	Liver	CYP2B↑
Citral	Liver	CYP4A1↑
Limonene	Liver	CYP2B1↑ CYP2B2↑
Safrole	Liver	CYP1A1↑ CYP1A2↑ CYP2B↑
Methoxsalen	Liver	CYP1A↑ CYP2B↑
Anthraflavic acid	Liver	CYP1A↑
Alcohol	Liver	CYP1A1↑ CYP2B↑ CYP2C7↑ CYP2E1↑ CYP4A1↑
	Colon	CYP2C7↑ CYP2E1↑
	Kidney	CYP1A1↑ CYP2E1↑
	Lung	CYP1A1↑ CYP2E1↑

ANUTRIENTS GENERATED DURING COOKING

Inducing agents present in food may be generated during cooking. In early human studies, volunteers fed for only four days diets containing high amounts of charcoal-broiled beef displayed increased metabolism of the two CYP1A substrates theophylline and phenacetin, attributed to higher activity of this subfamily in the liver (theophylline) and intestine (phenacetin) (Conney et al., 1976; Kappas et al., 1978). The agents mediating these effects are likely to be polycyclic aromatic hydrocarbons which are potent and specific inducers of the CYP1 family, and generated during the broiling of meat (Skog and Jägerstad, Chapter 3, this volume). Oven-cooked beef failed to modulate phenacetin metabolism (Heller et al., 1989). In more recent studies (Kall and Clausen, 1995), using caffeine as an in vivo probe for CYP1A2 activity, increased caffeine metabolism was seen when a diet supplemented with grilled hamburgers was fed for five days; however, marked interindividual differences were observed.

Using the same approach, Sinha et al. (1994) showed that pan-fried meat containing high levels of heterocyclic amines, but low levels of polycyclic aromatic hydrocarbons, stimulated the metabolism of caffeine, though once again, marked interindividual differences were evident. Moreover, prior studies in animals established the ability of heterocyclic amines to induce the CYP1A proteins in the liver and other tissues of the rat (Rodrigues et al., 1989; Kleman et al., 1990; Degawa et al., 1992).

Conclusions

It is apparent that the nature of the diet is an important factor in determining cytochrome P450 expression. Changes in the composition of the diet, such as the content of macronutrients and micronutrients, the presence of anutrients and caloric intake, can lead to significant, and toxicologically relevant alterations in the expression of cytochromes P450. Such changes appear to be manifested rapidly, and long-term intake of the diets is not a prerequisite. For example, concurrent intake of a single glass of grapefruit juice with certain drugs can alter their metabolism sufficiently to interfere with their clinical efficacy. The mechanism(s) through which diet and nutrition regulate cytochromes P450 has not yet been studied. Do these dietary and nutritional factors act directly or indirectly by impairing hormonal homeostasis and thus interfering with the hormonal regulation of the cytochromes? What is, however, evident is that the diet-induced changes in the levels of cytochromes P450 are selective, in that only a number of isoforms are influenced whereas others are resistant to a particular dietary change. Even in the small number of studies conducted so far, only a limited number of cytochrome P450 proteins were monitored so that the effect of diet and nutrition on the whole spectrum of cytochrome P450 proteins remains to be addressed.

Macronutrient composition of the diet has been shown to alter the profile of cytochromes P450, and in human studies the half-life of model drugs was modified when the diet was changed from high-protein, low-carbohydrate to low-protein, high-carbohydrate (Conney et al., 1977). The relevance of micronutrient deficiency is much more difficult to extrapolate to the human situation, as in the animal studies very marked long-term deficiencies were induced that are unlikely to be relevant to humans. What is perhaps more appropriate to investigate is whether chronic low micronutrient intake has any consequence on the activity of cytochromes P450. The most important effect of diet, however, is likely to be due to the presence of anutrients. Although to the layman the presence of chemicals in food is often synonymous with the presence of man-made chemicals such as food additives and pesticide contaminants, it is now recognised that naturally occurring chemicals are endowed with more biological activity than previously envisaged. In some studies unrealistic, high doses of individual food constituents have been used in isolation. It would be more relevant to utilise complete foods as chemicals present in the same type of food may interact, acting synergistically or antagonising each other's effects. For example high-fibre foods may prevent the absorption of chemicals capable of modulating cytochrome P450 activity.

An increasing number of people nowadays alter their dietary habits voluntarily for cosmetic reasons, or involuntarily for health reasons. It has become fashionable in affluent societies for people to manipulate their caloric intake and follow regimes which they believe will result in weight loss. The number of people eating vegetarian diets is rising whereas the consumption of red meat is decreasing. Patients suffering from chronic diseases such as diabetes receive specialised diets. It is possible that such diets modulate cytochrome P450 activity and other xenobiotic-metabolising systems and consequently alter response to the pharmacological effects of drugs and toxicity of chemicals. Although the number of studies carried out in humans is limited, in almost all cases observations made in animal studies were also evident in humans. Moreover, prolonged administration of the new diet was not required for the changes in cytochrome P450 expression to become evident. A frequent observation in human studies is the very marked difference in response of individuals to the same dietary manipulation, ranging from no effect to a very pronounced change. Why some people are prone to changes in the diet, as far as cytochrome P450 expression is concerned, whereas others are resistant is an important issue that merits clarification.

There are currently available a number of probes for individual cytochrome P450 proteins which can be used to study the effect of diet in vivo, e.g. caffeine for CYP1A2, chlorzoxazone for CYP2E1, debrisoquine for CYP2D6, etc., and such studies would be simple to conduct. It is feasible that changes in cytochrome P450 expression mediated by dietary changes may have a role in the aetiology and progression of disease. In animal studies, one of the initial effects of starvation was a rise in CYP2E1 expression, whose orthologous human protein has very similar substrate specificity to the animal protein. This enzyme is capable of generating reactive oxygen species, even in the absence of a substrate (Ronis *et al.*, 1996), which have been implicated in the aetiology of many degenerative diseases.

References

Alvarez AP, Anderson KE, Conney AH and Kappas A (1976) Interactions between nutritional factors and drug biotransformation in man. *Proceedings of the National Academy of Sciences USA*, **73**, 2501–2504.

Anderson KE, McCleery RB, Vesell ES, Vickers FF and Kappas A (1991) Diet and cimetidine induce comparable changes in theophylline metabolism in normal subjects. *Hepatology*, **13**, 941–946.

Arce DS and Keen CL (1992) Reversible and persistent consequences of copper deficiency in developing mice. *Reproductive Toxicology*, **6**, 211–221.

Astorg P, Gradelet S, Leclerc J, Canivenc M-C and Siess M-H (1994) Effects of β-carotene and canthaxanthin on liver xenobiotic-metabolizing enzymes in the rat. *Food and Chemical Toxicology*, **32**, 735–742.

Austin CA, Shephard EA, Pike SF, Rabin BR and Phillips IR (1988) The effect of terpenoid compounds on cytochrome P-450 levels in rat liver. *Biochemical Pharmacology*, **37**, 2223–2229.

Ayalogu EO, Phillipson CE, Preece N, Ioannides C and Parke DV (1988) Effect of vitamin A on rat hepatic mixed-function oxidases, glutathione transferase activity and generation of oxygen radicals. *Annals of Nutrition and Metabolism*, **32**, 75–82.

Ayalogu EO, Snelling J, Lewis DFV, Talwar S, Clifford MN and Ioannides C (1995) Induction of hepatic CYP1A2 by the oral administration of caffeine to rats: lack of association with the Ah locus. *Biochimica et Biophysica Acta*, **1272**, 89–94.

Ayrton AD, Ioannides C and Walker R (1988) Induction of rat hepatic cytochrome P-450 I proteins by the antimutagen anthraflavic acid. *Food and Chemical Toxicology*, **26**, 909–915.

Bacon BR, Healey JF, Brittenhan GM, Park CH, Nunnari J, Tavill AS and Bonkavsky HL (1989) Hepatic microsomal function in rats with chronic dietary overload. *Gastroenterology*, **90**, 1844–1853.

Bailey DG, Spence JD, Munoz C and Arnold JMO (1991) Interaction of citrus juices with felodipine and nifedipine. *Lancet*, **337**, 268–269.

Bailey DG, Arnold JMO, Strong HA, Munoz C and Spence JD (1993a) Effect of grapefruit and naringin on nisoldipine pharmacokinetics. *Clinical Pharmacology and Therapeutics*, **54**, 589–594.

Bailey DG, Arnold JMO, Munoz C and Spence JD (1993b) Grapefruit–felodipine drug interaction, mechanism, predictability and effect of naringin. *Clinical Pharmacology and Therapeutics*, **53**, 637–642.

Barcelo O, Gardiner JM, Gescher A and Chipman JK (1996) CYP2E1-mediated mechanism of anti-genotoxicity of the broccoli constituent sulforaphane. *Carcinogenesis*, **17**, 277–282.

Barnett CR, Flatt PR and Ioannides C (1988) Role of ketone bodies in the diabetes-induced changes in hepatic mixed-function oxidase activities. *Biochimica et Biophysica Acta*, **967**, 250–254.

Barnett CR, Flatt PR and Ioannides C (1990a) Induction of hepatic microsomal P450I and IIB proteins by hyperketonaemia. *Biochemical Pharmacology*, **40**, 393–397.

Barnett CR, Gibson GG, Wolf CR, Flatt PR and Ioannides C (1990b) Induction of cyto-chrome P450III and P450IV family proteins in streptozotocin-induced diabetes. *Biochemical Journal*, **268**, 765–769.

Barnett CR, Petrides L, Wilson J, Flatt PR and Ioannides C (1992) Induction of rat hepatic mixed-function oxidases by acetone and other physiological ketones: their role in diabetes-induced changes in cytochrome P450 proteins. *Xenobiotica*, **22**, 1441–1450.

Barone JJ and Roberts HR (1996) Caffeine consumption. *Food and Chemical Toxicology*, **34**, 119–129.

Becking GC (1972) Influence of dietary iron levels on hepatic drug metabolism in vivo and in vitro in the rat. *Biochemical Pharmacology*, **21**, 1585–1593.

Benton RE, Honig PK, Zamani K, Cantilena LR and Woosley RL (196) Grapefruit juice alters terfenadine pharmacokinetics, resulting in prolongation of repolarization on the electrocardiogram. *Clinical Pharmacology and Therapeutics*, **59**, 383–388.

Bjeldanes LF, Kim J-Y, Grose KR, Bartholomew JC and Bradfield CA (1991) Aromatic hydrocarbon responsiveness-receptor agonists generated from indole-3-carbinol *in vitro* and *in vivo*: comparisons with 2,3,7,8-tetrachlorodibenzo-*p*-dioxin. *Proceedings of the National Academy of Sciences USA*, **88**, 9543–9547.

Bradfield CA and Bjeldanes LF (1987) Structure–activity relationships of dietary indoles: a proposed mechanism of action as modifiers of xenobiotic metabolism. *Journal of Toxicology and Environmental Health*, **21**, 311–323.

Bradfield CA, Chang Y and Bjeldanes LF (1985) Effects of commonly consumed vege-tables on hepatic xenobiotic-metabolizing enzymes in the mouse. *Food and Chemical Toxicology*, **23**, 899–904.

Brady JF, Wang M-H, Hong J-Y, Xiao F, Li Y, Yoo J-S, Ning SM, Fukuto JM, Gapac JM and Yang CS (1991a) Modulation of rat hepatic microsomal monooxygenase activities and cytotoxicity by diallyl sulfide. *Toxicology and Applied Pharmacology*, **108**, 342–354.

Brady JF, Ishizaki H, Fukuto JM, Lin MC, Fadel A, Gapac JM and Yang CS (1991b) Inhibition of cytochrome P-450 2E1 by diallyl sulfide and its metabolites. *Chemical Research in Toxicology*, **4**, 642–647.

Brown BI, Allis JW, Simmons JE and House DE (1995) Fasting for less than 24 hours induces cytochrome P450 2E1 and 2B1/2 activities in rats. *Toxicology Letters*, **81**, 39–44.

Bu-Abbas A, Clifford MN, Walker R and Ioannides C (1994) Selective induction of rat hepatic CYP1 and CYP4 proteins and of peroxisomal proliferation by green tea. *Carcinogenesis*, **15**, 2575–2579.

Burk RF and Masters BSS (1975) Some effects of selenium deficiency on the hepatic microsomal cytochrome P-450 system in the rat. *Archives of Biochemistry and Biophysics*, **170**, 125–131.

Butler LE and Dauterman WC (1989) Sensitivity of selected drug biotransformation enzymes to dietary protein levels in adult F334 male rats. *Journal of Biochemical Toxicology*, **4**, 71–72.

Campbell TC and Hayes JR (1976) The effect of quantity and quality of dietary protein on drug metabolism. *Federation Proceedings*, **35**, 2470–2474.

Canivenc-Lavier M-C, Vernevaut M-F, Totis M, Siess M-H, Magdalou J and Suschetet M (1996a) Comparative effects of flavonoids and model inducers on drug-metabolizing enzymes in rat liver. *Toxicology*, **114**, 19–27.

Canivenc-Lavier M-C, Bentejac M, Miller M-L, Leclerc J, Siess M-H, Latruffe N and Suschetet M (1996b) Differential effects of nonhydroxylated flavonoids as inducers of cytochrome P450 1A and 2B isozymes in rat liver. *Toxicology and Applied Pharmacology*, **136**, 348–353.

Carpenter MR and Howard CN (1974) Vitamin E, steroids and liver microsomal hydroxylations. *American Journal of Clinical Nutrition*, **27**, 966–979.

Carporaso N, Whitehouse J, Monkman S, Boustead C, Issaq H, Fox S, Morse MA, Idle JR and Chung F-L (1994) In vitro but not in vivo inhibition of CYP2D6 by phenethyl isothiocyanate (PEITC), a constituent of watercress. *Pharmacogenetics*, **4**, 275–280.

Catz CS, Juchau MR and Yaffe SJ (1970) Effects of iron, riboflavin and iodide deficiencies on hepatic drug-metabolising enzyme systems. *Journal of Pharmacology and Experimental Therapeutics*, **174**, 197–205.

Chen L, Bondoc FY, Hussin AHJ, Thomas PE and Yang CS (1996) Caffeine induces cytochrome P4501A2: induction of CYP1A2 by tea in rats. *Drug Metabolism and Disposition*, **24**, 529–533.

Chou MW, Kong J, Chung K-T and Hart RW (1993) Effect of caloric restriction on the metabolic activation of xenobiotics. *Mutation Research*, **295**, 223–235.

Chung F-L, Morse MA and Eklind KI (1992) New potential chemopreventive agents for lung carcinogenesis of tobacco-specific nitrosamine. *Cancer Research*, **52**, 2719s–2722s.

Colby HD, Kramer RE, Greiner JW, Robinson DA, Krausse RF amd Canady WJ (1975) Hepatic drug metabolism in retinol-deficient rats. *Biochemical Pharmacology*, **24**, 1644–1646.

Conney AH, Pantuck EJ, Hsia KC, Garland WA, Anderson KE, Alvares AP and Kappas A (1976) Enhanced phenacetin metabolism in human subjects fed charcoal-broiled beef. *Clinical Pharmacology and Therapeutics*, **20**, 633–642.

Conney AH, Pantuck EJ, Kuntzman R, Kappas A, Anderson KE and Alvares AP (1977) Nutrition and chemical biotransformation in man. *Clinical Pharmacology and Therapeutics*, **22**, 707–719.

Correia MA and Burk RF (1978) Rapid stimulation of hepatic microsomal heme oxygenase in selenium-deficient rats. *Journal of Biological Chemistry*, **253**, 6203–6210.

de Kruif CA, Marsman JW, Venekamp JC, Noordhoek J, Blaauboer BJ and Wortelboer HM (1991) Structure elucidation of acid reaction products of indole-3-carbinol: detection in vivo and enzyme induction in vitro. *Chemico-Biological Interactions*, **80**, 303–315.

Degawa M, Kobayashi K-i, Miura S-i, Arai H, Esumi H, Sugimara T and Hashimoto Y (1992) Species difference among experimental rodents in induction of P450IA family enzymes by 2-amino-1-methyl-6-phenylimidazol[4,5-*b*]pyridine. *Japanese Journal of Cancer Research*, **83**, 1047–1051.

Deliconstantinos G, Anastasopoulou K and Karayannakos P (1983) Modulation of hepatic microsomal Ca^{2+}-stimulated ATPase and drug oxidase activities of guinea pigs by dietary cholesterol. *Biochemical Pharmacology*, **32**, 1309–1312.

Dhur A, Galan P and Hereberg S (1989) Effects of different degrees of iron deficiency on cytochrome P450 complex and pentose phosphate pathway dehydrogenases in the rat. *Journal of Nutrition*, **119**, 40–47.

Dragnev KH, Nims RW and Lubet RA (1995) The chemopreventive agent diallyl sulfide. A structurally atypical phenobarbital-type inducer. *Biochemical Pharmacology*, **50**, 2099–2104.

Ducharme MD, Warbasse LH and Edwards DJ (1995) Disposition of intravenous and oral cyclosporine after administration with grapefruit juice. *Clinical Pharmacology and Therapeutics*, **57**, 485–491.

Edes TE, Gysbers DG, Buckley CS and Thornton WH (1991) Exposure to the carcinogen benzopyrene depletes tissue vitamin A: β-carotene prevents depletion. *Nutrition and Cancer*, **15**, 159–166.

Edwards DJ, Bellevue III FH and Woster PM (1996) Identification of 6',7'-dihydroxy-bergamottin, a cytochrome P450 inhibitor, in grapefruit juice. *Drug Metabolism and Disposition*, **24**, 1287–1290.

Fagan TC, Walle T, Oexmann MJ, Walle UK, Bai SA and Gaffny TE (1987) Increased clearance of propranolol and theophylline by high-protein compared with high-carbohydrate diet. *Clinical Pharmacology and Therapeutics*, **41**, 402–406.

Furh U, Klittich K and Staib AH (1993) Inhibitory effect of grapefruit juice and the active component, naringetin, on CYP1A2-dependent metabolism of caffeine. *British Journal of Clinical Pharmacology*, **35**, 431–436.

Fuhr U, Maier A, Keller A, Steinjuans VW, Sauter R and Staib AH (1995) Lacking effect of grapefruit juice on theophylline pharmacokinetics. *International Journal of Clinical Pharmacology and Therapeutics*, **33**, 311–314.

Gillner M, Bergman J, Cambilau C, Fernström B and Gustafsson JÅ (1985) Interaction of indoles with binding sites for 2,3,7,8-tetrachlorodibenzo-*p*-dioxin in rat liver. *Molecular Pharmacology*, **28**, 357–363.

Glusker JP and Rossi M (1986) Molecular aspects of chemical carcinogens and bio-flavonoids. In *Plant Flavonoids in Biology and Medicine: Biochemical, Pharmacological, and Structure-Activity Relationships*, Cody V, Middleton E and Harbone JB (eds), A.R. Liss, New York, pp. 395–410.

Goasduff T, Dréano Y, Guillois B, Méndez J-F and Berthou F (1996) Induction of liver and kidney CYP1A1/1A2 by caffeine in rat. *Biochemical Pharmacology*, **52**, 1915–1919.

Gonzalez FJ and Gelboin HV (1994) Role of human cytochromes P450 in the metabolic activation of chemical carcinogens and toxins. *Drug Metabolism Reviews*, **26**, 165–183.

Gradelet S, Astorg P, Leclerc J and Siess M-H (1996a) *β*-apo-8'-carotenal, but not *β*-carotene, is a strong inducer of liver CYP1A1 and 1A2 in the rat. *Xenobiotica*, **26**, 909–919.

Gradelet S, Astorg P, Leclerc J, Chevalier J, Vernevaut MF and Siess M-H (1996b) Effects of canthaxanthin, astaxanthin, lycopene and lutein on liver xenobiotic-metabolizing enzymes in the rat. *Xenobiotica*, **26**, 49–63.

Grosse W and Wade AE (1971) The effect of thiamine consumption on liver microsomal drug-metabolizing pathways. *Journal of Pharmacology and Experimental Therapeutics*, **176**, 758–765.

Guengerich FP (1984) Effects of nutritive factors on metabolic processes involving bioactivation and detoxication of chemicals. *Annual Reviews of Nutrition*, **4**, 207–231.

Guengerich FP and Kim DH (1990) In vitro inhibition of dihydropyridine oxidation and aflatoxin B1 activation in human liver microsomes by naringetin and other flavonoids. *Carcinogenesis*, **11**, 2275–2279.

Guo Z, Smith TJ, Wang E, Sadrieh N, Ma Q, Thomas PE, and Yang CS (1992) Effects of phenethyl isothiocyanate, a carcinogenesis inhibitor, on xenobiotic-metabolizing enzymes and nitrosamine metabolism in rats. *Carcinogenesis*, **13**, 2205–2210.

Gwang JH (1996) Induction of rat hepatic cytochrome P4501A and P4502B by the methoxsalen. *Cancer Letters*, **108**, 115–120.

Haber D, Siess M-H, De Waziers I, Beaune P and Suschetet M (1994) Modification of hepatic drug-metabolizing enzymes in rats fed naturally occurring allyl sulphides. *Xenobiotica*, **24**, 169–182.

Hakkak R, Korounian S, Ronis MJ, Ingelman-Sundberg M and Badger TM (1996) Effects of diet and ethanol on the expression and localization of cytochromes P450 2E1 and P450 2C7 in the colon of male rats. *Biochemical Pharmacology* **51**, 61–69.

Hamilton SM and Teel RW (1996) Effects of isothiocyanates on cytochrome P-450 1A1 and 1A2 activity and on the mutagenicity of heterocyclic amines. *Anticancer Research*, **16**, 3597–3602.

Hamilton SM, Zhang Z and Teel RW (1994) Effects of isothiocyanate alkyl chain-length on hamster liver cytochrome P-450. *Cancer Letters*, **82**, 217–224.

Hammermueller JD, Bray TM and Bettger WJ (1987) Effect of zinc and copper deficiency on microsomal NADPH-dependent active oxygen generation in rat liver. *Journal of Nutrition*, **117**, 894–901.

Hartshorn RD, Demers LM, Sultatos LG, Vessell ES, MaxLang C and Hughes CH Jr. (1979) Effects of chronic parenteral carbohydrate administration on hepatic drug metabolism in the rat. *Pharmacology*, **18**, 103–111.

Hashmi R, Siddiqui AM, Kachole MS and Pawar SS (1986) Alterations in hepatic microsomal mixed-function oxidase system during different levels of food restriction in adult male and female rats. *Journal of Nutrition*, **116**, 682–688.

Heller RF, Henry DA and Brent PJ (1989) Enzyme induction by eating charcoal-grilled steak with no effect of blood lipids. *Clinical and Experimental Pharmacology and Physiology*, **16**, 783–788.

Hietanen E, Laitinen M, Vainio H and Hanninen O (1975) Dietary fats and properties of endoplasmic reticulum. II. Dietary lipid induced changes in activities of drug metabolising enzymes in liver and duodenum of rats. *Lipids*, **10**, 467–472.

Hietanen E, Ahotupa M, Bereziat J, Park SS, Gelboin HV and Bartsch H (1987) Monoclonal antibody characterization of hepatic and extrahepatic cytochrome P450 activities in rats treated with phenobarbital or methylcholanthrene and fed various cholesterol diets. *Biochemical Pharmacology*, **36**, 3973–3980.

Hoensch H, Woo CH and Schmid R (1975) Cytochrome P-450 and drug metabolism in intestinal villous and crypt cells of rats: effect of dietary iron. *Biochemical and Biophysical Research Communications*, **65**, 399–406.

Hong J, Pang J, Gonzalez FJ, Gelboin HV and Yang CS (1987a) The induction of a specific form of cytochrome P-450 (P-450j) by fasting. *Biochemical and Biophysical Research Communications*, **142**, 1077–1083.

Hong J-Y, Pan J, Dong Z, Ning SM and Yang CS (1987b) Regulation of N-nitrosomethylamine demethylase in rat liver and kidney. *Cancer Research*, **47**, 5948–5953.

Huang Q, Lawson TA, Chung FL, Morris CR and Mirvish SS (1993) Inhibition by phenylethyl and phenylhexyl isothiocyanates of metabolism of and DNA methylation by N-nitrosomethylamylamine in rats *Carcinogenesis*, **14**, 749–754.

Imaoka S, Terao Y and Funae Y (1990a) Changes in the amount of cytochromes P450 in rat hepatic microsomes with starvation. *Archives of Biochemistry and Biophysics*, **278**, 168–178.

Imaoka S, Yamaguchi Y and Funae Y (1990b) Induction and regulation of cytochrome P450 K-5 (lauric acid hydroxylase) in rat renal microsomes by starvation. *Biochimica et Biophysica Acta*, **1036**, 18–23.

Ioannides C (ed) (1996) *Cytochromes P450: Metabolic and Toxicological Aspects*, CRC Press, Boca Raton.

Ioannides C and Parke DV (1975) Mechanism of induction of hepatic drug metabolising enzymes by a series of barbiturates. *Journal of Pharmacy and Pharmacology*, **68**, 189–202.

Ioannides C and Parke DV (1990) The cytochrome P450I gene family of microsomal haemoproteins and their role in the metabolic activation of chemicals. *Drug Metabolism Reviews*, **22**, 1–85.

Ioannides C and Steele CM (1986) Hepatic microsomal mixed-function oxidase activity in ethanol treated hamsters and its consequences on the bioactivation of aromatic amines to mutagens. *Chemico-Biological Interactions*, **59**, 129–139.

Ioannides C, Delaforge M and Parke DV (1981) Safrole: its metabolism, carcinogenicity and interactions with cytochrome P-450. *Food and Cosmetics Toxicology*, **19**, 657–666.

Ioannides C, Delaforge M and Parke DV (1985) Interactions of safrole and isosafrole and their metabolites with cytochromes P-450. *Chemico-Biological Interactions*, **53**, 303–311.

Ioannides C, Barnett CR, Irizar A and Flatt PR (1996) Expression of cytochrome P450 proteins in disease. In *Cytochromes P450: Metabolic and Toxicological Aspects*, Ioannides C (ed), CRC Press, Boca Raton, pp. 301–327.

Irizar A and Ioannides C (1997) Marked inhibition of hepatic cytochrome P450 activity in cholesterol-induced atherosclerosis in rabbits. *Toxicology*, **126**, 179–193.

Ishizaki H, Brady JF, Ning SM and Yang CS (1990) Effect of phenethyl isothiocyanate on microsomal N-nitrosodimethylamine (NDMA) metabolism and other monooxygenase activities. *Xenobiotica*, **20**, 255–264.

Janeczko R, Waxman DJ, Le Blanc GA, Morville A and Adesnik M (1990) Hormonal regulation of levels of the messenger RNA encoding hepatic P450 2c (IIc11), a constitutive male-specific form of cytochrome P450. *Molecular Endocrinology*, **4**, 295–303.

Jellinck PH, Forkert PG, Riddick DS, Okey AB, Michnovicz JJ and Bradlow HL (1993) Ah receptor binding properties of indole carbinols and induction of hepatic estradiol hydroxylation. *Biochemical Pharmacology*, **45**, 1129–1136.

Jin L and Baillie TA (1997) Metabolism of the chemopreventive agent diallyl sulphide to glutathione conjugates in rats. *Chemical Research in Toxicology*, **10**, 318–327.

Johansson I, Ekström G, Scholte B, Puzycki B, Jornvall H and Ingelman-Sundberg M (1988) Ethanol-, fasting- and ethanol-inducible cytochromes P-450 in rat liver: Regulation and characteristics of enzymes belonging to the IIB and IIE gene sub-families. *Biochemistry*, **27**, 1925–1934.

Johansson I, Lindros KO, Eriksson H and Ingelman-Sundberg M (1990) Transcriptional control of *CYP2E1* in the perivenous liver region and during starvation. *Biochemical and Biophysical Research Communications*, **173**, 331–338.

Kall MA and Clausen J (1995) Dietary effect on mixed function P450 1A2 activity assayed by estimation of caffeine metabolism in man. *Human and Experimental Toxicology*, **14**, 801–807.

Kall MA, Vang O and Clausen J (1996) Effects of dietary broccoli in human *in vivo* drug metabolizing enzymes: evaluation of caffeine, oestrone and chlorzoxazone metabolism. *Carcinogenesis*, **17**, 793–799.

Kanazawa Y, Kitada M, Mori T, Inokai Y, Imaoka S, Funae Y and Kamataki T (1991) Ascorbic acid deficiency decreased specific forms of cytochrome P-450 in liver microsomes of guinea pigs. *Molecular Pharmacology*, **39**, 456–460.

Kappas A, Anderson KE, Conne AH and Alvares AP (1976) Influence of dietary protein and carbohydrate on antipyrine and theophylline metabolism in man. *Clinical Pharmacology and Therapeutics*, **20**, 643–653.

Kappas A, Alvares AP, Anderson KE, Pantuck EJ, Pantuck CB, Chang R and Conney AH (1978) Effect of charcoal-broiled beef on antipyrine and theophylline metabolism. *Clinical Pharmacology and Therapeutics*, **23**, 445–450.

Kato R and Gillette JR (1965) Effect of starvation on NADPH-dependent enzymes in liver microsomes of male and female rats. *Journal of Pharmacology and Experimental Therapeutics*, **150**, 279–284.

Kawata S, Tamura S, Matsuda Y, Ito N and Matsuzawa Y (1992) Effect of dietary fiber on cytochrome P450IA1 in rat colonic mucosa. *Carcinogenesis*, **13**, 2121–2125.

Kim RB and Wilkinson GR (1996) Watercress inhibits human CYP2E1 activity in vivo as measured by chlorzoxazone 6-hydroxylation. *Clinical Pharmacology and Therapeutics*, **59**, 170.

Kleman K, Övervik E, Mason G and Gustafsson J-Å (1990) Effects of the food mutagens MEIQx and PhIP on the expression of P450IA proteins in various tissues of male and female rats. *Carcinogenesis*, **11**, 2185–2189.

Kolars JC, Schmiedlin-Ren P, Schuetz JD, Fang C and Watkins PB (1992) Identification of rifampin-inducible P450IIIA4 (CYP3A4) in human small bowel enterocytes. *Journal of Clinical Investigation*, **90**, 1871–1878.

Kubota S, Lasker JM and Lieber CS (1988) Molecular regulation of ethanol-inducible cytochrome P-45-IIE1 in hamsters. *Biochemical and Biophysical Research Communications*, **150**, 304–310.

Kuenzig W, Tkaczevski V, Kamm JJ, Conney AH and Burns JJ (1977) The effects of ascorbic acid deficiency on extrahepatic metabolism of drugs and carcinogens in the guinea pig. *Journal of Pharmacology and Experimental Therapeutics*, **201**, 527–533.

Kupferschmidt H, Ha H, Ziegler W, Meier P and Krähenbühl S (1995) Interaction between grapefruit juice and midazolam in humans. *Clinical Pharmacology and Therapeutics*, **58**, 20–28.

Kwak MK, Kim SG, Kwak JY, Novak RF and Kim ND (1994) Inhibition of cytochrome P4502E1 expression by oroganosulfur compounds allylsulfide, allylmercaptan and allyl methylsulfide in rats. *Biochemical Pharmacology*, **47**, 531–539.

Leakey JEA, Cunny HC, Bazare P, Webb PJ, Feuers FJ, Duffy PH and Hart RW (1989) Effects of aging and caloric restriction on hepatic drug metabolizing enzymes in the Fischer 344 rat. I. The cytochrome P-450 dependent monooxygenase system. *Mechanisms of Ageing and Development*, **48**, 145–155.

Leo MA and Lieber CS (1982) Interaction of drugs and retinol. *New England Journal of Medicine*, **307**, 597–601.

Leo MA and Lieber CS (1985) New pathway for retinol metabolism in liver microsomes. *Journal of Biological Chemistry*, **260**, 5228–5231.

Leo MA, Iida S and Lieber CS (1984) Retinoic acid metabolism by a system reconstituted with cytochrome P-450. *Archives of Biochemistry and Biophysics*, **234**, 305–312.

Leo MA, Lasker JM, Kim C-I, Black M and Lieber CS (1989) Metabolism of retinol and retinoic acid by human liver cytochrome P450IIC8. *Archives of Biochemistry and Biophysics*, **269**, 305–312.

Lewis DFV, Ioannides C and Parke DV (1986) Molecular dimensions of the substrate binding site of cytochrome P-448. *Biochemical Pharmacology*, **35**, 2179–2185.

Li X-Y, Åstrom A, Duell EA, Qin L, Griffiths CEM and Voorhees JJ (1995) Retinoic acid antagonizes basal as well as coal tar and glucocorticoid-induced cytochrome P5401A1 expression in human skin. *Carcinogenesis*, **16**, 519–524.

Ma W, Dannan GA, Guengerich FP and Yang CS (1989) Similarities and differences in the regulation of hepatic cytochrome P-450 enzymes by diabetes and fasting in male rats. *Biochemical Pharmacology*, **38**, 3179–3184.

Ma X, Baraona E and Lieber CS (1993) Alcohol consumption enhances fatty acid ω-oxidation, with greater increase in male than in female rats. *Hepatology*, **18**, 1247–1253.

Maltzman TH, Christou M, Gould MN and Jefcoate CR (1991) Effects of monoterpenoids on *in vivo* DMBA-DNA adduct formation and on phase I hepatic metabolizing enzymes. *Carcinogenesis*, **12**, 2081–2087.

Manjgaladze M, Chen S, Frame LT, Seng JE, Duffy PH, Feuers RJ, Hart RW and Leakey JEA (1993) Effects of caloric restriction on rodent drug and carcinogen metabolizing-enzymes: implications for mutagenesis and cancer. *Mutation Research*, **295**, 201–222.

Mantyla E, Hietanen E and Ahotupa M (1982) The effect of dietary cholesterol on monooxygenation and glucuronidation reactions in control and 2,4,5,2',4', 5'-hexachlorobiphenyl-treated C57BL and DBA/JB mice. In *Cytochrome P450, Biochemistry, Biophysics and Environmental Implications*, Hietanen E, Laitinen M and Hanninen O (eds), Elsevier Biomedical Press, Amsterdam, pp. 161–164.

Martini R and Murray M (1993) Participation of P450 3A enzymes in rat hepatic microsomal retinoic acid 4-hydroxylation. *Archives of Biochemistry and Biophysics*, **303**, 57–66.

Martini R and Murray M (1994a) Retinal dehydrogenation and retinoic acid 4-hydroxylation in rat hepatic microsomes: developmental studies and effect of foreign compounds on the activities. *Biochemical Pharmacology*, **47**, 905–909.

Martini R and Murray M (1994b) Suppression of the constitutive microsomal cytochrome P450 2C11 in male rat liver during dietary vitamin A deficiency. *Biochemical Pharmacology*, **48**, 1305–1309.

Martini R, Butler AM, Jiang X-M and Murray M (1995) Pretranslational down regulation of cytochrome P450 2C11 in vitamin A-deficient male rat liver: prevention by dietary inclusion of retinoic acid. *The Journal of Pharmacology and Experimental Therapeutics*, **273**, 427–434.

McDanell R, McLean AM, Hanley AB, Heaney RK and Fenwick GR (1987) Differential induction of mixed-function oxidase (MFO) in rat liver and intestine by diets containing processed cabbage: correlation with cabbage levels of glucosinolates and glucosinolate hydrolysis products. *Food and Chemical Toxicology*, **25**, 363–368.

McDanell R, McLean AEM, Hanley AB, Heaney RK and Fenwick GR (1990) The effect of feeding Brassica vegetables and intact glucosinolates on mixed-function oxidase activity in the livers and intestines of rats. *Food and Chemical Toxicology*, **27**, 289–293.

McDanell RE, Henderson LA, Russell K and McLean AEM (1992) The effect of Brassica vegetable consumption on caffeine metabolism in humans. *Human and Experimental Toxicology*, **11**, 167–172.

Merkel U, Sigusch U and Hoffmann A (1994) Grapefruit juice inhibits 7-hydroxylation of coumarin in healthy volunteers. *European Journal of Clinical Pharmacology*, **261**, 1195–1199.

Miller KW and Yang CS (1984) Studies on the mechanism of induction of N-nitrosodimethylamine demethylase by fasting, acetone and ethanol. *Archives of Biochemistry and Biophysics*, **229**, 483–491.

Miller MS, Brendel K, Burks TF and Sipes IG (1983) Interactions of capsaicinoids with drug-metabolizing systems. *Biochemical Pharmacology*, **32**, 547–551.

Min DI, Ku Y-M, Geraets DR and Lee H-C (1996) Effect of grapefruit juice on the pharmacokinetics and pharmacodynamics of quinidine in healthy volunteers. *Journal of Clinical Pharmacology*, **36**, 469–476.

Miranda CL, Mukhtar H, Bend JR and Chhabra RS (1979) Effects of vitamin A deficiency on hepatic and extrahepatic mixed-function oxidase and epoxide-metabolizing enzymes in guinea pig and rabbit. *Biochemical Pharmacology*, **28**, 2713–2716.

Morgan ET, MacGeoch C and Gustafsson J-Å (1985) Hormonal and developmental regulation and expression of the hepatic microsomal steroid 16α-hydroxylase cytochrome P-450 apoprotein in the rat. *Journal of Biological Chemistry*, **260**, 11895–11898.

Mori T, Kitamura R, Imaoka S, Funae Y, Kitada M and Kamataki T (1992) Examination for lipid peroxidation in liver microsomes as causal factor in the decrease in the content of cytochrome P-450 due to ascorbic acid deficiency. *Research Communications in Chemical Pathology and Pharmacology*, **75**, 209–219.

Murray M (1991) In vitro and in vivo studies of the effect of vitamin E on microsomal cytochrome P-450 in rat liver. *Biochemical Pharmacology*, **42**, 2107–2114.

Murray M, Zaluzny L, Dannan GA, Guengerich FP and Farrell GC (1987) Altered regulation of cytochrome P-450 enzymes in choline-deficient cirrhotic male rat liver: impaired regulation and activity of the male-specific androst-4-ene-3, 17-dione 16α-hydroxylase, cytochrome P-450$_{UT-A}$, in hepatic cirrhosis. *Molecular Pharmacology*, **31**, 117–121.

Murray M, Cantrill E, Frost L, Mehta I and Farrell GC (1988) Effects of long-term choline deficiency on hepatic microsomal cytochrome P450-mediated steroid and xenobiotic hydroxylases in the female rat. *Biochemical Pharmacology*, **37**, 1187–1192.

Murray M, Cantrill R, Martini G and Farrell G (1991) Increased expression of cytochrome P450IIIA2 in male rat liver after dietary vitamin A supplementation. *Archives of Biochemistry and Biophysics*, **286**, 618–624.

Murray M, Butler AM and Agus C (1996) Restoration of cytochrome P450 2C11 in vitamin A-deficient rat liver by exogenous androgen. *FASEB Journal*, **10**, 1058–1063.

Nakahama T, Fukuhara M, Ohkubo C and Asano M (1992) Modulation of hepatic and pulmonary drug-metabolizing enzyme activities of rabbits by dietary cholesterol. *Research Communications in Chemical Pathology and Pharmacology*, **75**, 57–68.

Nanji AA, Zhao S, Lamb RG, Dennenberg AJ, Sadrzadeh SMH and Waxman DJ (1994) Changes in cytochromes P-450, 2E1, 2B1, and 4A, and phospholipases A and C in the intragastric feeding rat model for alcoholic liver disease: relationship to dietary fats and pathologic liver injury. *Alcoholism: Clinical and Experimental Research*, **18**, 902–908.

Norred WP and Wade AE (1972) Dietary fatty-induced alterations of hepatic microsomal drug metabolism. *Biochemical Pharmacology*, **21**, 2887–2897.

Olsson U, Lundgren B, Segura-Aguillar J, Messing-Erilsson, Andersson K, Becedas L and De Pierre JW (1993) Effects of selenium deficiency on xenobiotic-metabolizing and othe enzymes in rat liver. *International Journal of Vitamin and Nutrition Research*, **63**, 31–37.

O'Shea D, Davis SN, Kim RB and Wilkinson GR (1994) Effect of fasting and obesity in humans on the 6-hydroxylation of chlorzoxazone: a putative probe of CYP2E1 activity. *Clinical Pharmacology and Therapeutics*, **56**, 359–367.

Pantuck EJ, Hsiao K-C, Loub WD, Wattenberg LW, Kuntzman R and Conney AH (1976) Stimulatory effects of vegetables on intestinal drug metabolism in the rat. *Journal of Pharmacology and Experimental Therapeutics*, **198**, 278–283.

Pantuck EJ, Pantuck EB, Garland WA, Min BH, Wattenberg LW, Anderson KE, Kappas A and Conney AH (1979) Stimulatory effect of Brussel sprouts and cabbage on human drug metabolism. *Clinical Pharmacology and Therapeutics*, **25**, 88–95.

Parke DV (1991) Nutritional requirements for detoxication of environmental chemicals. *Food Additives and Contaminants*, **8**, 381–396.

Parke DV and Ioannides C (1981) The role of nutrition in toxicology. *Annual Review of Nutrition*, **1**, 207–234.

Parke DV and Ioannides C (1994) The effects of nutrition on chemical toxicity. *Drug Metabolism Reviews*, **26**, 739–765.

Pascoe GA, Sakai-Wond J, Soliven E and Correia MA (1983) Regulation of intestinal cytochrome P-450 and heme by dietary nutrients. Critical role of selenium. *Biochemical Pharmacology*, **32**, 3027–3035.

Periquet B, Periquet A, Bailly A, Ghisolfi J and Thouvenot J (1986) Effects of retinoic acid on hepatic cytochrome P450 dependent enzymes in rats under different vitamin A status. *International Journal of Vitamin and Nutrition Research*, **56**, 223–229.

Perrot N, Nalpas B, Yang CS and Beaune P (1989) Modulation of cytochrome P450 isozymes in human liver, by ethanol and drug intake. *European Journal of Clinical Investigation*, **19**, 549–555.

Pessayre D, Dolder A, Artigou JY, Wandscheer JC, Descotoire V, Degott C and Benhamou JP (1979) Effect of fasting on metabolite-mediated hepatotoxicity in the rat. *Gastroenterology*, **77**, 264–271.

Peterson FJ, Holloway DE, Diquette PH and Rivers JM (1983) Dietary ascorbic acid and hepatic mixed-function oxidase activity in the guinea pig. *Biochemical Pharmacology*, **32**, 91–96.

Pineau T, Daujat M, Pichard L, Girard F, Angevain J, Bonfils C and Maurel P (1991) Developmental expression of rabbit cytochrome P450 CYP1A1, CYP1A2 and CYP3A6 genes. *European Journal of Biochemistry*, **197**, 145–153.

Rashid J, McKinstry C, Renwick AG, Dirnhuber M, Waller DF and George CF (1993) Quercetin, an in vitro inhibitor of CYP3A, does not contribute to the interaction between nifedipine and grapefruit juice. *British Journal of Clinical Pharmacology*, **36**, 460–463.

Raucy JL (1995) Risk assessment: toxicity from chemical exposure resulting from enhanced expression of CYP2E1. *Toxicology*, **105**, 217–223.

Raucy JL, Lasker JM, Kraner JC, Salazar DE, Lieber CS and Corcoran GB (1991) Induction of cytochrome P450IIE1 in the obese overfed rat. *Molecular Pharmacology*, **39**, 275–280.

Reicks MM and Crankshaw DL (1996) Modulation of rat hepatic cytochrome P-450 activity by garlic organosulfur compounds. *Nutrition and Cancer*, **25**, 242–248.

Roberts AB, Nichols MD, Newton DL and Sporn MB (1979) In vitro metabolism of retinoic acid in hamster intestine and liver. *Journal of Biological Chemistry*, **254**, 6296–6302.

Roberts BJ, Shoaf SE, Jeong K-S and Song BJ (1994) Induction of CYP2E1 in liver, kidney, brain and intestine during chronic ethanol administration and withdrawal: evidence that CYP2E1 possesses a rapid phase half-life of 6 hours or less. *Biochemical and Biophysical Research Communications*, **205**, 1064–1071.

Roberts ES, Vaz ADN and Coon MJ (1992) Role of isozymes of rabbit microsomal cytochrome P-450 in the metabolism of retinoic acid, retinol and retinal. *Molecular Pharmacology*, **41**, 427–433.

Rodrigues AD, Ayrton AD, Williams EJ, Lewis DFV, Walker R and Ioannides C (1989) Preferential induction of the rat hepatic P450 I proteins by the food carcinogen 2-amino-3-methylimidazo[4,5-f] quinoline. *European Journal of Biochemistry*, **181**, 627–631.

Roffey SJ, Walker R and Gibson GG (1990) Hepatic peroxisomal and microsomal enzyme induction by citral and linalool in rats. *Food and Chemical Toxicology*, **28**, 403–408.

Rompelberg CJM, Verhagen H and van Bladeren PJ (1993) Effects of the naturally occurring alkenylbenzenes eugenol and trans-anethole on drug-metabolizing enzymes in the rat liver. *Food and Chemical Toxicology*, **31**, 637–645.

Ronis MJ, Lindros K and Ingelman-Sundberg M (1996) The CYP2E subfamily. In *Cytochromes P450: Metabolic and Toxicological Aspects*, Ioannides C (ed), CRC Press, Boca Raton, FL, pp. 211–239.

Roomi MW, Ogg M, Tsao CS and Gibson GG (1997) Ascorbic acid deficiency decreases the expression of CYP4A1 in liver microsomes of guinea pigs. *Research Communications in Chemical Pathology and Pharmacology*, **95**, 3–10.

Rubin E, Hutterer F and Lieber CS (1968) Ethanol induces hepatic smooth endoplasmic reticulum and drug-metabolising enzymes. *Science*, **156**, 1469–1470.

Sachan D (1982) Modulation of drug metabolism by food restriction in male rats. *Biochemical and Biophysical Research Communications*, **104**, 984–989.

Sachan DS and Su PK (1986) Effects of levels of feed restriction on in vivo and in vitro alterations in drug metabolism and associated enzymes. *Drug-Nutrient Interactions*, **4**, 363–370.

Seng JE, Gandy J, Turturro A, Lipman R, Bronson RT, Parkinson A, Johnson W, Hart RW and Leakey JA (1996) Effects of caloric restriction on expression of testicular cytochrome P450 enzymes associated with the metabolic activation of chemical carcinogens. *Archives of Biochemistry and Biophysics*, **335**, 42–52.

Shertzer HG (1982) Indole-3-carbinol and indole-3-acetonitrile influence on hepatic microsomal metabolism. *Toxicology and Applied Pharmacology*, **64**, 353–361.

Sinha R, Rothman R, Brown ED, Mark SD, Hoover RN, Caporaso NE, Levander OA, Knize MG, Lang NP and Kadlubar FF (1994) Pan-fried meat containing high levels of heterocyclic aromatic amines but low levels of polycyclic aromatic hydrocarbons induces cytochrome P4501A2 activity in humans. *Cancer Research*, **54**, 6154–6159.

Smith TJ, Guo Z, Guengerich FP and Yang CS (1996) Metabolism of 4-(methylnitrosamino)-1-(3-pyridyl)-1-butanone (NNK) by human cytochrome P450 1A2 and its inhibition by phenethyl isothiocyanate. *Carcinogenesis*, **17**, 809–813.

Sohn Ho, Lim HB, Lee YG, Lee DW and Lee KB (1994) Modulation of cytochrome P-450 induction by long-term food restriction in male rats. *Biochemistry and Molecular Biology International*, **32**, 889–896.

Sohn OS, Surace A, Fiala ES, Richie Jr JP, Colosimo S, Zang E and Weisburger JH (1994) Effects of green and black tea on hepatic xenobiotic metabolizing systems in male F344 rats. *Xenobiotica*, **24**, 119–127.

Song BJ, Veech RL, Park SS, Gelboin HV and Gonzalez FJ (1989) Induction of rat hepatic N-nitrosomethylamine demethylase by acetone is due to protein stabilization. *Journal of Biological Chemistry* **264**, 3568–3572.

Spear PA, Garcin H and Narbonne JF (1988) Increased retinoic acid metabolism following 3,3′,4,4′,5,5′-hexachlorobiphenyl injection. *Canadian Journal of Physiology and Pharmacology*, **66**, 1181–1186.

Spence JD (1997) Drug interactions with grapefruit: whose responsibility is to warn the public? *Clinical Pharmacology and Therapeutics*, **61**, 395–400.

Steele CM and Ioannides C (1986) Differential effects of chronic ethanol administration to rats on the activation of aromatic amines to mutagens in the Ames test. *Carcinogenesis*, **7**, 825–829.

Stresser DM, Bailey GS and Williams DE (1994) Indole-3-carbinol and β-naphthoflavone induction of aflatoxin B_1 metabolism and cytochromes P-450 associated with bioactivation and detoxication of aflatoxin B_1 in the rat. *Drug Metabolism and Disposition*, **22**, 383–391.

Stresser DM, Williams DE, Griffin DA and Bailey GS (1995) Mechanism of tumor modulation by indole-3-carbinol: disposition and excretion in male Fischer 344 rats. *Drug Metabolism and Disposition*, **23**, 965–974.

Strother A, Throckmorton JK and Herzer C (1971) The influence of high sugar consumption by mice on the duration of action of barbiturates and the in vitro metabolism of barbiturates, aniline and *p*-nitroanisole. *Journal of Pharmacology and Experimental Therapeutics*, **179**, 490–498.

Strother S and Chau LSK (1980) Influence of glucose (*in vivo* or *in vitro*) on duration of narcotic analgesics and on the kinetics of drug metabolism. *Pharmacology*, **21**, 161–166.

Surh Y-J, Lee RC-J, Park K-K, Mayne ST, Liem A and Miller JA (1995) Chemoprotective effects of capsaicin and diallyl sulfide against mutagenesis and tumorigenesis by vinyl carbamate and N-nitrosodimethylamine. *Carcinogenesis*, **16**, 2467–2471.

Suzuki H, Torii Y, Hitomi K and Tsukagoshi N (1993) Ascorbate-dependent elevation of mRNA levels for cytochrome P450s induced by polychlorinated biphenyls. *Biochemical Pharmacology*, **46**, 186–189.

Takahashi H, Johansson I, French SW and Ingelman-Sundberg M (1992) Effects of dietary fat composition on activities of the microsomal ethanol oxidizing system and ethanol-inducible cytochrome P450 (CYP2E1) in the liver of rats chronically fed ethanol. *Pharmacology and Toxicology*, **70**, 347–352.

Tannebaum GS, Porstad O and Brazeau P (1979) Effects of prolonged food deprivation on the ultradian growth hormone rhythm and immunoreactive somatostatin tissue levels in the rat. *Endocrinology*, **104**, 1733–1738.

Tassaneeyakul W, Birkett DJ, Veronese ME, McManus ME, Tikey RH, Quatrochi LC, Gelboin HV and Miners JO (1993) Specificity of substrate and inhibitor probes for human cytochromes P450 1A1 and 1A2. *Journal of Pharmacology and Experimental Theapeutics*, **265**, 401–407.

Ueng T-H, Ueng Y-F, Tsai JN, Chao I-C, Chen T-L, Park SS, Iwasaki M and Guengerich FP (1993a) Induction and inhibition of cytochrome P450 dependent monooxygenases in hamster tissues by ethanol. *Toxicology*, **81**, 145–154.

Ueng T-H, Ueng Y-FM, Chen T-L, Park SS, Iwasaki M and Guengerich FP (1993b) Induction of cytochrome P450-dependent monooxygenases in hamster tissues by fasting. *Toxicology and Applied Pharmacology*, **119**, 66–73.

Ushio F, Fukuhara M, Bani M-H and Narbonne J-F (1996) Expression of cytochrome P450 isozymes in Syrian hamster after vitamin A supplementation and deficiency. *International Journal for Vitamin and Nutrition Research*, **66**, 197–202.

Vang O, Jensen MB and Autrup H (1990) Induction of cytochrome P450IA1 in rat colon and liver by indole-3-carbinol and 5,6-benzoflavone. *Carcinogenesis*, **11**, 1259–1263.

Vang O, Jensen MB and Autrup H (1991) Induction of cytochrome P-450IA1, IA2, IIB1 and IIE1 by broccoli in rat liver and colon. *Chemico-Biological Interactions*, **78**, 85–96.

Verhoeven DTH, Verhagen H, Goldbohm RA, van den Brandt PA and van Poppel G (1997) A review of mechanisms underlying anticarcinogenicity of brassica vegetables. *Chemico-Biological Interactions*, **103**, 79–129.

Vistisen K, Poulsen HE and Loft S (1992) Foreign compound metabolism capacity in man measured from metabolites of dietary caffeine. *Carcinogenesis*, **13**, 1561–1568.

Wade AE and Evans JS (1977) Influence of norethindrone on drug-metabolizing enzymes of female rat liver in various B-vitamin deficiency states. *Pharmacology*, **15**, 298–301.

Wade AE, White RA, Walton LC and Bellows JT (1985) Dietary fat – a requirement for induction of mixed-function oxidase activities in starved-refed rats. *Biochemical Pharmacology*, **34**, 3747–3754.

Watteberg LW (1993) Chemoprevention of carcinogenesis by minor non-nutrient constituents of the diet. In *Food, Nutrition and Chemical Toxicity*, Parke DV, Ioannides C and Walker R (eds), Smith-Gordon Nishimura, London, pp. 287–300.

Westin S. Mode A, Murray M, Chen R and Gustafsson J-Å (1993) Growth hormone and vitamin A induce P450 2C7 mRNA expression in primary rat hepatocytes. *Molecular Pharmacology*, **44**, 997–1002.

Wortelboer HM, de Kruif CA, van Israel AJJ, Noordhoek J, Blaauboer BJ, van Bladeren PJ and Falke HE (1992a) Effects of cooked Brussels sprouts on cytochrome P-450 profile and phase-II enzymes in liver and small intestinal mucosa of the rat. *Food and Chemical Toxicology*, **30**, 17–27.

Wortelboer HM, van der Linden ECM, de Kruif CA, Noordhoek J, Blaauboer BJ, van Bladeren PJ and Falke HE (1992b) Effects of indole-3-carbinol on biotransformation enzymes in the rat: *in vivo* changes in liver and small intestinal mucosa in comparison with primary hepatocyte cultures. *Food and Chemical Toxicology*, **30**, 598–599.

Wrighton SA and Elswick B (1989) Modulation of the induction of rat hepatic cytochromes P450 by selenium deficiency. *Biochemical Pharmacology*, **38**, 3767–3771.

Xu Z and Bray TM (1992) Effects of increased microsomal oxygen radicals on the function and stability of cytochrome P450 in dietary zinc deficient rats. *Journal of Nutritional Biochemistry*, **3**, 326–332.

Yamada H, Fujisaki H, Kaneko H, Ishii Y, Hamaguchi T and Oguri K (1993) Picrotoxin as a potent inducer of rat hepatic cytochrome P450, CYP2B1 and CYP2B2. *Biochemical Pharmacology*, **45**, 1783–1789.

Yang CS (1974) Alterations of the aryl hydrocarbon hydroxylase system during riboflavin depletion and repletion. *Archives of Biochemistry and Biophysics*, **160**, 623–630.

Yang CS and Wang Z-Y (1993) Tea and cancer. *Journal of the National Cancer Institute*, **85**, 1038–1049.

Yang CS and Yoo J-SH (1988) Dietary effects on drug metabolism by the mixed-function oxidase system. *Pharmacology and Therapeutics*, **38**, 53–72.

Yang CS, Brady JF and Hong J-Y (1992) Dietary effects on cytochromes P450, xenobiotic metabolism and toxicity. *FASEB Journal*, **6**, 737–744.

Yee GD, Stanley DL, Pessa L, Dalla Costa T, Beltz SE, Ruiz J and Lowenthal DT (1995) Effect of grapefruit juice on blood cyclosporin concentration. *Lancet*, **345**, 955–956.

Yoo J-SH, Hong J-Y, Ning SM and Yang CS (1990a) Roles of dietary corn oil in the regulation of cytochromes P450 and glutathione S-transferases in the rat liver. *Journal of Nutrition*, **120**, 1718–1726.

Yoo J-SH, Park H-S, Ning SM, Lee M-J and Yang CS (1990b) Effect of thiamine deficiency on hepatic cytochromes P450 and drug metabolizing enzyme activities. *Biochemical Pharmacology*, **39**, 519–525.

Yoo J-SH, Ming SM, Pantuck CB, Pantuck EJ and Yang CS (1991) Regulation of hepatic microsomal cytochrome P450IIE1 level by dietary lipids and carbohydrates in rats. *Journal of Nutrition*, **121**, 959–965.

Yoo J-SH, Smith TJ, Ming SM, Lee M-J, Thomas PE and Yang CS (1992) Modulation of the levels of cytochromes P450 in rat liver and lung by dietary lipid. *Biochemical Pharmacology*, **43**, 2535–2542.

Yu T-S, Wu C-M and Liou Y-C (1989) Volatile compounds from garlic. *Journal of Agriculture and Food Chemistry*, **37**, 243–250.

Yun Y-P, Casazza JP, Sohn DH, Veech RL and Song BJ (1992) Pretranslational activation of cytochrome P450IIE during ketosis induced by a high fat diet. *Molecular Pharmacology*, **41**, 474–479.

Zannoni VG, Flynn EJ and Lynch M (1972) Ascorbic acid and drug metabolism. *Biochemical Pharmacology*, **21**, 1377–1392.

6 Interactions between Drugs and Diet

John A Thomas[1], W Wayne Stargel[2] and Christian Tschanz[2]

[1]University of Texas Health Science Center, San Antonio, TX, USA
[2]Monsanto Company, 5200 Old Orchard Road Skokie, IL 60077, USA

Introduction

The ingestion of food along with the administration of a therapeutically active drug can profoundly affect the rate and degree of drug and nutrient absorption (Welling, 1984; D'Arcy, 1985). Numerous interactions take place between medications and nutrients (food, beverages, vitamins, etc.) (Kirk, 1995; Thomas, 1995; Tschanz et al., 1996). Surveys by Welling (1980, 1996) disclosed that 51 of 55 and 100 of 130 drugs tested, exhibited abnormal absorption patterns when taken with food. Some clinical conditions, where prolonged medication is prescribed, can enhance such potential interactions between foods and drugs (Stiefeld et al., 1991). Increasing attention is being focused upon patient counselling programmes involving potential drug–food interactions (Wix et al., 1992; Thomas, 1995). Both the pharmacist and the dietitian should assist in identifying food–drug interactions and should be involved in patient education and counselling programmes, particularly at the time of hospital discharge though unfortunately, the majority of US teaching hospitals do not have such facilities (Wix et al., 1992).

It is possible that the introduction of some genetically engineered foods will also impact on the incidence of drug–food interactions. However, most attention to recombinant DNA-derived food has focused on their safety (Kessler et al., 1992). There is no reason to believe that genetically engineered foods differ significantly from natural foodstuffs with regard to drug–nutrient interactions. As yet, it is too early to know the impact of plant genetic engineering on foods and nutrition (Comai, 1993). Indeed, while the technique can improve agronomic and quality traits, including nutritional value, virtually nothing is known about potential drug–nutrient interactions.

Nutrition and Chemical Toxicity. Edited by Costas Ioannides. © John Wiley & Sons Ltd. ISBN 0 471 97453 6

Increasing interest in drug–nutrient interactions is related to the fact that drugs are becoming increasingly potent and possess greater specificity. Potent drugs with extended duration of action have also led to an increased incidence of drug–nutrient interactions. In an ageing population using an increasing number of prescription drugs, there is a greater likelihood of affecting the nutritional status of the geriatric patient (Chen et al., 1985; Munro et al., 1987; Smith, 1995). In addition to the elderly, conditions such as pregnancy, malnourishment and infant nursing can be predisposed to food–drug interactions. Among other factors, the biodisposition of drugs can be modified by malnutrition (Mehta et al., 1982).

Drugs and nutrients have many similar characteristics including physicochemical properties that may affect biochemical actions and other dose-related toxicities. Often, the mechanism of action of a drug may involve a nutrient(s) in a manner comparable with a non-nutrient component(s). The cellular site(s) of nutrient–drug interactions can occur in the gastrointestinal tract, in the blood, or at the drug's receptor(s). Furthermore, some drugs may modify body composition, as evidenced by cationic amphophilic drugs affecting phospholipid storage (Kodavanti and Mehendale, 1990).

The clinical relevance of nutrient–drug interactions is not always completely understood. Interactions depend mainly upon the specific drug and may increase, delay or reduce a particular pharmacological event. Not all patients experience the same incidence of risk for nutrient–drug interactions (Skaar, 1991). Several factors are included in assessing the potential for nutrient–drug interactions including restrictive diets, eating habits, chronic wasting diseases, renal/hepatic dysfunction and multiple medications (Skaar, 1991). While many contributing factors are involved in nutrient–drug interactions, the elderly are at particular risk (Roe, 1993) with special nutrient–drug interactions also important in diabetes mellitus (Roe, 1998a), cardiovascular disease (Roe, 1988b) and certain genetic disorders (Montgomery et al., 1991; Kitler, 1994). Pathophysiological changes associated with ageing, endocrine changes, alcoholism and those patients on restricted diets are also at risk for drug–nutrient interactions (Lee et al., 1991).

Factors affecting gastrointestinal absorption

The majority of clinically significant nutrient–drug interactions involve the absorption process. Adrenergic mechanisms have a significant modulating action upon gut motility, blood flow and mucosal transport (De Ponti et al., 1996). Both α and β-subtypes of adrenoceptors have been recognised at different levels of the gastrointestinal tract and are involved in the regulation of motility and secretion; thus, they may influence drug–nutrient interactions. α_1-Adrenoceptors are located post-junctionally on mostly smooth muscle cells, while α_2-adrenoceptors can be found both at pre- and post-synaptic sites. Several agents can act selectively as agonists as well as antagonists (Table 6.1).

Table 6.1 Receptors modulating gastrointestinal motility and secretion

	Receptor type				
	α_1	α_2	β_1	β_2	β_3
Distribution in the gut	Smooth muscle; Gastric neurons	Adrenergic neurons (autoreceptors); Myenteric neurons (heteroceptors)	Smooth muscle; Enteric neurons (?)	Smooth muscle; Peripheral noradrenergic neurons (?)	Smooth muscle
Functional response	Smooth muscle contraction or relaxation; neuronal depolarisation (gastric neurons)	Smooth muscle presynaptic-inhibition; Smooth muscle contraction	Smooth muscle relaxation	Smooth muscle relaxation; Facilitation of transmitter release	Smooth muscle relaxation
Selective agonists	Phenylephrine, methoxamine, cirazoline	Clonidine, azepexole	Xamoterol, prenalterol	Terbutaline, salbutamol, ritrodrine	
Selective antagonists	Prazosin, corynanthine	Yohimbine, idazoxan, rauwolscine	Betaxolol, atenolol		

[a]Modified from Hussar (1988).

With the exception of ethanol, few drugs are absorbed to any significant degree in the stomach, most acidic or basic drugs being absorbed in the small intestine. Thus, gastric function has a major effect upon both the rate and degree of drug absorption, as changes in gastric motility can affect the residence time of the food and/or drug in the gastrointestinal tract. The composition of the diet and the timing of meals can also influence drug absorption; for example, delays in gastric emptying time may be caused by fatty foodstuffs and thus affect a drug's absorption. In addition, foods can enhance drug absorption (Table 6.2) (Randle, 1987; Kirk, 1995), can delay drug absorption (Table 6.3) (Smith and Bidlack, 1984; Randle, 1987; Garabedian-Ruffalo et al., 1988), or can decrease drug absorption (Table 6.4) (Smith and Bidlack, 1984; Randle, 1987; Garabedian-Ruffalo et al., 1988; Kirk, 1995). Several mechanisms whereby foodstuffs and drugs can interact can result in an altered pharmacological response (Tables 6.2–6.4). Such mechanisms involve physiological changes in blood levels of the drub as a result of the food either increasing or decreasing its rate of absorption.

Table 6.2 Drugs–nutrient interactions causing enhanced absorption[a]

Drug	Mechanism
Atovaquone	High fat meal facilitates absorption
Carbamazepine	Increased bile production; enhanced dissolution and absorption
Cyclosporin	Increased bioavailability
Diazepam	Food enhances enterohepatic recycling of drug; increased dissolution secondary to gastric acid secretion
Dicumerol	Increased bile flow; delayed gastric emptying permits dissolution and absorption
Erythromycin	Unknown
Griseofulvin	Drug is lipid-soluble, enhanced absorption
Hydralazine	Food reduces first-pass extraction and metabolism, blocks enzymic transformation in gastrointestinal tract
Hydrochlorothiazide	Delayed gastric emptying enhances absorption from small bowel
Labetalol	Food may reduce first-pass extraction and metabolism
Lithium citrate	Purgative action decreases absorption
Lovastatin	Unknown
Metoprolol	Food may reduce first-pass extraction and metabolism
Misoprostol	Food decreases its side effects
Nitrofurantoin	Delayed gastric emptying permits dissolution and increased absorption
Phenytoin	Delayed gastric emptying and increased bile production improves dissolution and absorption
Propoxphene	Delayed gastric emptying improves dissolution and absorption
Propranolol	Food may reduce first-pass extraction and metabolism
Spironolactone	Delayed gastric emptying permits dissolution and absorption; bile may solubilise

[a]Modified from Anderson (1988); Katz and Dejean (1985).

Table 6.3 Drugs–nutrient interactions causing delayed absorption[a]

Drug	Mechanisms
Paracetamol (Acetaminophen)	High pectin foods act as absorbent and protectant
Ampicillin	Reduction in stomach fluid volume
Amoxicillin	Reduction in stomach fluid volume
Aspirin	Direct interference; change in gastric pH
Atenolol	Mechanism unknown, possibly physical barrier
Cephalosporins	Mechanism unknown
Cimetidine	Mechanism unknown
Digoxin	High-fibre, high-pectin foods bind drug
Frusemide	Mechanism unknown
Glipizide	Unknown
Metronidazole	Mechanism unknown
Piroxicam	Mechanism unknown
Quinidine	Possibly protein binding
Sulphonamides	Mechanism unknown; may be physical barrier
Valproic acid	Mechanism unknown

[a]Modified from Katz and Dejean (1985); Kessler *et al.* (1982); Kirk (1995).

Table 6.4 Drugs–nutrient interactions causing decreased absorption[a]

Drug	Mechanism
Ampicillin	Reduction in stomach fluid volume
Atenolol	Mechanism unknown; possibly physical barrier
Azithromycin	Reduces bioavailability
Captopril	Mechanism unknown
Chlorpromazine	Drug undergoes first-pass metabolism in gut; delayed gastric emptying affects bioavailability
Erythromycin	Mechanism unknown
Isoniazid	Food raises pH preventing dissolution and absorption; also delayed gastric emptying
Levodopa	Drug competes with amino acids for absorption and transport
Lincomycin	Mechanism unknown
Methyldopa	Competitive absorptions
Nafcillin	Mechanisms unknown; may be alteration of gastric fluid on pH
Penicillamine	May form chelates with calcium or iron
Penicillin G	Delayed gastric emptying, gastric acid degradation; impaired dissolution
Propantheline	Mechanism unknown
Tetracyclines	Binds with calcium ions or iron salts forming insoluble chelates
Zidovudine	Food decreases concentration of drug

[a]Modified from Anderson (1988); Katz and Dejean (1985); Kessler *et al.* (1992); Kirk (1995).

Interactions between drugs and nutrients involve several physiological factors whereby a drug affects processes related to eating, sensory appreciation of food, swallowing, digestion, gastric emptying, nutrient absorption, nutrient metabolism or renal excretion of nutrients (Roe, 1993). Hence, physiological interactions can also include reactions in which the absorption, metabolism or elimination of a drug is changed by food ingestion. The mechanisms of food–drug interactions are not well characterised, but involve both direct and indirect factors (Table 6.5). While the exact number of drugs which influence gastrointestinal absorption is not known, estimates reveal that 100–150 separate agents can elicit such actions. Realistically, this number probably represents a very small fraction of the total marketed drug products.

Oral administration of drugs is most convenient, and associating drug doses with daily routines such as mealtimes usually improves patient compliance. However, this association can result in an increased incidence of nutrient–drug interactions, with certain foods able to decrease, delay of increase the absorption of drugs, hence altering their bioavailability, solubility in gastric fluid and gastric emptying time (Trovato et al., 1991). Delayed drug absorption does not necessarily imply that less total drug is actually absorbed, but that peak blood levels of the drug may be achieved over a longer period of time. Drugs that bind or complex to nutrients are often unavailable for absorption, or at least their absorption is delayed.

Food (and food components) can affect the bioavailability of drugs by binding directly to the drug, or by changing luminal pH, gastric emptying, intestinal transit, mucosal absorption and splanchnic–hepatic blood flow (Anderson and Kappas, 1987; Anderson, 1988). Food-induced changes in the bioavailability of some drugs may be partially dependent upon hepatic biotransformation, as evidenced by absorbed nutrients competing with drugs for first-pass metabolism in the intestine or the liver. Many drugs undergo metabolic transformation by enteric microorganisms that may in turn be affected by nutrients; thus, the drug's metabolism may also be modified.

Table 6.5 Drug–food/drug–fluid interactions affecting absorptive processes

Indirect mechanisms
    Drug-induced alterations in gastrointestinal motility (e.g. anticholinergics)
    Drug-induced malabsorption syndromes (e.g. Neomycin)

Direct mechanisms
    Drug-induced pH alterations in gastrointestinal tract (e.g. antacids)
    Drug-induced changes in bioavailability (e.g. absorption to drug-kaolin/pectin)
    Drug-induced retardation of absorption (e.g. charcoal)
    Drug-binding/chelation (e.g. anionic exchange resins-Cholestyramine; metal ions-iron, calcium)

Modified from Ama et al. (1986).

Drugs may be metabolised by two basic reactions, referred to as Phase I and Phase II. Phase I reactions include oxidation, hydroxylation, reduction or hydrolysis and result in changes to a functional group on the drug molecule (Table 6.6). The mixed function oxidase system (MFOS) is an inducible enzyme system that catalyses the oxidation of a wide variety of drugs. The MFOS is found primarily in the endoplasmic reticulum of the liver and other tissues. Phase II reactions include conjugation to glucuronate or glutathione, and acetylation of sulphonation to functional group(s) on the drug molecule. Modifications of functional groups frequently renders the drug more water-soluble (or polar) and thus more readily excreted by the kidney. Conjugation enzymes are present in the endoplasmic reticulum of the cytoplasm. Several oxidised products of the MFOS are substrates for conjugating enzymes.

The metabolism of drugs by Phase I and Phase II reactions is catalysed by various enzymes, and the formation of metabolites necessitates that other substances be provided by the body through nutrition. Several nutrients and micronutrients (e.g. vitamins) exert significant roles in Phase I oxidation reactions (Table 6.6) (Hoyumpa and Schenker, 1982). Phase II reactions involving conjugation depend upon the body to provide carbohydrates, amino acids, fats and proteins. Acute starvation may depress the MFOS; thus, nutritional status has a major influence on drug metabolism.

Metabolism and bioavailability

Bioavailability describes that fraction of the drug's dosage that reaches the systemic circulation metabolically unchanged (Winstanley and Orme, 1989). Many factors affect a drug's disposition including diet, genetic traits, age, sex and pregnancy (Hoyumpa and Schenker, 1982). Bioavailability can be

Table 6.6 Nutrients in Phase I (oxidation) metabolic reactions[a]

Nutrients	Component of reaction requiring nutrient
Ascorbic acid (vitamin C)[b]	?
Nicotinic acid	NADPH
Riboflavin (vitamin B$_2$)	FMN and FAD in NADPH-cytochrome c reductase
Glycine	Haem (cytochrome P-450)
Pantothenic acid	CoA (ALA synthesis)
Iron	Haem
Copper	Ferrochelatase in haem synthesis
Protein	Apo-enzymes
Calcium	Maintenance of membranes
Magnesium	Maintenance of membranes
Zinc	Maintenance of membranes

[a]Modified from Lee *et al.* (1991).
[b]Some species.

modified by food, and thus result in a drug's pharmacokinetics and pharmacodynamics being altered. Food can influence drug bioavailability as a result of physiocochemical or chemical interactions between a specific nutrient or other food component(s) and the drug molecule in the gastrointestinal tract, while grastrointestinal processes can also affect a drug's bioavailability.

Excretion

Drugs are excreted from the body either unchanged or as metabolites. The organs of excretion (e.g. kidney, skin, liver and lungs) eliminate polar compounds (i.e. water-soluble) more efficiently than drugs that are lipid-soluble. Lipid-soluble drugs are usually poorly excreted unless they have undergone some degree of biotransformation to render them more water-soluble.

The kidney plays a major role in the excretion of drugs and their metabolites. Renal excretion of drugs involves three processes: glomerular filtration, active tubular secretion and passive tubular reabsorption. Drugs excreted in the faeces are primarily unabsorbed orally ingested drugs (or their metabolites) or are excreted into the bile and not reabsorbed from the gastrointestinal tract.

Organic acid and organic base renal transport mechanisms exert important roles in the elimination of non-filterable molecular species. Many drugs undergo such elimination processes via these organic acid and organic base systems (Table 6.7) (Bennett and Porter, 1993). The mechanism of action of some drugs may be dependent upon these transport systems, yet other drugs involve proximal tubular transport systems as a major route of elimination from the body. Drugs transported by the organic ion system may cause nephrotoxicity either directly or indirectly.

Drugs that are rapidly metabolised or otherwise undergo conjugation are generally more readily excreted. The degree of protein binding to a drug (i.e. bound versus free or unbound) can affect its rate of metabolism. Drugs that modify electrolytes can also change the excretion of a drug (Table 6.8) (Bennett

Table 6.7 Some drugs eliminated by organic transport systems[a]

Organic acid system	Organic base system
Phenylbutazone	Isoproterenol
Salicylate	Quinidine
Cephalothin	Morphine
Sulphonamides	Procaine
Chlorothiazide	Tolazoline
Frusemide	Macanylamine
Penicillin	Piperidine
Methotrexate	
Probenecid	

[a]Modified from Lieber (1994).

Table 6.8 Drug-induced electrolyte disturbances[a]

Sodium
Hyponatraemia – drugs that impair water excretion
Hypernatraemia – saline
Anti-inflammatory steroids
Potassium
Cardiac glycosides
Anti-inflammatory steroids
Hypokalaemia
Diuretics
Antibiotics
Tocolytic agents
Liquorice
Hyperkalaemia
Potassium supplements
Potassium-sparing diuretics
Selected antihypertensive drugs
Calcium
Hypocalcaemia
Aminoglycoside antibiotics
Thiazide diuretics
Vitamin D supplements
Phosphorus
Hypophosphataemia
Parenteral nutrition
Hyperphosphataemia
Cytotoxic drugs

[a]Modified from Lieber (1994).

and Porter, 1993). Loop (of Henle) and thiazide diuretics increase urinary excretion of sodium, potassium and magnesium. So-called 'loop' diuretics increase the urinary excretion of calcium, while thiazides may exert an opposite action. Cardiac glycosides can also facilitate potassium excretion. Conversely, anti-inflammatory steroids and certain antihypertensive agents can lead to sodium retention.

Many major clinical syndromes in nephrology caused by drugs (and by other chemicals) can ultimately affect drug–nutrient interactions (Bennett and Porter 1993). The magnitude of nephrotoxicity depends upon the dose, duration of treatment/exposure, and several other factors known to affect pharmacological activity (e.g. age, sex, hepatic function, etc.). Aminoglycoside antibiotics commonly lead to proximal tubular injury in 10–15% of therapeutic regimens. Likewise, nephrotoxicity is seen following amphotericin-B and *cis*-platinum therapy.

Although hepatotoxicity or liver damage may vary depending on the type, severity and duration of injury, there are only a few mechanisms that alter a drug's excretion (Hoyumpa and Schenker, 1982). Drug elimination may be modified due to decreased enzyme activity resulting from hepatic parenchymal cell disease, altered hepatic blood flow, hypoalbuminaemia or a combination of these factors or conditions. Hypoalbuminaemia can affect the protein binding of a drug in the serum and change its pharmacodynamics. In cirrhosis, reduced functional hepatic cell mass may lead to diminished enzyme complement.

Special interactions/conditions

ANTICOAGULANTS

Many drugs and foods interact with anticoagulants, particularly warfarin (Wells et al., 1994). Warfarin may interact with antibiotics, cardiac medications and central nervous system-acting drugs. The potential for warfarin to interact with other drugs, resulting in a change in its anticoagulant effect, is widely recognised among health professionals and informed patients. Drug–food interactions involving warfarin can lead to potentiation, inhibition or no effect (Table 6.9) (Wells et al., 1994). Agents cited represent those where there is a high probability of interaction. Other drugs may also interact, but generally are less likely to do so (Wells et al., 1994; Harris, 1995). Vitamin K content in foods and the quantity of vitamin K supplementation may affect the action(s) of oral anticoagulant therapy. Further, supplements of vitamins A, E and C may affect the

Table 6.9 Drug–food interactions with anticoagulants (warfarin)[a]

Potentiation	Inhibition	No effect
Alcohol[b]	Barbiturates	Alcohol
Amiodarone	Carbamazine	Antacids
Cimetidine	Chlordiazepoxide	Atenolol
Clofibrate	Cholestryramine	Bumetanide
Co-trimoxazole	Griseofuliven	Diflunisal
Erythromycin	Nafcillin	Enoxacin
Fluconazole	Rifampin	Famotidine
Isoniazid	Sucralphate	Felodipine
Metronidazole	Vitamin K (foods)	Fluoxetine
Miconazole	Dicloxacillin	Ketorolac
Omeprazole		Metoprolol
Phenylbutazone		Moricizine
Piroxicam		Naproxen
Propafenone		Nitrazepam
Propranolol		Nizatidine
Sulphinpyrazone		Psillium
		Ranitidine

[a]Modified from Mehta et al. (1982).
[b]Concomitant liver disease.

efficacy of oral anticoagulant therapy. Drugs that do exhibit a high probability of affecting anticoagulating properties are not necessarily contraindicated, but may necessitate an increased awareness or more prudent therapeutic approach.

ANTIMICROBIALS

Relationships between circulating levels of antibiotics and their therapeutic efficacy have been studied extensively relative to other classes of drugs (Welling, 1980). The importance of food on the absorption of antimicrobials is well documented. The effects of food and fluid volumes on the absorption of ingested antimicrobials has clinical relevancy as they are related to the drug's efficacy (Toothaker and Welling, 1980; Royer *et al.*, 1984). Certain classes of antibiotics may be affected differently by the presence of food. Certain antibiotics have their absorption reduced by foods (e.g. selected penicillins and tetracyclines), some may be delayed by food (e.g. sulphonamides), some may be unaffected by food (e.g. ampicillin, amoxycillin), and some may actually have their absorption enhanced by food (e.g. griseofulvin, nitrofurantoin) (Table 6.10) (Welling, 1980). Different formulations of erythromycin are affected differently by the presence of food (*viz.* delayed, reduced, increased or unaffected). The bioavailability of oral erythromycin is affected by the chemical derivative, the dosage formulation and the timing of the meal relative to the administration of the antibiotic.

Table 6.10 Effect of food on the absorption of antibiotics[a]

Reduced	
Penicillin G	Amoxycillin[b]
Penicillin V(K)	Tetracycline(s)
Ampicillin	Isoniazid
Delayed	
Cephalexin	Sulphonamide(s)
Cephradine	Metronidazole
Unaffected	
Penicillin V(acid)[b]	Amoxycillin[b]
Ampicillin[b]	Clarithromycin
Increased	
Griseofulvin	Nitrofurantoin
Variable	
(i.e. formulations reduced, increased, delayed or unaffected)	
Erythromycin(s)	

[a]Modified from Cardinale (1988); Mooradian (1988).
[b]Literature studies not in complete agreement.

There may be conditions where the food–antiobiotic interaction may diminish absorption of the antimicrobial yet the presence of the food may lessen drug side effects associated with the gastrointestinal tract. Nevertheless, these special conditions need not compromise the therapeutic efficacy of the antibiotics.

DRUG–ETHANOL INTERACTIONS

The ingestion of ethanol with other drugs can produce clinically significant interactions, these being more frequent in heavy users of alcohol than in persons who imbibe only small amounts (Liever, 1994).

Chronic alcoholism is a major aetiology of liver disease leading to altered drug metabolism. The use of therapeutic agents in alcoholics is complicated by underlying hepatic disease and by acute and chronic ethanol–drug interactions. Drug metabolism is affected by both acute and chronic use of ethanol. Chronic alcoholism results in hepatic enzyme induction; this tends to increase metabolism and leads to larger doses being required in order to achieve the desired therapeutic effect. Depending on the class of drugs (e.g. sedatives), many alcoholics exhibit a tolerance or lack of effect. The acute use of alcohol can overwhelm metabolic enzymes and leads to a diminution of normal hepatic metabolism.

Several classes of drugs can be affected by the use of alcohol (Table 6.11) (Hoyumpa and Schenker, 1982; Chu *et al.*, 1992; Lieber, 1994). The acute

Table 6.11 Effect of ethanol on degradation of drugs[a]

Drugs	Acute administration	Chronic ingestion	Alcohol withdrawal
Sedatives and tranquilisers			
Chlordiazepoxide	Decreased		Decreased
Diazepam	Decreased		Decreased
Lorazepam	Decreased		
Clorazepate	Decreased		
Oxazepam	No effect (?)		
Meprobamate	Decreased	Increased	
Pentobarbital	Decreased	Increased	
Chlorpromazine	Decreased		
Chloral hydrate	Decreased		
Miscellaneous drugs			
Tolbutamide	Decreased	Increased	
Phenytoin	Decreased	Increased	
Warfarin	Decreased	Increased	
Antipyrine	Decreased	Increased	
Chlormethiazole	Decreased		Decreased
Acetaminophen	Decreased	Increased	
Rifamycin		Increased	

[a]Modified from Lee *et al.* (1991); Mooradian (1988); Munro *et al.* (1987).

ingestion of ethanol and agents with sedative action leads to greater psycho-motor impairment than that produced by each agent separately. Several mechanisms may explain these interactions including a combined central ner-vous system–depressant action, altered drug metabolism by ethanol, or acute impairment of the degradation process of the sedative(s). Lieber (1994) has described several possible anatomical or cellular sites (e.g. liver, stomach) of ethanol–drug interactions. The majority of ethanol is catalysed by alcohol deyhydrogenase (ADH) in the liver, yet ADH is only marginally involved in alcohol–drug interactions.

Chronic alcohol–drug interactions produce accelerated hepatic drug meta-bolism (e.g. metabolic drug tolerance) such that alcoholics display tolerance to other drugs. Such tolerances may be partially due to adaptation of the central nervous system and to metabolic adaptation. The induction of the microsomal ethanol-oxidising system (MEOS) following chronic ethanol consumption affects various other drug-metabolising systems in hepatic microsomes, leading to a generalised acceleration of metabolism.

Large amounts of ethanol ingested in a brief time (i.e. binges) or small quan-tities in the individual who seldom drinks can result in an additive or synergistic effect in the presence of other central nervous system depressants. A well-known interaction of a drug with ethanol is that of disulfiram, which inhibits acetaldehyde dehydrogenase and results in an accumulation of acetaldehyde, the result being nausea and vomiting within minutes after the ingestion of alcohol.

Transethnic differences also occur in the metabolism of ethanol and thus there are genetic differences in its disposition or metabolism (Kitler, 1994). Chinese, Japanese and Native Americans exhibit a higher rate of alcohol meta-bolism compared with Caucasians. Jewish men and women have reduced incidence of severe alcohol-related problems, reputedly due to a heightened sensitivity to relatively low doses of alcohol. Hence, transethnic differences in ethanol metabolism may ultimately affect drug–ethanol interactions.

DRUG–VITAMIN INTERACTIONS

Several drugs can change the body's requirements for vitamins (Christakis and Christakis, 1983; Katz and DeJean, 1985; Munro et al., 1987). Such vitamin–drug interactions can occur with either water-soluble or fat-soluble vitamins (Table 6.12). The principal mechanism of interaction usually involves impaired absorption of the vitamin by a drug. Some antibiotics can modify enteric organisms and thus affect the absorption of fat-soluble vitamins. Drugs may also induce enzyme systems that can accelerate the metabolism of a vitamin. Ethanol consumption can depress hepatic levels of vitamin A and can affect the clearance of β-carotene. Physiologically, glutathione can spare and potentiate vitamin E, yet ethanol can interfere with such metabolic events

Table 6.12 Some drug–vitamin interactions

Vitamin	Drug	Interaction
Vitamin B_{12}	K^+ supplements	Gastric pH slows vitamin B_{12} absorption
	Colchicine	Vitamin B_{12} absorption impaired
VitaminB$_6$ (pyridoxine)	Oral contraceptives Hydralazine Isoniazid Penicillamine	Increased requirement for vitamin B_6
Vitamin C	Salicylates	Decreased uptake of vitamin C
	Tetracyclines	Depletion of vitamin C
Fat-soluble vitamins (A, D, E and K)	Mineral oil	Retards absorption of fat-soluble vitamins
Vitamin A, D and K	Cholestyramine	Retards absorption of vitamins A, D and K
Vitamin D	Cathartics (irritants)	Retards absorption of vitamin D
Vitamin A	Neomycin	Retards absorption
	Ethanol	Hepatotoxicity causing hypervitaminosis A
	Tetracycline	Intracranial hypertension
Vitamin D	Glutethimide	Produces vitamin D deficiency
Vitamin E	Dicutmarol	Enhances anticoagulant action
	Digoxin	Hypercalcaemia and arrhythmias
Vitamin K	Anticonvulsants	Induces enzymic inactivation
	Dicumarol	Inhibits hypoprothrombin action

[a]Modified from D'Arcy and McElnay (1985), Kessler *et al.* (1992), Murray and Healy (1991) and Randle (1987).

(Lieber 1994). Glutathione, which acts as one of the scavenging mechanisms for toxic free radicals, can be reduced by ethanol.

Several mechanisms of drug–folate interaction have been reported (Roe, 1974). The mechanism of action varies considerably, ranging from impaired absorption, to competitive binding to serum proteins, to enzyme inhibition. Folate intake exhibits wide variation, particularly in the elderly (Munro *et al.*, 1987). Folate absorption is strongly pH dependent; gastric atrophy and atrophic gastritis with achlorhydria and hypochlorhydria lead to malabsorption of folate and vitamin B_{12}. Folic acid supplementation in folate-deficient patients with epilepsy changes the pharmacokinetics of phenytoin, usually leading to lower serum levels and possible seizure breakthroughs (Lewis *et al.*, 1995). Ethanol can change the kinetic of folate metabolism and increases its excretion.

Folate antagonism diminishes the availability of substrates required for the synthesis of nucleic acids. The inhibition of nucleic acid synthesis is a possible mechanism responsible for developmental toxicity caused by drugs such as methotrexate and aminopterin (Farrar and Blumer, 1991; Thomas and Markovac, 1994).

DRUG–MINERAL INTERACTIONS

Several important classes of drugs have their pharmacological action modified by minerals (Smith and Bidlack, 1984). Calcium, iron, magnesium and zinc can interfere with the gastrointestinal absorption of tetracyclines, while iron can reduce the absorption of penicillamine. It is evident that a very diverse group of pharmacological agents can have their actions modified by minerals (see also Table 6.8).

There are three types of drug–mineral interactions: (i) malabsorption of the mineral and/or drug; (ii) mineral depletion and retention; and (iii) drug–mineral interactions induced by simultaneous antacid ingestion (Murray and Healy, 1991). Many drug–mineral interactions have little clinical importance, though they are considered increasingly important in conditions such as malnutrition, the elderly, and patients with chronic diseases (Randle, 1987; Hussar, 1988; Hansten and Horn, 1989).

Due to the relative abundance of mineral and trace elements in foods, minerals such as sodium, potassium, magnesium, calcium and phosphorus are involved in drug interactions (Hazell, 1985). Sodium restriction can enhance the renal tubular reabsorption of lithium, producing toxic blood levels. Calcium antagonists exhibit enhanced efficacy in the salt-repleted hypertensive patient (Bennett, 1997). Other minor elements include arsenic, cobalt, chromium, copper, fluorine, iron, iodine, manganese, molybdenum, nickel, selenium, silicon, tin, vanadium and zinc. While these trace elements have important physiological functions, most are not important contributors to drug–mineral interactions.

Drugs cause malabsorption of minerals in two ways: First, by primary drug-induced malabsorption whereby the drug directly prevents the absorption of one or more minerals. Primary malabsorption involves direct binding with the nutrient through chemical complexing (e.g. chelation) and through direct adverse action by the drug on the mucosa of the small intestine, thus preventing the mineral from being absorbed. In secondary malabsorption, drugs influence the mineral's absorption, disposition and metabolism. While drugs may cause mineral depletion through primary and secondary malabsorption processes, depletion can also be caused by diuretics.

Perhaps the largest group of agents producing interaction upon the gastro-intestinal tract are gastric antacids. Antacids may alter a drug's solubility characteristics by modifying gastric pH and even through chelation (Royer et al., 1984; Cardinale, 1988; Hussar, 1988). Hence, antacids are capable of interfering with a drug's absorption. In addition, aluminium-containing preparations can cause a relaxing action on gastric smooth muscle, thus delaying gastric emptying time. Antacids exert two actions, namely effect changes in gastric pH and to chelate with minerals to prevent their absorption. Alkalinity, or increasing gastric pH, will lead to diminished absorption of calcium, iron, magnesium and zinc (D'Arcy, 1985).

GENETIC DIFFERENCES

Differences in response to drug action among various ethnic and racial sub-populations have long been recognised, and have been accentuated by specific drugs producing exaggerated biological effects. Altered drug metabolism has been studied extensively among different populations (Kitler, 1994). Among the many conditions to which the human body must adapt is the nutritional environment (Childs, 1988).

Ethnic differences can be related to individual variations in response to drugs (Ghoneim et al., 1981), but variations are frequently controlled genetically in addition to other, environmental, factors. There are marked inter-ethnic differences with groups exhibiting the ability to metabolise drugs rapidly whereas others metabolise them slowly. There are also racial differences in body fat composition, lean tissue density and adipose tissue metabolism (Ama et al., 1986) each of which can affect a drug's pharmacodynamics.

Different classes of drugs exhibit transethnic differences (Table 6.13). Genetic differences are evident in absorption, distribution and elimination processes. Other physiological endpoints are marked by genetic differences, including pain threshold (higher in Orientals), immune responsiveness and metabolic parameters. These ethnic and racial differences in response to pharmacological agents have the potential to involve drug–nutrient interactions.

Lactose intolerance is a common form of carbohydrate malabsorption which affects all ages. Lactose, a disaccharide of glucose and galactose, is present in

Table 6.13 Transethnic responsiveness to selected pharmacological agents[a]

Drug/agent	General ethnic biological response[b]
Ethanol	Exaggerated in Orientals
Analgesics	Higher pain threshold in Asians
Benzodiazepines	Lower dosages required in Asian populations
Insulin	Hyperinsulinaemia in Native Americans
Diuretics (thiazides)	More effective in Blacks than Whites
Propranolol	Renal clearance in Chinese twice that of Caucasians
Phenytoin (DPH)	Eliminated faster in Eskimos
Lithium	Lower doses required in Japanese populations
Dermatological preparations	Reduced absorption in Blacks
Haloperidol	Asians exhibit more extra-pyramidal symptoms
Immunosuppressive agents	Reduced allograph survival in Blacks
Tissue plasminogen activators (rt-PA)	Enhanced thrombolytic activity in Blacks

[a]Modified from Hoyumpa and Schenker (1982).
[b]Individual pharmacological responses may vary.

human milk, in cow's milk, and in standard infant formulas and many dairy products. Lactose is also an additive in foodstuffs including baked goods, cereals, and soft drinks (Montes and Perman, 1991).

Lactose intolerance can be genetically related to lactase phenotypes, as evidenced by differences among various subpopulations worldwide (Montgomery et al., 1991). Lactase-phlorizin hydrolase plays an important role in neonatal nutrition. There are transethnic differences in lactase activity and in lactase mRNA.

Several drugs can induce lactose intolerance (Roe, 1985), notably those that cause malabsorption. Unlike mineral oil, which can produce malabsorption at luminal sites, drugs such as methotrexate, neomycin and colchicine interact at mucosal sites and cause lactose intolerance. Drugs that induce lactose intolerance are often also cytotoxic (e.g. neomycin, colchicine, methotrexate), which contributes to the malabsorption.

GERIATRICS

Elderly people are more at risk from adverse and clinically important outcomes of drug–nutrient interactions (Roe, 1984) mainly as their gastrointestinal tracts are often more vulnerable to such events. These increased risks are likely due to multiple drug usage, age-related modifications in drug disposition, geriatric pathologies which might impair drug clearance, and simply because subgroups of the elderly may suffer from nutritional inadequacies.

Drug–nutrient interactions in the elderly can be categorised as physicochemical, physiological or pathophysiological (Roe, 1993). Physicochemical interactions would be represented by chelation or chelation complexes and modifications in the stability of the nutrient. Physiological interactions include drug-induced changes in appetite, digestion, gastric emptying, biotransformation and renal, excretion. Pathophysiological interactions occur when a drug impairs nutrient absorption or its toxicity causes an inhibition of metabolic processes.

The elderly frequently are taking more drugs due to various biological status in their deteriorations. Often, the elderly consume over-the-counter (OTC) drug products such as laxatives, vitamin/minerals and antacids and it has been estimated that by the year 2000, about 50% of all chronic care drugs will be OTC products (Cardinale, 1988). Perhaps the most common form of drug–nutrient interaction in the elderly is a mineral deficiency caused by the frequent use of diuretics, leading to potassium and magnesium loss (Lamy, 1982; Roe 1984).

Nutritional modulation in the elderly indicates that alterations in the macronutrient and micronutrient constituents of the diet can be affected by gene expression (Mooradian, 1988). Nutritional problems in the elderly are related not only to multiple drug use, but also to the consumption of specialised diets for one or more chronic illnesses. Several major mechanisms are involved in

Table 6.14 Mechanism of drug–nutrient interaction in the elderly

Appetite suppression (anorexic)
Appetite stimulation
Diminished nutrient absorption; toxicity to mucosal cells
Facilitated renal elimination
Decreased nutrient use
Antagonism/competitive (e.g. coumarin and Vitamin K)
Inhibition or facilitation with metabolism or transport system(s)
Hormonal effects of nutrients
Indirect effect due to components of drug formulation

[a]Modified from Thomas and Tschanz (1994).

drug-nutrient interactions in the elderly (Table 6.14) (Mooradian, 1988). Side effects such as nausea, vomiting and diarrhoea can secondarily affect drug–nutrient interactions. Cytotoxic drugs can damage mucosal cells in the gastrointestinal tract while the activity of enteric microflora can be suppressed by certain antibiotics, thus altering digestion.

Certain diseases in the elderly, including hypertension, cardiac failure and renal insufficiency, indicate particular concerns about selected classes of drugs and to what extent they affect nutrition. Drug-induced adverse outcomes can complicate the therapy by affecting nutritional status. Digoxin, while effective for congestive heart disease, possesses inherent anorexic properties including nausea and vomiting. Loop diuretics not only facilitate the loss of sodium but also potassium, magnesium, calcium and thiamine. Thus, osteoporosis can be exacerbated in the elderly post-menopausal patient undergoing therapy with loop diuretics.

It should be evident that the elderly represents a particular at-risk population with respect to drug–nutrient interactions, especially as the ageing process can profoundly affect the pharmacokinetics of a drug.

HYPOGLYCAEMICS

Insulin can provoke a sensation of hunger. Insulin-induced hypoglycaemia, however, can also be associated with nausea and a sensation of weakness, rather than the desire for food (Roe, 1979). Since diabetic patients with renal and/or hepatic disease are often more vulnerable to hypoglycaemia, certain of the oral antidiabetic agents must be used with clinical discretion. The co-administration of sulphonylurea drugs with thiazide diuretics can exacerbate the diabetic condition. A decreased alcohol tolerance may also be manifest in patients ingesting sulphonylurea agents. Still other drugs may enhance the hypolgycaemic actions of the sulphonylurea drugs including propranolol, salicylates, phenylbutazone, chloramphenicol, probenecid and the sulphonamides (Thomas and Thomas, 1994). Tolbutamide and chlorpropamide may stimulate appetite by enhancing the release of pancreatic insulin.

Some antibiotics can affect hypoglycaemia (Stiefeld *et al.*, 1991). Co-trimoxazole of fluconazole can interact with oral hypoglycaemic agents, leading to an increased hypoglycaemia. Rifampicin can antagonise the action(s) of oral hypoglycaemics. While there is continuing interest in developing new hypoglycaemic agents, some recent focus has been devoted to compounds that act directly upon the gastrointestinal tract (Hulin, 1994). The absorption of both simple and complex carbohydrates from the intestine is mediated by a family of enzymes called α-glucosidases, which hydrolyse oligo- or polysaccharides to monosaccharides. The inhibition of α-glucosidases leads to a delay in the absorption of carbohydrates. A number of α-glucosidase inhibitory drugs are under development as new hypoglycaemic agents, including acarbose and miglitol. Acarbose is a reversible competitive inhibitor of glucoamylase and sucrase (Saperstein *et al.*, 1990). Miglitol appears to mimic glucose, but also inhibits α-glucoamylase and sucrase (Hulin, 1994). These compounds can reduce postprandial hyperglycaemia and diminish insulin secretion.

PARENTERAL NUTRITION

Total parenteral nutrition (TPN) can affect the metabolism of drugs (Anderson, 1988). Experimental evidence suggests that TPN can reduce the hepatic clearance of barbiturates, while antipyrine pharmacokinetics can be altered by intravenous nutritional regimens leading to increased renal clearance and a shortened plasma half-life. Accordingly, antipyrine metabolism can be increased by nutritional repletion (Anderson, 1988).

Alcohol interferes with a variety of nutritional factors including the type and amount of dietary fat, protein and amino acids. Such interactions provide the rationale for the parenteral administration of complete amino acid mixtures to patients with severe alcoholic liver disease (Lieber, 1994). Although dietary deficiencies (i.e. reduced food intake) may play a role in alcoholic liver injury, supplementation with S-adenosyl-L-methionine (SAM) and polyunsaturated lecithin may significantly offset some of the toxic manifestations of alcohol.

Short-chain peptides have been considered as candidates for parenteral nutrition (Furst *et al.*, 1990). Their use is based on the assumption that specially concocted amino acid solutions will enhance the therapeutic benefits to patients receiving parenteral nutrition. Dipeptide-based parenteral solutions exhibit low osmolarity, thus enabling them to fulfil the nitrogen requirements of patients with severe fluid restriction. Synthetic peptides are rapidly eliminated and amounts of these solutes do not significantly accumulate in biological fluids. L-Alanyl-L-glutamine has undergone clinical evaluation, and other dipeptides are certain to be tested for their potential efficacy. It is difficult to predict any clinical significant drug–dipeptide interactions.

Summary

Nutritional status has a significant role in a drug's response. Certain disease states and other special subpopulations may have unique nutritional requirements that affect a drug's therapeutic efficacy. Some classes of drugs like the antimicrobials have their absorption modified by the presence of food in the gastrointestinal tract. Although a drug's pharmacokinetic profile can usually be predicted, it can be changed by nutrients and by certain disease states, as well as ageing.

References

Ama PFM, Poehlman ET, Simoneau JA, Boulay MR, Theriault G, Tromblay A and Bouchard C (1986) Fat distribution and adipose tissue metabolism in non-obese male black African and Caucasian subjects. *International Journal of Obesity*, **10**, 503–514.

Anderson KE (1988) Influences of diet and nutrition on clinical pharmacokinetics. *Clinical Pharmacokinetics*, **14**, 325–346.

Anderson KE and Kappas A (1987) How diet affects drug metabolism. *Hospital Therapy*, **April**, 93–102.

Bennett WM (1997) Drug interactions and consequences of sodium restriction. *American Journal of Clinical Nutrition*, **65**, 6785–6815.

Bennett WM and Porter GA (1993) Overview of clinical nephrotoxicity. In *Toxicology of the Kidney*, 2nd edn, Hook JB and Goldstein RS (eds), Target Organ Toxicity Series, Raven Press, New York, Chapter 3, 61–97.

Cardinale V (1988) Stemming the tide of polymedicine. *Drug Topics*, 132, 36–41.

Chen LH, Liu S, Cook Newell ME and Barnes K (1985) Survey of drug use by the elderly and possible impact of drugs on nutritional status. *Drug–Nutrient Interactions*, **3**, 73–86.

Childs B (1988) Genetic variation and nutrition. *American Journal of Clinical Nutrition*, **48**, 1500–1504.

Christakis P (1983) Part II: Drug interactions – nutrients, vitamins, foods. *Pharmacy Times*, **November**, 68–79.

Chu S, Park Y, Locke C, Wilson DS and Cavanaugh JC (1992) Drug-food interaction potential of clarithromycin, a new macrolide antimicrobial. *Journal of Clinical Pharmacology*, **32**, 32–36.

Comai L (1993) Impact of plant genetic engineering on foods and nutrition. *Annual Reviews of Nutrition*, **13**, 191–215.

D'Arcy PF (1985) Nutrient–drug interactions. *Adverse Drug Reactions and Toxicological Reviews*, **14**, 233–254.

D'Arcy PF and McElnay JC (1985) Drug interactions in the gut involving metal ions. *Reviews on Drug Metabolism and Drug Interaction*, **5**, 83–99.

De Ponti F, Giaroni C, Cosentino M, Lecchini S and Frigo G (1996) Adrenergic mechanisms in the control of gastrointestinal motility: from basic science to clinical applications. *Pharmacology and Therapeutics*, **69**, 59–78.

Farrar HC and Blumer JL (1991) Fetal effects of maternal drug exposure. *Annual Reviews of Pharmacology and Toxicology*, **31**, 525–547.

Furst P, Albers S and Stehle P (1990) Dipeptides in clinical nutrition. *Proceedings of the Nutritional Society*, **49**, 343–359.

Garabedian-Ruffalo SM, Syrja-Farber M, Lanius PM and Plucinski A (1988) Monitoring of drug–drug and drug–food interactions. *American Journal of Hospital Pharmacy*, **45**, 1530–1534.

Ghoneim MM, Kortilla K, Chiang CH, Jacobs L, Schoenwald RD, Medwaldt SP and Kayala KO (1981) Diazepam effects and kinetics in Caucasians and Orientals. *Clinical Pharmacology and Therapeutics*, **29**, 749–756.

Hansten PD and Horn JR (1989) *Drug Interactions*, 6th edn, Lea & Febiger, Philadelphia, PA.

Harris JE (1995) Interaction of dietary factors with oral anticoagulants: review and applications. *Journal of the American Dietetic Association*, **95**, 580–584.

Hazell T (1985) Minerals in foods: dietary sources, chemical forms, interactions, bioavailability. *World Review of Nutrition and Diet*, **46**, 1–123.

Hoyumpa Am and Schenker S (1982) Major drug interactions: effect of liver disease, alcohol, and malnutrition. *Annual Reviews of Medicine*, **33**, 113–149.

Hulin B (1994) New hypoglycaemic agents. *Progress in Medicinal Chemistry*, **31**, 1–58.

Hussar DA (1988) Drug interactions in the older patient. *Geriatrics*, **43**, 20–30.

Katz NL and Dejean A (1985) Interrelationships between drugs and nutrients. *Pharm Index*, **December**, 9–15.

Kessler DA, Taylor MR, Maryanski JH, Flamm EL and Kahl LS (1992) The safety of foods developed by biotechnology. *Science*, **256**, 1747–1832.

Kirk JK (1995) Significant drug–nutrient interactions. *American Family Physician*, **51**, 1175–1182.

Kitler ME (1994) Clinical trials and transethnic pharmacology. *Drug Safety*, **11**, 378–391.

Kodavanti UP and Mehendale HM (1990) Cationic amphophilic drugs and phospholipid storage disorder. *Pharmacological Reviews*, **42**, 427–351.

Lamy PP (1982) Effects of diet and nutrition on drug therapy. *Journal of the American Geriatric Society*, **30**, S99–S112.

Lee CR, McKenzie CA and Mantooth R (1991) Food and drug interactions. *U.S. Pharmacist*, **May**, 44–58.

Lewis DP, Van Dyke DC, Willhite LA, Stumbs PJ and Berg MJ (1995) Phenytoin-folic acid interaction. *Annals of Pharmacotherapy*, **29**, 726–735.

Lieber CS (1994) Mechanisms of ethanol-drug-nutrition interactions. *Clinical Toxicology*, **32**, 631–681.

Mehta S, Nain CK, Sharma B and Mathur VS (1982) Disposition of four drugs in malnourished children. *Drug–nutrient Interactions*, **1**, 205–211.

Montes RG and Perman JA (1991) Lactose intolerance. *Postgraduate Medicine*, **89**, 175–184.

Montgomery RK, Buller HA, Rings EHHM and Grand RJ (1991) Lactose intolerance and the genetic regulation of intestinal lactase-phlorizin hydrolase. *FASEB Journal*, **5**, 2824–2832.

Mooradian AD (1988) Nutritional modulation of life span and gene expression. *Annals of Internal Medicine*, **109**, 891–892.

Munro HN, Suter PM and Russell RM (1987) Nutritional requirements of the elderly. *Annual Reviews of Nutrition*, **7**, 23–49.

Nurray JJ and Healy MD (1991) Drug–mineral interactions: a new responsibility for the hospital dietitian. *Journal of the American Diet Association*, **91**, 66–70, 73.

Randle NW (1987) Food or nutrient effects on drug absorption: a review. *Hospital Pharmacy*, **22**, 694–697, 718.

Roe DA (1974) Effects of drugs on nutrition. *Life Sciences*, **15**, 1219–1234.

Roe DA (1979) Interactions between drugs and nutrients. *Medical Clinics of North America*, **63**, 985–1007.

Roe DA (1984) Therapeutic significance of drug–nutrient interactions in the elderly. *Pharmacological Reviews,* **36,** 109S–122S.

Roe DA (1985) Prediction of the cause, effects, and prevention of drug–nutrient interactions using attributes and attribute values. *Drug–Nutrient Interactions,* **3,** 187–189.

Roe DA (1988a) Drug and nutrient interactions in the elderly diabetic. *Drug–nutrient Interactions,* **5,** 195–203.

Roe DA (1988b) Drug and nutrient interactions in elderly cardiac patients. *Drug–nutrient Interactions,* **5,** 205–212.

Roe DA (1993) Drug and food interactions as they affect the nutrition of older individuals. *Aging: Clinical Experimental Research,* **5,** 51–53.

Royer RJ, Debry G, Ulmer M and Bannwarth B (1984) Food and drug interactions. *World Review of Nutritional Diet,* **43,** 117–128.

Saperstein R, Chapin EW, Brady EJ and Slater EE (1990) Effects of an α_2- adrenoceptor antagonist on glucose tolerance in the genetically obese mouse. *Metabolism,* **39,** 445–451.

Skaar DJ (1991) Drug–nutrient interactions: implications for pharmaceutical care. *Partners in Pharmaceutical Care,* **October,** 11–19.

Smith CH (1995) Drug–food/food–drug interactions In *Geriatric Nutrition,* 2nd edn, Raven Press, New York, pp. 311–328.

Smith CH and Bidlack WR (1984) Dietary concerns associated with the use of medications. *Journal of the American Diet Association,* **84,** 901–914.

Stiefeld SM, Graziani AL, MacGregor RR and Esterhai JL (1991) Toxicities of antimicrobial agents used to treat osteomyelitis. *Orthopedic Clinics North America,* **22,** 439–465.

Thomas JA (1995) Drug–nutrient interactions. *Nutritional Reviews,* **53,** 271–282.

Thomas JA and Markovac J (1994) Aspects of neural tube defects: a minireview. *Toxic Substances Journal,* **13,** 303–312.

Thomas JA and Thomas MJ (1994) Insulin, glucagon, somatostatin, and orally effective hypoglycemic drugs. In *Modern Pharmacology,* 4th edn, Little Brown & Co., New York, pp. 797–808.

Thomas JA and Tschanz C (1994) Nurtient–drug interactions, In *Nutritional Toxicology,* Kotsonis FN, Mackey M and Hjelle JJ (eds), Target Organ Toxicity Series, Raven Press, New York, pp. 139–148.

Toothaker RD and Welling PG (1980) The effect of food on drug bioavailability. *Annual Reviews of Pharmacology and Toxicology,* **20,** 173–199.

Trovato A, Nuhlicek DN and Midtling JE (1991) Drug–nutrient interactions. *American Family Physician,* **44,** 1651–1658.

Tschantz C, Stargel WW and Thomas JA (1996) Interactions between drugs and nutrients. *Advances in Pharmacology,* **35,** 1–26.

Welling PG (1980) Effect of food on bioavailability of drugs. *Pharmacy International,* **1,** 14–18.

Welling PG (1984) Interactions affecting drug absorption. *Clinical Pharmacokinetics,* **9,** 404–434.

Welling PG (1996) Effects of food on drug absorption. *Annual Reviews of Nutrition,* **16,** 383–415.

Wells S, Holbrook AM, Crowther NR and Hirsh J (1994) Interactions of warfarin with drugs and food. *Annals of Internal Medicine,* **121,** 676–683.

Winstanley PA and Orme ML'E (1989) The effects of food on drug bioavailability. *British Journal of Clinical Pharmacology,* **28,** 621–628.

Wix AR, Doering PL and Hatton RC (1992) Drug–food interaction counseling programs in teaching hospitals. *American Journal of Hospital Pharmacy,* **49,** 8555–860.

7 Glutathione, Sulphur Amino Acids and Chemical Detoxication

Tammy M Bray, Emily Ho and Mark A Levy

Department of Human Nutrition, The Ohio State University, Columbus, OH 43210, USA

Introduction

There has been an increased interest in the potential clinical or therapeutic use of glutathione (GSH, L-γ-glutamyl-L-cysteinyl-glycine) or its precursors for treatment of toxicity or disease, especially those believed to be free radical-mediated and which are characterised by depleted tissue GSH stores. These interests stem primarily from studies which have demonstrated that: (i) supplementation of GSH precursors concomitantly with exposure to drugs or toxins reduces chemical toxicity (Hazelton *et al.*, 1986); and (ii) decreased tissue GSH concentrations are associated with the clinical onset of chemical toxicity (Stevens and Anders, 1981). However, the success of any clinical or therapeutic approach in preventing toxicity or disease will depend not only upon an understanding of the metabolism and regulation of GSH, but also on the molecular mechanisms by which GSH protects against chemical toxicity.

GSH is the most abundant non-protein thiol in mammalian cells. The most recognised function of GSH is its role as a substrate for GSH-S transferases [EC 2.5.1.18] and GSH peroxidase [EC 1.11.1.9], enzymes which catalyse reactions for the detoxication of xenobiotic compounds and for the antioxidation of reactive oxygen species (ROS) and free radicals. Other physiological roles of GSH, such as storage and transport of cysteine, regulation of leukotriene and prostaglandin metabolism, deoxyribonucleotide synthesis, immune function and cell proliferation have also been acknowledged. Recently, the involvement of GSH in cellular redox balance was demonstrated when several enzymes involved in intermediary metabolism were found to be regulated by thiol: disulphide exchange between protein thiols and low-molecular-weight disulphides (GSSG) (Weis *et al.*, 1993). Thiol:disulphide exchanges provide a

Nutrition and Chemical Toxicity. Edited by Costas Ioannides. © John Wiley & Sons Ltd. ISBN 0 471 97453 6

mechanism for maintaining the oxidation state of protein sulphydryl groups in equilibrium with the thiol status of the cellular environment. Many cellular processes, including signal transduction and gene transcription, are dependent on the redox status of critical sulphydryl groups for interactions among proteins and between transcription factors and DNA. In addition, the molecular basis for cell survival or cell death induced by xenobiotics or oxidative stress is dependent upon cellular redox balance, and GSH plays an important role in both the metabolism of toxins and regulation of cellular redox state. Figure 7.1 summarises the involvement of GSH and GSH-dependent enzymes in multiple cellular functions. Due to its multiple functions in various tissues and its involvement in many diseases and malnutrition, a clear understanding of the interrelationships among tissue glutathione, nutrition and chemical toxicity can be clinically relevant. The focus of this review is to highlight the important role of diet and nutrition in modulating tissue GSH levels, the rate-limiting amino acids as substrates for the *in vivo* synthesis of GSH, and the interrelationships between cellular GSH and the expression of chemical toxicity.

Regulation of GSH synthesis

GSH synthesis *in vivo* is tightly regulated and takes place in two steps as illustrated in Figure 7.2. The initial rate-limiting step is catalysed by γ-glutamylcysteine synthetase to form γ-glutamylcysteine from glutamate and cysteine. Because plasma cysteine concentrations are relatively low, cysteine may also be supplied by cleavage of the disulphide cystine, synthesis of cysteine from methionine via the cystathionine pathway or, alternatively,

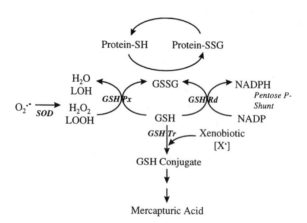

Figure 7.1 Multiple cellular functions of GSH and GSH-dependent enzymes. GSH, reduced glutathione; GSSG, oxidised glutathione; GSH-Px, glutathione peroxidase; GSH-Rd, glutathione reductase; SGH-Tr, glutathione transferase; SOD, superoxide dismutase; $O_2 \cdot^-$, superoxide.

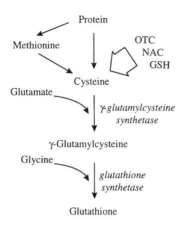

Figure 7.2 Enzymes and substrates in GSH synthesis. OTC, 2-oxothiazolidine-4-carboxylate; NAC, N-acetylcysteine.

through supplementation of cysteine precursors such as N-acetylcysteine (NAC) or 2-oxothiazolidine-4-carboxylate (OTC). In the second step, GSH synthetase catalyses the reaction between glycine and γ-glutamylcysteine to form GSH. The rate-limiting step catalysed by γ-glutamylcysteine synthetase is regulated by feedback inhibition of GSH in *in vitro* systems (Richman and Meister, 1975). This appears to be an important regulatory mechanism which limits the maximum tissue concentration of GSH *in vivo*. The relative importance of cysteine as the rate-limiting amino acid for GSH synthesis is often debated (*vide infra*).

The structural uniqueness of GSH, conferred by the γ-glutamyl bond, contributes to its intracellular stability and determines tissue specificity for uptake of extracellular GSH. The intracellular stability of GSH can be attributed to the resistance of the γ-glutamyl bond to intracellular peptidases and by the resistance of the C-terminal glycine to intracellular γ-glutamyl cyclotransferase (DeLeve and Kaplowitz, 1990).

However, the γ-glutamyl bond can be cleaved by γ-glutamyltranspeptidase, an enzyme located on the external surface of cell membranes of various tissues, and thus the locational specificity of γ-glutamyltranspeptidase determines the tissue specificity of GSH uptake (Hah *et al.*, 1978; Griffith and Meister, 1979). For example, although the liver is the major organ for synthesis and export of GSH (Lauterburg *et al.*, 1984), hepatic uptake of plasma GSH is very low due to the relative absence of γ-glutamyltranspeptidase activity in the liver. On the other hand, extrahepatic tissues such as the lung and kidney have γ-glutamyltranspeptidase for extracellular degradation of GSH to cysteinyl glycine and γ-glutamyl amino acids. After uptake into the cell, these dipeptides are further metabolised to the amino acid constituents of GSH by dipetidases, γ-glutamyl cyclotransferase and oxoprolinase, and are available for intracellular GSH or protein synthesis. Thus, uptake of plasma GSH via γ-glytamyl transpeptidase contributes to the intracellular GSH concentration in extrahepatic tissues.

Nutritional status regulates tissue GSH concentration

The availability of sulphur amino acids in the diet can influence tissue GSH concentrations. This was first demonstrated in rat studies when hepatic GSH concentrations were decreased during consumption of low-protein diets or diets deficient in sulphur amino acids, but hepatic GSH concentrations were returned to normal when the rats were placed on low-protein diets supplemented with sulphur amino acids or adequate protein diets (Edward and Westerfield, 1952; Boebel and Baker, 1983; Cho et al., 1984). This was further confirmed when hepatic GSH concentration was decreased in rats fed 4% and 7.5% protein diets compared with rats fed a diet adequate in protein (15%) (Bauman et al., 1988a). When rats fed 7.5% protein diets were supplemented with cysteine, methionine or hydroxy-methionine at a concentration equivalent to the sulphur amino acid content of the 15% protein diet, hepatic GSH levels increased to the concentration observed in rats fed the 15% protein diet (Bauman et al., 1988a).

Hepatic GSH levels are tightly regulated. For example, hepatic GSH concentrations did not fall below 3 μmol/g of tissue when rats were fasted for 24 hours or fed a diet containing almost no protein (0.5%) for two weeks (Taylor et al., 1992). When rats were fed high-protein (30% or 45%) diets with a sulphur amino acid content two or three times higher than normal hepatic GSH concentrations did not exceed the normal physiological maximum of 8 μmol/g (Bauman et al., 1998a). Figure 7.3 illustrates how tissue GSH and cysteine

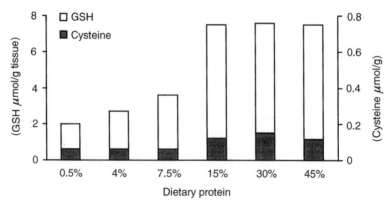

Figure 7.3 Effect of various dietary protein levels on hepatic GSH and cysteine concentrations. (Adapted from Bauman et al., 1988a and Taylor et al., 1992.)

levels responded to dietary protein levels when the dietary protein concentration was below the requirement. However, tissue concentrations of GSH were not enhanced when dietary protein was adequate or above the requirement level (Williamson *et al.*, 1982; Hazelton *et al.*, 1986).

Previous dietary protein status affects the diurnal response of hepatic GSH concentration to sulphur amino acid supplementation. Figure 7.4 provides an example of sulphur amino acid supplementation to rats previously fed a normal protein (15%) diet for two weeks. The rate of increase or the peak concentration of hepatic GSH of the diurnal cycle did not change compared with the unsupplemented group. However, in rats which were previously fed a low-protein (7.5%) diet for two weeks and then supplemented with the sulphur amino acid, the hepatic GSH concentration increased more rapidly and was sustained at a higher concentration than in rats which were previously fed a normal protein (15%) diet for two weeks (Bauman *et al.*, 1988b). In rats, previously fed a 0.5% protein diet for two weeks, this initial increase was even more pronounced than in rats fed the 7.5% protein diet and the peak concentration exceeded the physiological maximum (Taylor *et al.*, 1992). The difference in response to sulphur amino acids between rats fed low-protein diets and rats fed adequate diets is not readily explained, even though hepatic GSH concentration was similar before sulphur amino acid supplementation (i.e. the feedback inhibition mechanism is not involved) and the amount of supplementation was identical for both low and normal protein groups.

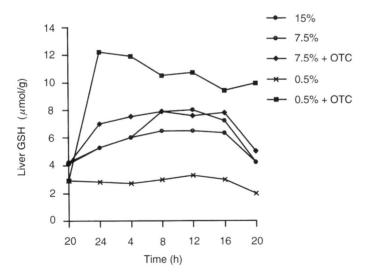

Figure 7.4 Effect of dietary protein status and sulphur amino acid (OTC) supplementation on the diurnal response of hepatic GSH concentrations. (Adapted from Bauman *et al.*, 1988b and Taylor *et al.*, 1992.)

Nutritional status may also influence tissue GSH concentrations by affecting the uptake of extracellular GSH into extrahepatic tissues via γ-glutamyl transpeptidase and by affecting the transport of plasma amino acids into tissues. The influence of nutritional status on extrahepatic tissue GSH concentrations was demonstrated in studies where lung GSH concentration was decreased by long-term severe dietary protein restriction, i.e. 0.5% protein diet for two weeks (Taylor et al., 1992), but there was no difference in lung GSH concentrations between rats fed 7.5% and 15% protein diets. Supplementation of a cysteine prodrug to the 0.5% protein group increased lung GSH levels but the concentration was not affected as dramatically as in the liver, and it was not restored to the lung concentration of rats fed the 15% protein diet (Taylor et al., 1992). However, the enzyme activity of γ-glutamyltranspeptidase was not measured in any of these studies, and the role of this enzyme in the relationship between the protein status and the uptake of GSH is still unknown. In addition to the uptake of GSH via the γ-glutamyltranspeptidase mechanism, amino acid transport mechanisms for substrates of GSH synthesis such as cysteine, cystine, methionine and glutamate may also affect the extrahepatic tissue concentration of GSH. An imbalance of the plasma amino acid profile may influence the uptake of these amino acids since they compete for some of the same transport systems (Christensen, 1990). It has been demonstrated that cystine uptake into cultured endothelial cells is inhibited competitively by glutamate and that the GSH concentration in these cells decreases when they are cultured in a glutamate-enriched medium (Miura et al., 1992). However, the specific effects of the balance of dietary amino acids and nutritional status on amino acid transport for GSH synthesis are unknown.

The relative importance of cysteine and glutamate as the limiting amino acid for GSH synthesis

To maintain tissue GSH concentrations, each of the amino acids needed for the synthesis of GSH must be simultaneously present in sufficient amounts. If a given amino acid is present only to a limited extent, then GSH can be formed only as long as the supply of that amino acid lasts: the amino acid in short supply is the limiting amino acid. The candidates for the limiting amino acids during in vivo GSH synthesis are cysteine and glutamate. Glutamine, the precursor of glutamate, is considered the limiting amino acid for GSH synthesis only when cellular glutamate levels are limited or exhausted.

Since the key enzyme controlling GSH synthesis is γ-glutamylcysteine synthetase, the intracellular availability of cysteine and glutamate become the critical factors in GSH synthesis. The apparent K_m values of γ-glutamyl cysteine synthetase for cysteine and glutamate are 0.3 and 1.8 mM, respectively (Richman and Meister, 1975). This reflects the high affinity of cysteine and low affinity of glutamate for this enzyme and the relative intracellular concentrations of these two substrates under normal metabolism. Generally, glutamate and glutamine are in large excess in the cell whereas cysteine concentrations are low (Bannai and Tateishi, 1986; Tateishi et al., 1989). Plasma cysteine levels are also low, although cysteine can also be supplied by cleavage of the disulphide cystine and by synthesis from methionine via the cystathionine pathway. Even when the dietary sulphur amino acid is in excess (Bauman et al., 1988a), intracellular cysteine levels are tightly regulated and maintained at a limited concentration. As dietary protein or sulphur amino acid increases, cysteine dioxygenase, the enzyme which degrades excess cysteine intracellularly, is induced (Birnbaum et al., 1957; Wong et al., 1986). A 20-fold decrease in hepatic cysteine dioxygenase activity was found in rats fed a protein-deficient diet compared with rats fed a protein-adequate diet. Also, hepatic cellular cysteine concentrations are maintained at a level approximately 50 times lower than that of tissue GSH. In protein-deficient diets (4%), cellular cysteine is maintained at a concentration of 0.05 μmol/g compared with GSH which is 2–3 μmol/g. In protein-excess diets (35%), hepatic cysteine is maintained at 0.2 μmol/g compared with 8–10 μmol/g for GSH (Bauman et al., 1988a). Therefore, it is probable that the rate of GSH synthesis and consequently, the GSH concentration, is significantly influenced by the availability of intracellular cysteine. This suggests that cysteine is the rate-limiting substrate in GSH synthesis.

Evidence to support the hypothesis that cysteine, and not glutamate, is the rate-limiting substrate in GSH synthesis has been provided in several studies. Using primary rat hepatocytes, the intracellular and extracellular levels of cysteine and methionine become exhausted during culture (Tateishi et al., 1989). In contrast, the intracellular content of glutamate and glycine were preserved at relatively high levels. At the same time, supplementation of cysteine and methionine, but not glutamate, resulted in prolonged increases in the intracellular GSH levels of depleted hepatocytes. Hepatocytes have a large pool of glutamate that is difficult to reduce to a rate-limiting level for GSH synthesis, and omission of glutamate from the medium had no effect on either glutamate pool size or the rate of GSH synthesis during cell culture studies (Thor et al., 1979). Therefore the supply of cysteine and not glutamate appears to be critical for the synthesis of GSH. Furthermore, if GSH synthesis is dependent on the availability of the cysteine, then increases in cysteine concentration should result in the enhancement of intracellular GSH. This has been demonstrated in several in vitro and in vivo models. For example, supplementation of cysteine to isolated hepatocytes, incubated in a complete medium resulted in an increase in intracellular GSH (Beatty and Reed, 1981). In models where hepatocytes had been stressed with oxidants, GSH concentrations were depleted. Supplementation of cysteine increased GSH concentration and protected cells from oxidant damage (Dalhoff and Poulsen, 1993; Goss et al., 1994). When hepatocytes isolated from protein-energy malnourished rats were incubated with cysteine alone, total GSH in the cells increased and even exceeded that of controls (Deneke et al., 1983; Bauman et al., 1988a).

The protective effect of cysteine on GSH depletion has been seen in many other culture models as well, including gastric cells, human retinal pigment epithelium and human endothelial cells (Cotgreave *et al.*, 1991; Hiraishi *et al.*, 1994). In all of these *in vitro* models, addition of exogeneous cysteine alone to various culture systems resulted in an increase in intracellular GSH and protection from oxidant damage.

The beneficial effects of cysteine supplementation on GSH concentration can also be observed *in vivo*. Intravenous supply of cysteine to GSH-depleted rats caused marked increases in hepatic GSH *in vivo* (Aebi and Lauterberg, 1992). The effect of cysteine supplementation in total parenteral nutrition (TPN) has also to be investigated. Beagle pups fed TPN solutions supplemented with cysteine had significantly greater hepatic GSH levels than unsupplemented controls (Malloy and Rassin, 1984).

Using cysteine derivatives, other studies reinforce the hypothesis that cysteine availability is the critical rate-limiting step in GSH synthesis. For example, NAC has been shown to safely increase intracellular GSH and protect tissues from paracetamol (acetaminophen) toxicity (Wong *et al.*, 1986; Witschi *et al.*, 1995). OTC, a stable derivative of cysteine, produces sustained and efficient intracellular delivery of cysteine for GSH synthesis (Nishina *et al.*, 1987; Bauman *et al.*, 1998b). Oral administration of OTC can evaluate hepatic GSH in protein-deficient rats and in addition gives protection against pulmonary oxygen toxicity during hyperoxia exposure (Taylor *et al.*, 1992). Because of the limiting nature of cysteine, introduction of any cysteine source to cells results in GSH synthesis.

Although most evidence suggests that cysteine is the limiting amino acid for GSH synthesis, glutamine supplementation may be beneficial for maintaining tissue GSH in situations of high energy and nutrient demand such as severe trauma (Hong *et al.*, 1990, 1992; Zeigler *et al.*, 1992; Welbourne *et al.*, 1993). However, glutamine is not a rate-limiting substrate for GSH synthesis under normal conditions since the synthesis of GSH does not require glutamine directly. However, it may be rate-limiting amino acid for GSH synthesis when intracellular glutamate has been depleted, therefore making glutamine the primary source of glutamate formation. Nonetheless, during normal *in vivo* metabolism, intracellular glutamate is formed primarily from amination of α-ketoglutarate catalysed by glutamate dehydrogenase. This reaction occupies a central position in nitrogen balance and energy homeostasis. Evidence shows that intracellular glutamate rarely becomes limiting and consequently does not influence GSH biosynthesis (Bannai and Tateishi, 1986; Tateishi *et al.*, 1989). In human fibroblasts, intracellular glutamate cannot be exhausted even if the cells are cultured in media lacking in glutamate (Bannai and Tateishi, 1986). In isolated hepatocytes, exclusion of glutamate from the medium does not affect the rate of GSH synthesis.

However, there are extreme situations where glutamate may become conditionally limiting. Rats infused with glutamine-free TPN solution for 5 days exhibited increased mortality after administration of a large dose of paracetamol (Hong *et al.*, 1992). However, rats receiving glutamine-supplemented TPN solutions had higher concentrations of hepatic GSH and showed improved survival rates. In a similar model, patients receiving glutamine-free parenteral nutrition after bone marrow transplantation had a negative nitrogen balance, increased incidence of clinical infection, higher rates of microbial colonisation and a longer hospital stay compared with patients receiving glutamine-supplemented parenteral nutrition (Hong *et al.*, 1990; Zeigler *et al.*, 1992). It has been postulated that the beneficial effects of glutamine supplementation in TPN are attributed to the ability of glutamine to maintain hepatic GSH concentrations. This hypothesis stems from studies that showed supplementation of glutamine in rats exposed to lethal doses of paracetamol attenuated the fall in hepatic GSH levels when compared with unsupplemented controls (Hong *et al.*, 1992). However, hepatic GSH concentrations before and after paracetamol administration in both groups were still within the normal physiological range. In addition, the slightly higher concentration of GSH in glutamine-supplemented compared with control animals could be caused by several other factors. For example, severe oedematous liver in the glutamine-free group would cause a lower GSH concentration when it is expressed as μmol GSH per gram of wet weight of liver rather than dry weight of liver. It is possible that there is no actual difference in the total amount of GSH in the liver between the two groups.

The beneficial effects of glutamine supplementation may also be attributed to factors other than increased GSH synthesis. It is known that 85–90% of paracetamol is normally metabolised by glucuronide and sulphate conjugation, leaving a relatively small amount to be metabolised via glutathione conjugation (Black, 1980). The formation of the conjugating agent, glucuronic acid depends on the availability of glucose in the system (Mandel, 1971). Glutamine supplementation may act as an alternative energy source and provide a sparing effect on glucose utilisation. In addition, glutamine synthesis and release by skeletal muscle during trauma, sepsis, surgery and burns are important for the functioning of the immune system because lymphocytes and macrophages have a high rate of glutamine utilisation for the production of energy (Newsholme *et al.*, 1988). In fact, glutamate and glutamine play a central role in energy metabolism and nitrogen balance independent of GSH synthesis. Therefore, the beneficial effects of glutamine supplementation during severe trauma may include increased substrate availability and provision of energy for protein or immune function.

TPN formulations often contain methionine as the source of sulphur amino acids, glycine and glutamate, but they do not include glutamine. However, it is clear that glutamine supplementation of TPN solutions may be beneficial for patients in severe catabolic states, but glutamine is not the limiting factor in GSH synthesis. A large body of evidence instead suggests that cysteine is the critical rate-limiting factor in GSH synthesis. Therefore, cysteine levels in the diet are consequential in maintaining GSH status and become important in both disease prevention and health promotion.

GSH, xenobiotic toxicity and cell signalling

The mechanism of toxicity for most xenobiotics usually involves the interaction of many different factors. In addition, the ability of cells and tissues to compensate for and adapt to environmental stresses makes it difficult to discern or describe a mechanism of toxicity which encompasses most or all xenobiotics. Nevertheless, toxins generally initiate a sequence of events which exhibit many common features. Figure 7.5 summarises the putative molecular mechanisms by which xenobiotics cause tissue damage and indicates possible metabolic sites at which GSH may inhibit these processes.

Most xenobiotics are enzymically activated by enzymes of the cytochrome P-450 system (mixed function oxidases, MFO) to a reactive intermediate which can be more readily excreted following conjugation than as the parent compound. However, the reactive intermediate also has greater potential to react with cellular macromolecules and thus poses a potential threat to the integrity and functioning of the cell. This is perhaps the most recognised mechanism of xenobiotic toxicity. For example, reactive intermediates oxidise cell membrane lipids and modify the structure and function of proteins through covalent binding. Each of these events is a measurable parameter considered prerequisite for chemical toxicity. In addition, RNA and DNA are often the targets of activated xenobiotics which may lead to many deleterious effects including mutagenicity. Interaction of xenobiotics with any or all of these macromolecules is considered as a possible mechanism for xenobiotic toxicity.

In addition, the reactive intermediates of some xenobiotics may be indirectly toxic by reacting with oxygen to form ROS. Paraquat and alloxan, which are toxic in the lung and pancreas, respectively, are two examples of compounds which may be indirectly toxic. The cytotoxicity of these compounds has been associated with increased ROS generation (i.e. $O_2 \cdot {}^-$) following their activation to reactive intermediates by MFO. As with reactive intermediates, ROS may be directly cytotoxic by oxidising cellular lipids, proteins, DNA and RNA (Pinkus *et al.*, 1996; Sen and Packer, 1996).

Normally, the harmful effects of xenobiotics and ROS are minimised by cellular defence systems which counteract their toxicity. GSH, because of its role in both xenobiotic detoxication and free radical metabolism, plays a critical role in this defence mechanism. For example, GSH serves as a substrate for the glutathione-S-transferases (GSH-Tr). This family of enzymes catalyse the addition of the thiol group of GSH to the activated intermediate of various xenobiotics, thereby facilitating their excretion from the cell (Habig and Jakoby, 1981). In addition, GSH is also utilised by glutathione peroxidase (GSH-Px) to reduce hydrogen peroxide (H_2O_2) and other hydroperoxides to less destructive metabolites (Eklow *et al.*, 1984). Thus, it is generally accepted

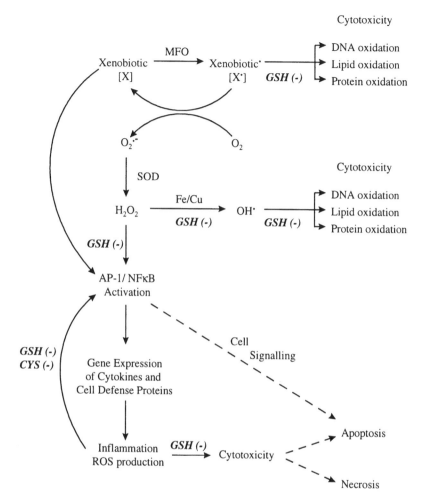

Figure 7.5 Putative molecular mechanisms of xenobiotic toxicity. MFO, mixed function oxidases; SOD, superoxide dismutase; GSH (-), GSH-inhibited pathway; AP-1, activator protein 1; NFκB, nuclear factor κB; ROS, reactive oxygen species; O$_2$·$^-$, superoxide; OH·, hydroxyl radical.

that GSH plays a central role in the cellular defence against chemical and ROS injury (Bellomo *et al.*, 1997).

More recently, there has been growing interest in the role of GSH in cell signalling pathways. In addition to its roles in amino acid transport and defence against xenobiotics and intracellular ROS generation, GSH is the major intra-cellular redox buffer in almost all cell types (Meister, 1989; Staal *et al.*, 1994). The redox status of the cell has been shown to regulate signal transduction, gene transcription and post-translational modification of proteins (Sies, 1991, Anderson *et al.*, 1994; Sen and Packer, 1996). The ability of cells to maintain appropriate GSH levels is, therefore, critically important in maintaining cellular function and integrity (Shi *et al.*, 1994).

Two transcription factors in particular, nuclear factor kappa beta (NFκB) and activator protein-1 (AP-1), are regulated by the intracellular redox status and xenobiotic electrophiles (Sen and Packer, 1996). Both NFκB and AP-1 are activated by oxidative stress and xenobiotics and induce the expression of a variety of proteins which function in the immune system and/or cellular detox-ication systems (Pinkus *et al.*, 1993; Janssen *et al.*, 1995; Sen and Packer, 1996).

NFκB, in its most common form, is a heterodimer of p50 and p65, two of the five-member family of NFκB DNA-binding subunits, which also includes p52, c-Rel and Rel-B (Muller *et al.*, 1997). Normally, NFκB is found in an inactive form, bound to IkB, an inhibitory subunit which localises NFκB to the cyto-plasm and prevents it from binding to DNA (Schreck *et al.*, 1991). Recently, a mechanism for NFκB activation has been proposed. Activation requires the cytokine-activated protein kinase complex, IKK, which phosphorylates IkB, targeting it for ubiquitinylation and subsequent proteolytic degradation (DiDonato *et al.*, 1997). Loss of the IkB subunit allows NFκB to migrate to the nucleus where it induces genes involved in the immune response (Mihm *et al.*, 1995).

Many different stimuli including ROS, toxins, bacterial lipopolysaccharide (LPS) and various cytokines have been identified which can induce NFκB activity (Shreck *et al.*, 1991; Janssen *et al.*, 1995). ROS-mediated activation of NFκB was first proposed by Schreck *et al.*, (1991). This hypothesis was supported by the observation that tumour necrosis factor-α (TNF-α), interleu-kin-1 (IL-1), phorbol myristic acid (PMA), UV light and γ rays, known inducers of oxidative stress, induce NFκB activity (Sies, 1991). Later experiments also implicate H_2O_2 in NFκB activation. For example, TNF and okadaic acid expo-sure did not activate NFκB in JB6 cells which overexpressed catalase, but NFκB activation returned following the administration of aminotriazole, a catalase inhibitor (Schmidt *et al.*, 1995). Also, overexpression of superoxide dismutase (SOD), which leads to an accumulation of H_2O_2 in the cytosol, increased NFκB activation. These results indicate that H_2O_2, or a by-product of H_2O_2 metabo-lism, may be responsible for NFκB activation.

Activation of NFκB leads to increased expression of cytokines and other chemotactic factors involved in inflammation. This then leads to infiltration of immune cells such as macrophages and leukocytes which produce ROS as a killing or defence mechanism. Hence, an initial activation of NFκB by xenobiotics or ROS leads to increased cytokine activation. This could poten-tially increase NFκB activity through cytokine-mediated degradation of the IkB inhibitory unit. It is therefore conceivable that dysregulation of this cycle could lead to an environment in the targeted tissue where increasing amounts of ROS are produced which further induce NFκB. Thus, the inflammatory and auto-immune reactions initiated by ROS would be amplified via a positive feedback loop with NFκB, and it is possible that this may underlie the cytotoxic effect of certain xenobiotics (Mihm et al., 1995).

Droge et al. (1994) have reported several lines of evidence which suggest that GSH plays a role in inhibiting NFκB activation or that GSSG may function to activate NFκB. A series of experiments have demonstrated that: (i) in some cell lines 12-O-tetradecanoylphorbol-13-acetate (TPA) induces NFκB activation and also increases GSSG levels as well as the ratio of GSSG to GSH; (ii) depletion of intracellular GSH and GSSG with buthionesulphoximine (BSO) inhibits TPA-induced activation of NFκB; and (iii) TPA-induced activation of NFκB is enhanced by 1,3-bis (2-chloroethyl-1-nitrosourea) (BCNU), an agent that elevates intracellular GSSG concentrations by inhibiting GSH reductase. Thus, although a direct link between GSH and NFκB activity has not yet been established, it is readily apparent that manipulation of GSH and/or ROS levels can have a dramatic effect on NFκB activation and points to the importance of GSH in maintaining cellular homeostasis. It also provides some insight to the potential use of GSH for therapeutic applications.

There is also evidence that ROS and xenobiotic compounds activate AP-1 and lead to the increased expression of xenobiotic and ROS-metabolising enzymes such as glutathione-S-transferase, NAD(P)H:quinone reductase and glucuronosyltransferases (Janssen et al., 1995; Pinkus et al., 1996). A molecular mechanism by which AP-1 induces the expression of cellular defence enzymes has been proposed. It has been shown that the gene of each of these enzymes contains in its promoter region an antioxidant response element (ARE), other-wise known as the electrophile response element (EpRE) (Friling et al., 1992). The ARE region contains one or more AP-1-like binding regions that bind and are activated by AP-1 (Bergelson et al., 1994). Activation of the promoter region by AP-1 leads to an increased expression of these enzymes (Xie et al., 1995). It is speculated that increased AP-1 activation may serve as the common pathway leading to signal an increased expression of antioxidant and xenobiotic meta-bolising enzymes (Pinkus et al., 1996).

The precise mechanism by which ROS stimulate AP-1 activation and there-fore increase expression of xenobiotic metabolising enzymes is not yet clear. However, a number of studies have demonstrated that both $O_2\cdot^-$ and H_2O_2 induce the expression of Jun and Fos proteins, the major components of AP-1 (Amstad et al., 1990; Nose et al., 1991). In addition, ROS have also been implicated in the activation of AP-1 by ionising radiation (Datta et al., 1992). More recently, there has been speculation that intracellular redox status may play a role in the activation of these genes. For example, chemicals which generate ROS or oxidise thiol-containing structures, and therefore shift the intracellular redox state towards a more oxidative environment, induce GSH-S-transferase activity (Pinkus et al., 1996). In fact, similar to NFκB activation, high intracellular GSSG concentrations have been associated with increased AP-1 activation (Galter et al., 1994).

It was also shown that tyrosine kinase-dependent induction of Jun, the component of AP-1 responsible for DNA binding, was inhibited by increasing intracellular thiol status with the GSH precursor N-acetylcysteine (NAC) (Devary et al., 1993). NAC has also been observed to inhibit AP-1 activation in cells challenged with phenobarbital (Pinkus et al., 1993) or asbestos-induced oxidative stress (Janssen et al., 1995). Thus it appears that cellular redox may be a critical determinant of AP-1 activation as it is induced by oxidative stress but inhibited when the oxidative burden is low. GSH, because it is the primary intracellular redox buffer in almost all cell types, may also be critically important in regulating AP-1, a transcription factor associated with the expression of a wide variety of enzymes involved in xenobiotic and antioxidant metabolism.

In summary, intracellular GSH plays a critical role in chemical detoxication and antioxidant defence, two intimately related protective mechanisms involved in cellular defence against xenobiotic insults and oxidative stress. In addition to these functions, recent advances have revealed that GSH and sulphur amino acids may also play a critical role in signal transduction and gene transcription. By maintaining cellular redox balance and protecting critical sulphydryl groups, GSH may determine interactions not only among proteins, but also between transcription factors and DNA. The involvement of ROS in the activation of oxidative stress response transcription factors, particularly NFκB and AP-1, begins to reveal another dimension in the control and regulation of cellular homeostasis. The regulation of gene expression by GSH has promising clinical and therapeutic implications, though our knowledge of the influence of nutritional status on these complicated processes remains at a rudimentary level. Strategies which utilise GSH or its precursors for disease prevention and treatment of toxicity need to be based upon a sound understanding of the interrelationships between nutrition, GSH, signal transduction and the mechanisms of chemical toxicity.

References

Aebi S and Lauterburg BH (1992) Divergent effects of intravenous GSH and cysteine on renal and hepatic GSH. American Journal of Physiology, 263, R348–R352.

Amstad P, Crawford D, Muehlematter D, Zbinden I, Larsson R and Cerutti P (1990) Oxidants stress induces the proto-oncogenes, C-fos and C-myc in mouse epidermal cells. Bulletin du Cancer, 77, 501–502.

Anderson MT, Staal FJ, Gitler C, Herzenberg LA and Herzenberg LA (1994) Separation of oxidant-initiated and redox-regulated steps in the NF-kappa B signal transduction pathway. Proceedings of the National Academy of Sciences of the United States of America, 91, 11527–11531.

Bannai S and Tateishi N (1986) Role of membrane transport in metabolism and function of glutathione in mammals. Journal of Membrane Biology, 89, 1–8.

Bauman PF, Smith TK and Bray TM (1988a) Effect of dietary protein deficiency and L-2-oxothiazolidine-4-carboxylate on the diurnal rhythm of hepatic glutathione in the rat. *Journal of Nutrition*, **118**, 1048–1054.

Bauman PF, Smith TK and Bray TM (1988b) The effect of dietary protein and sulfur amino acids on hepatic glutathione concentration and glutathione-dependent enzyme activities in the rat. *Canadian Journal of Physiology and Pharmacology*, **66**, 1048–1052.

Beatty P and Reed DJ (1981) Influence of cysteine upon the glutathione status of isolated rat hepatocytes. *Biochemical Pharmacology*, **30**, 1227–1230.

Bellomo G, Palladini G and Vairetti M (1997) Intranuclear distribution, function and fate of glutathione and glutathione-S-conjugate in living rat hepatocytes studied by fluorescence microscopy. *Microscopy Research and Technique*, **36**, 243–252.

Bergelson S, Pinkus R and Daniel V (1994) Induction of AP-1 (Fos/Jun) by chemical agents mediates activation of glutathione S-transferase and quinone reductase gene expression. *Oncogene*, **9**, 565–571.

Birnbaum SM, Winitz M and Greenstein JP (1957) Quantitative nutritional studies with water-soluble, chemically defined diets. III. Individual amino acids as sources of "non-essential" nitrogen. *Archives of Biochemistry and Biophysics*, **72**, 428–436.

Black M (1980) Acetaminophen hepatoxicity. *Gastroenterology*, **78**, 382–392.

Boebel KP and Baker DH (1983) Blood and liver concentrations of glutathione, and plasma concentrations of sulfur-containing amino acids in chicks fed deficient, adequate, or excess levels of dietary cysteine. *Proceedings of the Society of Experimental Biology and Medicine*, **172**, 498–501.

Cho ES, Johnson N and Snider BC (1984) Tissue glutathione as a cyst(e)ine reservoir during cystine depletion in growing rats. *Journal of Nutrition*, **114**, 1853–1862.

Christensen HN (1990) Role of amino acid transport and countertransport in nutrition and metabolism. *Physiological Reviews*, **70**, 43–77.

Cotgreave IA, Constantin-Teodosiu D and Moldeus P (1991) Nonxenobiotic manipulation and sulfur precursor specificity of human endothelial cell glutathione. *Journal of Applied Physiology*, **70**, 1220–1227.

Dalhoff K and Poulsen HE (1993) Synthesis rates of glutathione and activated sulphate (PAPS) and response to cysteine and acetaminophen administration in glutathione-depleted rat hepatocytes. *Biochemical Pharmacology*, **46**, 1295–1297.

Datta R, Hallahan DE, Kharbanda SM, Rubin E, Sherman ML, Huberman E, Weichselbaum RR and Kufe DW (1992) Involvement of reactive oxygen intermediates in the induction of c-*jun* gene transcription by ionizing radiation. *Biochemistry*, **31**, 8300–8306.

DeLeve LD and Kaplowitz N (1990) Importance and regulation of hepatic glutathione. *Seminars in Liver Disease*, **10**, 251–266.

Deneke SM, Gershoff SN and Fanburg BL (1983) Potentiation of oxygen toxicity in rats by dietary protein or amino acid deficiency. *Journal of Applied Physiology*, **54**, 147–151.

Devary Y, Rosette C, DiDonato JA and Karin M (1993) NF-kappa B activation by ultraviolet light not dependent on a nuclear signal. *Science*, **261**, 1442–1445.

DiDonato JA, Hayakawa M, Rothwarf DM, Zandi E and Karin M (1997) A cytokine-responsive I kappa B kinase that activates the transcription factor NF-kappa B. *Nature*, **388**, 548–554.

Droge W, Schultze-Osthoff K, Mihm S, Galter D, Schenk H, Eck HP, Roth S and Gmunder H (1994) Functions of glutathione and glutathione disulfide in immunology and immunopathology. *FASEB Journal*, **8**, 1131–1138.

Edward S and Westerfield WW (1952) Blood and liver glutathione during protein deprivation. *Proceedings of the Society for Experimental Biology and Medicine*, **79**, 57–59.

Eklow L, Moldeus P and Orrenius S (1984) Oxidation of glutathione during hydroperoxide metabolism. A study using isolated hepatocytes and the glutathione reductase inhibitor 1,3-bis(2-chloroethyl)-1-nitrosourea. *European Journal of Biochemistry*, **138**, 459–463.

Friling RS, Bergelson S and Daniel V (1992) Two adjacent AP-1-like binding sites form the electrophile-responsive element of the murine glutathione S-transferase Ya subunit gene. *Proceedings of the National Academy of Sciences of the United States of America*, **89**, 668–672.

Galter D, Mihm S and Droge W (1994) Distinct effects of glutathione disulphide on the nuclear transcription factor kappa B and the activator protein-1. *European Journal of Biochemistry*, **221**, 639–648.

Goss PM, Bray TM and Nagy LE (1994) Regulation of hepatocyte glutathione by amino acid precursors and cAMP in protein-energy malnourished rats. *Journal of Nutrition*, **124**, 323–330.

Griffith OW and Meister A (1979) Glutathione: interorgan translocation, turnover and metabolism. *Proceedings of the National Academy of Sciences of the United States of America*, **76**, 5606–5610.

Habig WH and Jakoby WB (1981) Assays for differentiation of glutathione S-transferases. *Methods in Enzymology*, **77**, 398–405.

Hahn R, Wendel A and Flohe L (1978) The fate of extracellular glutathione in the rat. *Biochimica et Biophysica Acta*, **539**, 324–337.

Hazelton GA, Hjelle JJ and Klaassen CD (1986) Effects of cysteine pro-drugs on acetaminophen-induced hepatotoxicity. *Journal of Pharmacology and Experimental Therapeutics*, **237**, 341–349.

Hiraishi H, Terano A, Ota S, Mutoh H, Sugimoto T, Varada T, Razandi MV and Ivey KJ (1994) Protection of cultured rat gastric cells against oxidant-induced damage by exogenous glutathione. *Gastroenterology*, **106**, 1199–1207.

Hong RW, Helton WS, Robinson MK and Wilmore DW (1990) Glutamine-supplemented TPN preserves hepatic glutathione and improves survival following chemotherapy. *Surgical Forum*, **41**, 9–11.

Hong RW, Rounds JD, Helton WS, Robinson MK and Wilmore DW (1992) Glutamine preserves liver glutathione after lethal hepatic injury. *Annals of Surgery*, **215**, 114–119.

Janssen YM, Barchowsky A, Treadwell M, Driscoll KE and Mossman BT (1995) Asbestos induces nuclear factor kappa B (NF-kappa B) DNA-binding activity and NF-kappa B-dependent gene expression in tracheal epithelial cells. *Proceedings of the National Academy of Sciences of the United States of America*, **92**, 8458–8462.

Lauterburg BH, Adams JD and Mitchell JR (1984). Hepatic glutathione homeostasis in the rat: efflux accounts for glutathione turnover. *Hepatology*, **4**, 586–590.

Malloy MH and Rassin DK (1984) Cysteine supplementation of total parental nutrition: the effect in beagle pups. *Pediatric Research*, **18**, 747–751.

Mandel HG (1971) Pathways of drug biotransformation: biochemical conjugations. In *Fundamentals of Drug Metabolism and Drug Disposition*, La Du B, Mandel H and Way E (eds), The Williams & Wilkins Company, Baltimore, pp. 149–185.

Meister A (1989) On the biochemistry of glutathione. In *Glutathione Centennial: Molecular Perspectives and Clinical Implications*, Taniguchi N, Higashi T, Sakamoto Y and Meister A (eds), Academic Press, New York, pp. 3–22.

Mihm S, Galter D and Droge W (1995) Modulation of transcription factor NF kappa B activity by intracellular glutathione levels and by variations of the extracellular cysteine supply. *FASEB Journal*, **9**, 246–252.

Miura K, Ishii T, Sugita Y and Bannai S (1992) Cystine uptake and glutathione level in endothelial cells exposed to oxidative stress. *American Journal of Physiology*, **262**, C50–C58.

Muller JM, Rupec RA and Baeuerle PA (1997) Study of gene regulation by NF-kappa B and AP-1 in response to reactive oxygen intermediates. *Methods*, **11**, 301–312.

Newsholme EA, Newsholme P, Curi R, Challoner E and Ardawi MSM (1988) A role for muscle in the immune system and its importance in surgery, trauma, sepsis and burns. *Nutrition*, **4**, 261–268.

Nishina H, Ohta J and Ubuka T (1987) Effect of L-2-oxothiazolidine-4-carboxylate administration on glutathione and cysteine concentrations in guinea pig liver and kidney. *Physiological Chemistry and Physics and Medical Nuclear Magnetic Resonance*, **19**, 9–13.

Nose K, Shibanuma M, Kikuchi K, Kageyama H, Sakiyama S and Kuroki T (1991) Transcriptional activation of early-response genes by hydrogen peroxide in a mouse osteoblastic cell line. *European Journal of Biochemistry*, **201**, 99–106.

Pinkus R, Bergelson S and Daniel V (1993) Phenobarbital induction of AP-1 binding activity mediates activation of glutathione S-transferase and quinone reductase gene expression. *Biochemical Journal*, **290**, 637–640.

Pinkus R, Weiner LM and Daniel V (1996) Role of oxidants and antioxidants in the induction of AP-1, NF-kappaB, and glutathione S-transferase gene expression. *Journal of Biological Chemistry*, **271**, 13422–13429.

Richman PG and Meister A (1975) Regulation of γ-glutamyl-cysteine synthetase by nonallosteric feedback inhibition by glutathione. *Journal of Biological Chemistry*, **250**, 1422–1426.

Schmidt KN, Traenckner EB, Meier B and Baeuerle PA (1995) Induction of oxidative stress by okadaic acid is required for activation of transcription NF-kappa B. *Journal of Biological Chemistry*, **70**, 27136–27142.

Schreck R, Rieber P and Baeuerle PA (1991) Reactive oxygen intermediates as apparently widely used messengers in the activation of the NF-kappa B transcription factor and HIV-1. *EMBO Journal*, **10**, 2247–2258.

Sen CK and Packer L (1996) Antioxidant and redox regulation of gene transcription. *FASEB Journal*, **10**, 709–720.

Shi MM, Kugelman A, Iwamoto T, Tian L and Dorman HJ (1994) Quinone-induced oxidative stress elevates glutathione and induces gamma-glutamylcysteine synthetase activity in rat lung epithelial L2 cells. *Journal of Biological Chemistry*, **269**, 26512–26517.

Sies H (1991) Hydroperoxides and thiol oxidants in the study of oxidative stress in intact cells and organs. In *Oxidative Stress: Oxidants and Antioxidants*, Sies H (ed), Academic Press, London, pp. 73–90.

Staal FJ, Anderson MT, Staal GE, Herzenberg LA, Gitler C and Herzenberg LA (1994) Redox regulation of signal transduction: tyrosine phosphorylation and calcium influx. *Proceedings of the National Institutes of Science, USA*, **91**, 3619–3622.

Stevens JL and Anders MW (1981) Effect of cysteine, diethyl maleate, and phenobarbital treatments on the hepatotoxicity of 1[H] chloroform. *Chemico-Biological Interactions*, **37**, 207–217.

Tateishi N, Sakamoto Y, Takada A and Bannai S (1989) Regulation of glutathione level in primary cultured hepatocytes. In *Glutathione Centennial: Molecular Perspectives and Clinical Implications*, Taniguchi N, Higashi T, Sakamoto Y and Meister A (eds), Academic Press, New York, pp. 57–72.

Taylor CG, Bauman PF, Sikorski B and Bray TM (1992) Elevation of lung glutathione by oral supplementation of L-2-oxothiazolidine-4-carboxylate protects against oxygen toxicity in protein-energy malnourished rats. *FASEB Journal*, **6**, 3101–3107.

Thor H, Moldeus P and Orrenius S (1979) Metabolic activation and hepatotoxicity. Effect of cysteine, N-acetylcysteine, and methionine on glutathione biosynthesis and bromobenzene toxicity in isolated rat hepatocytes. *Archives of Biochemistry and Biophysics*, **192**, 405–413.

Weis M, Cotgreave IC, Moore GA, Norbeck K and Moldeus P (1993) Accessibility of hepatocyte protein thiols to monobromobimane. *Biochimica et Biophysica Acta*, **1176**, 13–19.

Welbourne TC, King AB and Horton K (1993) Enteral glutamine supports hepatic glutathione efflux during inflammation. *Journal of Nutritional Biochemistry*, **4**, 236–242.

Williamson JM, Boettcher B and Meister A (1982) Intracellular cysteine delivery system that protects against toxicity by promoting glutathione synthesis. *Proceedings of the National Academy of Sciences of the United States of America*, **79**, 6246–6249.

Witschi A, Junker E, Schranz C, Speck RF and Lauterberg BH (1995) Supplementation of N-acetylcysteine fails to increase glutathione in lymphocytes and plasma of patients with AIDS. *AIDS Research and Human Retroviruses*, **11**, 141–143.

Wong BK, Chan HC and Corcoran GB (1986) Selective effects of N-acetylcysteine stereoisomers on hepatic glutathione and plasma sulfate in mice. *Toxicology and Applied Pharmacology*, **86**, 421–429.

Xie, T, Belinsky M, Xu Y and Jaiswal AK (1995) ARE- and TRE-mediated regulation of gene expression. Response to xenobiotics and antioxidants. *Journal of Biological Chemistry*, **270**, 6894–6900.

Zeigler TR, Young LS, Benfell K, Scheltinga M, Hortos K, Bye R, Morrow FD, Jacobs DO, Smith RJ, Antin JH and Wilmore DW (1992) Clinical and metabolic efficacy of glutamine-supplemented parenteral nutrition after bone marrow transplantation. *Annals of Internal Medicine*, **116**, 821–828.

8 Modulation of the Carcinogenic Response by Caloric Restriction

Angelo Turturro[1], William T Allaben[2], Julian E Leakey[3] and
Ronald W Hart[4]

[1]*Divisionof Biometry and Risk Assessment*
[2]*Associate Director for Scientific Coordination*
[3]*Division of Microbiology and Chemistry*
[4]*Office of the Director*
*National Center for Toxicological Research, Food and Drug
Administration, Jefferson, Arkansas 72079, USA*

Introduction

Cancer is a multistep process which, if left unchecked, results in death. A number of biochemical, cellular and molecular processes and mechanisms have been implicated in the induction of cancer including various steps in intermediary metabolism, free radical formation/inactivation, xenobiotic activation/inactivation, induction of DNA damage, DNA repair, fidelity of DNA replication, gene expression, DNA methylation, cellular proliferation, apoptosis, modification of receptor site activity and altered cell–cell communication. At the organismic level cancer occurrence has been associated with altered immune function, changes in hormonal receptor-site activity, failure in immune function, changes in central neuroendocrine control systems, induction of stress proteins and various other physiological dysfunctions (Hart *et al.*, 1995a). As science and our understanding of these processes has continued to evolve, we have come to appreciate the involvement of these same systems in certain other degenerative diseases including the ageing process (Hart *et al.*, 1995b). The reason that the term 'modulation' is used in the title of this chapter is that both over and under consumption of calories and certain rate-limiting nutrients can modulate the expression of many, if not all, of the above processes associated with cancer. For example, a change in the number of calories consumed can alter each of the aforementioned processes in the absence of

Nutrition and Chemical Toxicity. Edited by Costas Ioannides. © John Wiley & Sons Ltd. ISBN 0 471 97453 6

malnutrition (Hart *et al.*, 1995a). Many of these processes are associated with the onset of various forms of cancer, are modulated by diet, and directly related to an organism's ability to maintain homeostasis. Loss of this ability can lead, in replicative cells, to uncontrolled replication of an individual cell.

The relationship among energy availability, the time to occurrence of various degenerative diseases and the age at and/or the frequency of reproduction may be interrelated via a process which permits those individuals processing such a mechanism to survive periods of food deprivation via up-regulation of those systems that maintain the information content of an organism and down-regulation of reproductive capacity until time of food availability, at which time the reverse may occur. This concept is one which has itself evolved over a number of years (Brash and Hart, 1977; Hart *et al.*, 1979; Hart and Stephens, 1980) coming to its present state in the late 1980s and early 1990s (Turturro and Hart, 1991; Turturro *et al.*, 1994; Hart and Turturro 1998). In this concept there exists a series of processes between the exposure of an organism to agents which may induce macromolecular damage and its pathological expression. These processes are termed longevity-assurance processes. This concept further suggests that these systems are multigenic and can be influenced by exogenous factors such as diet. Many of these 'longevity-assurance processes' and their failure or lack of response are or have recently become associated with the frequency of occurrence of a number of age-associated degenerative diseases, including cancer, heart disease and arthritis. Such a mechanism could have been selected for in evolution so that individuals could survive periods of food scarcity until times of food availability, at which time they could again successfully reproduce. An added advantage of this speculation is that it may in part explain the difference observed across mammalian species in the risk for spontaneous malignant transformation per cell per unit time. Although the aforementioned system presumably functions to preserve the integrity of the individual gene pools over prolonged periods of food deprivation until reproduction is again beneficial, it is also possible either that not all individuals uniformly down-regulate these homeostatic processes (back to prenutrient stress levels) or that changes in the germ cell DNA occur and result in a partial, but permanent, up-regulation of one of more of these processes. In either case, the individual (or its offspring) might prove to be more resistant to environmental stress and able to either live longer (shift its average and maximum achievable life span) or achieve a larger body size without influencing its risk for spontaneous malignant transformation per cell per unit time.

If indeed the above speculations are correct, one would expect to see very specific changes in certain cellular defence mechanisms as a consequence of changes in caloric intake. Some of the systems one would expect to be affected, if indeed this speculation were correct, might be oxidative metabolism, inactivation of free radicals and other electrophilic agents, DNA repair, fidelity of DNA replication, gene expression, apoptosis, cell–cell communication, cell replication and immune competency. Each of these are examined below with respect to the effect of caloric restriction on their expression.

Intermediary metabolism and oxidative stress

Intermediary or energy metabolism is central to cellular function. Dependent upon the activity state of the cell (proliferating, quiescent, actively secreting, etc.) and its hormonal control, a variety of the key regulatory enzymes associated with glycolysis decrease, whereas, those associated with gluconeogenesis increase (Table 8.1). For instance, with caloric restriction, many of the enzymes associated with gluconeogenesis, such as glutamate dehydrogenase, tyrosine amino transferase and malate dehydrogenase increase (Feuers *et al.*, 1989). In addition, those enzymes associated with lipid metabolism, such as malic enzyme and glycerol kinase decrease, as does the formation of fatty acids epoxides (Allaben *et al.*, 1990; Figure 8.1). The modulatory effect of caloric intake on intermediary metabolism appears to be implemented by the effect of caloric intake on a few key regulatory enzymes within selected metabolic pathways, with both sets of enzymes being under hormonal control (Feuers *et al.*, 1995).

Oxygen is a substrate for those reactions that generate reactive oxygen free radicals (i.e. superoxide anion, hydroxyl radical, singlet oxygen and hydrogen peroxide). If allowed to accumulate, oxygen radical damage occurs in all macromolecules including lipids, protein and DNA. As caloric intake decreases, it appears that the production of oxygen free radicals may decrease (Weindruch and Walford, 1988). A number of defence mechanisms have evolved to inactivate free radicals before their interaction with macromolecules, including the inducible enzymes superoxide dismutase, glutathione peroxidase, catalase and heam oxygenase. As carloric intake decreases, the efficiency of these enzymes appears to increase (Feuers *et al.*, 1995). For

Table 8.1 Mean activities of selected enzymes of intermediary metabolism in F-344 rats

Enzyme	*Ad libitum*	Restricted	% Change
Gluconeogenic			
Glutamate dehydrogenase	4742	6736	+42
Glucose-6-phosphatase	0.22	0.33	+50
Amino acid oxidase	645	647	–
Glycolytic			
Alcohol dehydrogenase	540	294	−46
Lactate dehydrogenase	1457	772	−47
Sorbitol dehydrogenase	1639	1308	−20
Pyruvate kinase (V_{max})	6621	3413	−48

Values are units/l, except glucose-6-phosphatase, which are μmol/min/mg microsomal protein. Methods are from Feuers *et al.* (1989) from which the table is adapted.

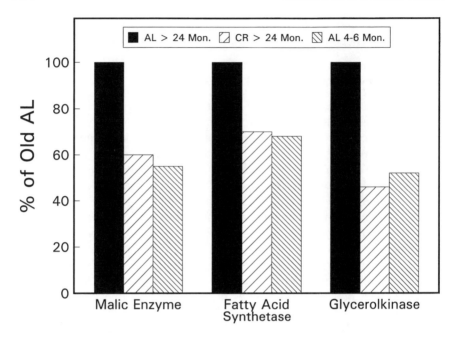

Figure 8.1 Diet effects on activities of enzymes important in fatty acid metabolism. Percentage of old *ad libitum* (AL) activities in B6C3F1 mice when a 40% caloric restriction (CR) is imposed. Age effects are shown by comparing the young (4–6-month) versus old (> 24-month-old) animals. Fatty acid metabolism in older animals is similar to that of younger animals when CR is used.

example, caloric restriction increases the effective concentration of catalase, thus increasing its efficiency (Figure 8.2). Also important in the inactivation of free radicals are essential nutrients such as vitamin C, vitamin E and β-carotene as well as essential minerals such as zinc, copper, manganese and selenium which are required for activation of the antioxidant enzymes. The importance of these factors is exemplified by the observation that as caloric intake decreases in the absence of proper nutrition (i.e. malnutrition) the susceptibility of the organism to disease is increased (Surgeon-General, 1988) while, as caloric intake decreases in the presence of a nutrient adequate diet, resistance to toxic and disease insult increases (Allaben *et al.*, 1990; Hart *et al.*, 1995a; Figure 8.3). Also important are the levels of metabolic free radical scavengers such as melatonin and bile pigments (Joeschke, 1995; Poeggeler *et al.*, 1993). While free radical formation may have a beneficial role to play in recruitment of polymorphonuclear leukocytes and other phagocytes important in the inactivation of pathogens, they have also been implicated in the development of many diseases including ischaemia–reperfusion injury in heart attacks, stroke, cancer, emphysema, immune and neurodegenerative disorders, and ageing

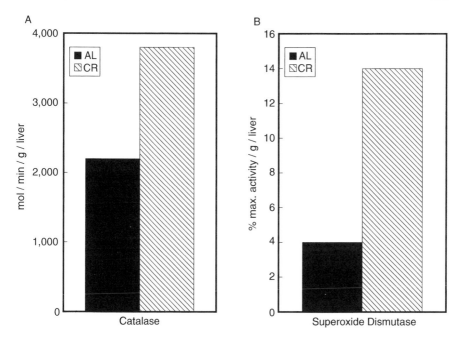

Figure 8.2 Modulation of catalase and superoxide dismutase activities by diet. Cytosols from 1-month-old male Fischer 344 rats show the catalase (A) and superoxide dismutase (B) activity as a function of whether the rats were fed either an *ad libitum* (AL) or a 40% restricted (CR) diet. Data from Feuers *et al.* (1995).

(McCord, 1995; Spitzer, 1995). As caloric intake is reduced in the absence of malnutrition, the time to occurrence or severity of each of these diseases is decreased (Weindruch and Walford, 1988; Turturro and Hart, 1992; Hart *et al.*, 1995a). Since caloric intake in the absence of malnutrition is proportional to free radical generation and inversely proportional to the efficiency of the inducible antioxidant enzymes, it would be expected that this should indeed be the case. Likewise, it would be expected from a molecular standpoint that there should be a corresponding decrease in macromolecular damage. It has been shown (Djuric *et al.*, 1992; 1995) that reduced caloric intake significantly decreases 5-hydroxymethyluracil levels in the DNA of both liver and mammary gland tissue.

The expression of drug-metabolising-enzymes

A number of degenerative diseases including cancer are age-dependent. The multistep hypothesis of cancer stipulates that exogenous and endogenous compounds can be activated to initiate a primary lesion in the DNA and that those cells that cannot repair such damage may, under appropriate conditions,

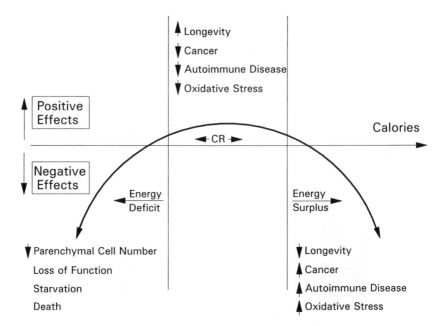

Figure 8.3 Optimal range of energy intake. Too few (i.e. malnutrition) or too many calories can have adverse effects. Caloric restriction (CR) under certain conditions seems to optimize the positive effects of calories. Figure adapted from James-Gaylor *et al.* (1998).

proliferate and expand into focal lesions that develop into cancers (Ogawa *et al.*, 1980; Baron *et al.*, 1986). In chemical carcinogenesis, metabolic activation is often the key to this process. Caloric restriction has been shown to alter the expression of several isoforms of drug metabolising enzymes (Manjgaladze *et al.*, 1993; Hart *et al.*, 1996; Table 8.2). Since these enzymes are primarily responsible for the activation and detoxication of many carcinogens and mutagens, modulation of xenobiotic toxicity, biotransformation and metabolic clearance of many endogeneous compounds as well as microsomal production of oxygen radicals, it is reasonable to assume that changes in this system, induced by variations in caloric intake, might be expected to impact on the rate of tumour occurrence (Leakey *et al.*, 1995). In rodents, the largest direct effect of caloric intake appears to be an apparent de-differentiation of sex-specific enzyme expression with decreasing caloric intake, including a 70% decrease in cytochrome CYP2C11 expression in male F-344 rats (Figure 8.4) and a 30% reduction of corticosterone sulphotransferase activity (Figure 8.5) in females at 40% caloric reduction from *ad libitum* (Manjgaladze et al., 1993). These differences are closely correlated with the extent of DNA damage induced by 2-acetylaminofluorene (2-AAF) or aflatoxin B_1, as a function of caloric intake

Table 8.2 Effects of caloric reduction on the drug-metabolising enzyme isoform selective activities in rats[a]

	Males	Females
Direct effects	(CYP2A2 ↓)?	Androgen 5α-reductase ↓
	CYP2A2 ↓	Corticosterone
		sulphotransferase ↓
	(CYP2C13 ↓)?	(CYP2C12 ↓)?
	(Arylsulphotransferase IV ↓)?	CYP2D ↔
	Androgen 5α-reductase ↑	Phenol UGT ↔
	Corticosterone	
	sulphotransferase ↑	
	CTP3A2 ↔	
	CYP2D ↔	
	Phenol UGT ↔	
Ageing-related effects	CYP2C11 ↑	
	CYP3A2 ↑	
	CYP2E ↑	
	Bilirubin UGT ↑	
	Androgen 5α-reductase ↓	
	Corticosterone	
	sulphotransferase ↓	
Circadian effects	CYP1A1 ↑	CYP1A1 ↑
	CYP2A1 ↑	CYP2A1 ↑
	CYP2B1 ↑	CYP2B1 ↑
	CYP2E1 ↑	CYP2E1 ↑
	CYP2A1 ↓ (testis)	

[a]Table adapted from Hart *et al.* (1996). These studies used 40% caloric restriction in Fischer 344 rats. Listed isoforms are hepatic unless stated otherwise. ↑, ↓ and ↔ denote increased, decreased and unchanged activities, respectively. ? denotes predicted effect from what is known about isoform's regulation. UGT, UDP-glucuronosyltransferase.

(Table 8.3). Both of these compounds are metabolically activated and deactivated through the above pathways (Chou *et al.*, 1993).

With regards to the modulatory effects of caloric intake on the drug metabolising enzyme system it would appear that, dependent upon the enzyme function investigated, differing effects are observed. Overall, most changes result in either the production of either fewer DNA lesions or less mutagenic ones as a consequence of reduced caloric intake.

DNA repair, replication, methylation and expression

Dependent upon the compound studied, strong relationships have been established between DNA-adduct formation and tumorigenesis. Recent among these studies were those of Poirier and Beland (1994), in which DNA-adduct levels were measured in the livers and bladders of mice during chronic exposure to several different doses of 2-AAF. An increase in DNA-adduct formation

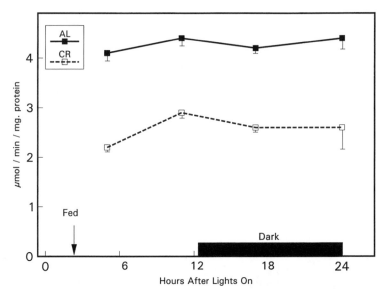

Figure 8.4 Levels of hepatic cytochrome CYP2C11 activity as a function of time after lights on. This isoform can metabolically activate some carcinogens, such as AFB_1 and produce other forms of DNA damage. 'Fed' indicates when animals (F-344 male rats) are fed; the black bar indicates when lights are off. Error bars are standard deviation. Data from Leakey *et al.* (1995).

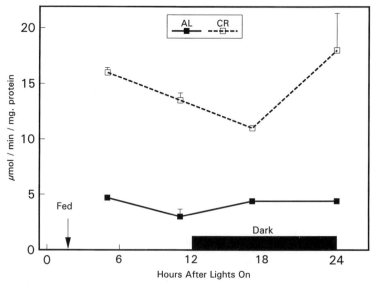

Figure 8.5 Levels of hepatic corticosterone sulphotransferase as a function of time after lights on. This isoform is involved in detoxication of certain metabolites. 'Fed' indicates when animals (F-344 male rats) are fed; the black bar indicates when lights are off. Error bars are standard deviation. Data from Leakey *et al.* (1995).

Table 8.3 Effect of caloric resriction on *in vitro* hepatocyte-carcinogen DNA binding[a]

Carcinogen	AL rats	CR rats
Aflatoxin B_1 (AFB_1)	90	66
Benzo(a)pyrene (BaP)	6.0	3.7
7, 12-Dimethylbenz(a)anthracene (DMBA)	4.1	4.6
2-Acetylaminofluorene (2-AAF)	42	30

[a]Values are in pmol carcinogen/mg DNA/30 min. Hepatocytes were isolated from AL (*ad libitum*) and CR (40% calorically restricted) F-344 rats and incubated with either 0.25 μM of [^{3}H]AFB$_1$ at 200 μCi/μmol, 15 μM of [^{3}H]BaP at 560 μCi/μmol, 4 μM of [^{3}H]DMBA at 200 μCi/μmol, or 20 μM of [^{3}H]2-AAF at 980 μCi/μmol. Adapted from Chou *et al.* (1993).

occurred during the first two weeks, followed by a plateau phase which was assumed to represent steady state and be proportional to dose. In live, a linear correlation existed between steady-state DNA-adduct levels and tumorigenesis. In bladder, a correction had to be made for proliferative capacity. Both of these findings are consistent with the earlier work of Hart and Setlow who showed that UV-induced thyroid cancer could be directly and proportionally reversed by the photoreactivation of 254 mm light-induced cyclobutane-type pyrimidine dimers (Hart *et al.*, 1977) and work by Chang *et al.*, (1981) showing that failure to correct for proliferative capacity would result in a miscall of the carcinogenic potential of chemical adducts. In addition to these effects on tumorigenesis Hart and Setlow clearly demonstrated as early as 1974 a strong correlation between DNA repair and species maximal lifespan within placental mammals. These observations have been repeated in a number of laboratories and are among the most consistent findings on the mechanism of ageing across species thus far reported (Turturro and Hart, 1984). Further evidence for a role of both DNA damage and the modulatory impact of DNA repair on cancer comes from the observation that many of the human syndromes defective in DNA repair exhibit accelerated rates of tumour induction (Tice and Setlow, 1985). As a consequence, a number of laboratories have tried to identify means to enhance DNA repair, but with little success.

Interestingly, various forms of DNA repair appear to be increased by caloric intake. For example, in cells isolated from the kidney and liver of Fischer 344 rats, there was a decline (Table 8.4) in UV-stimulated DNA repair with age (Weraarchakull *et al.*, 1989). This was consistent with earlier work by Licastro *et al.*, (1988) demonstrating that reduced caloric intake slowed the rate of loss of DNA repair capacity as a function of age. Concurrently, studies by Lipman *et al.*, (1989) showed that reduced caloric intake increased the level of excision repair in two rat strains following exposure to either methyl-methane sulphonate or UV (254 nm) light (Table 8.5). Additionally, this study also reported an increased level of O^6-methylguanine acceptor protein activity. Interestingly this response exhibited a strong circadian dependency, suggesting its dependence upon other factors. Another example of this circadian effort is the effect of the oestrous cycle on DNA repair in mammary gland and uterine DNA repair of

Table 8.4 Effect of caloric restriction and age on UV-induced DNA repair[a]

Age (months)	Hetpatocytes[b]		Kidney cells[c]	
	AL	CR	AL	CR
5	5.78	–	–	–
13	4.90	5.72	–	–
22	3.05	4.03	2.01	2.36
28	2.65	3.31	1.34	1.83
34	–	3.02	–	1.33

[a]Values are the ratio of dpm/μg DNA for irradiated to control cells after 1 hour for cells isolated from AL (*ad libitum*) and 40% calorically restricted (CR) male F-344 rats. AL and CR animals are significantly different (at $P < 0.01$ level) at all ages and in both cell types. Adapted from Weraarchakull *et al.* (1989).
[b]Irradiated at 877 J/m^2.
[c]Irradiated at 100 J/m^2.

Table 8.5 Effect of caloric restriction and age on UV-induced DNA repair[a]

Agent	Brown–Norway		BN X F-344 F1		B6C3F1	
	AL	CR	AL	CR	AL	CR
MMS (0.5 mM)	1.156	1.180	1.404	1.608	–	–
UV (20 J/m^2)	1.375	1.412	2.072	2.750	–	–
Spontaneous (MGAP)	0.38	0.65	–	–	0.34	0.46

[a]Values are the ratio of dpm/μg DNA for irradiated to control cells after 1 hour except O^6-methyl guanine acceptor protein activity (MGAP) levels which are fmol/μg DNA for cells isolated from AL (*ad libitum*) and 40% calorically restricted (CR) rats (Brown-Norway and BN X F-344F1) and mice (B6C3F1). Adapted from Lipman *et al.* (1989).

damage induced by *N*-methyl-nitrosamine, a non-metabolically activated carcinogen. This study showed that when oestrogen is lowest (dioestrus) DNA repair is highest. Likewise, as caloric intake, is reduced oestrogen decreases and DNA repair is elevated (Turturro and Hart, 1991).

Even in the absence of DNA damage, infidelity in DNA replication can lead to mutagenic changes in cellular DNA. As a function of increased age, there is a decrease in DNA polymerase α(pol α) expression and specific activity derived from either human diploid fibroblasts or the livers of C57BL/6N mice. These changes have been used to explain the increase in cancer observed with age (Srivastava *et al.*, 1993). The rate of loss of fidelity in pol α as a function of age (Table 8.6) is significantly slowed by reduced caloric intake (Srivastava *et al.*, 1993). These data are consistent with information suggesting that transient loss of polymerases in the cellular pool may contribute to impaired base selection and decreased accuracy of DNA synthesis. If this occurs, then caloric intake may influence this process, in part, by altering the rate and fidelity of DNA replication (Table 8.6). Also important is the observation by Busbee *et al.*, (1995) that the rate of loss of DNA pol α expression and loss of fidelity of

Table 8.6 Nucleotide misincorporation frequencies for hepatic DNA polymerase fractions from 6- and 26-month-old AL or CR C57BL/6N mice using synthetic template-primer[a]

Age (months)	Diet	Template	Polymerase fraction	dTMP	dGMP	Error rate
6	AL	[poly d(A-T)]	α	32.4	11.3	1/2880
6	CR	[poly d(A-T)]	α_1	38	10	1/3800
			α_2	31	8.5	1/3600
6	AL	[poly (dA).poly (dT)]	α	31.8	9	1/4600
6	CR	[poly (dA).poly (dT)]	α_1	41	10	1/4000
			α_2	32	12.5	1/3100
26	AL	[poly d(A-T)]	α_1	7	11.5	1/610
			α_2	5.5	7	1/790
26	CR	[poly d(A-T)]	α_1	13.5	15	1/900
			α_2	12	14	1/860
26	AL	[poly (dA).poly (dT)]	α_1	4.5	10	1/450
			α_2	3.5	6	1/580
26	CR	[poly (dA).poly (dT)]	α_1	11	12	1/960
			α_2	13.5	14	1/960

[a]dTMP is in pmols; dGMP in fmol. Polymerases were purified through the DNA affinity chromatography step for *ad libitum* (AL) or 40% calorically restricted (CR) mice. Adapted from Srivastava *et al.* (1993) and Busbee *et al.* (1995).

DNA replication are significantly slowed as caloric intake is decreased and that this appears to be associated with the appearance of an α-accessory protein with ATP-dependent helicase activity. The role of the α-accessory protein appears to be the stabilisation of the DNA replication process, thereby enhancing fidelity of replication by reducing the probability of misinsertion.

The expression of oncogenes was initially linked to the level of caloric intake by the work of Nakamura *et al.* (1989) who showed that c-*myc* expression in cells from B6C3F1 was inversely proportional to caloric intake. These findings were extended to the long-lived rodent species *Peromyscus*, where a relationship between body temperature and c-*myc* expression was established (Nakamura *et al.*, 1990) (Figure 8.6). Himeno *et al.* (1992) found a similar effect in rat for c-Ha-*ras*, c-K_1-*ras* and c-*Fos*, but not for c-*myc*. However, it should be pointed out that the procedures and conditions used by Himeno *et al.* (1992) were somewhat different than those used by other investigators (Table 8.7). Lyn-Cook and co-workers (1995) subsequently confirmed the findings of Nakamura *et al.* (1989) and the finding of Himeno *et al.* (1992) that caloric intake was inversely proportional to the expression of c-Ha-*ras* and a c-K_1-*ras* in rat (Table 8.7). Hass *et al.* (1993) and Lyn-Cook *et al.* (1995) have shown that caloric intake is inversely related to DNA methylation and directly related to *in vitro* transformation (Table 8.8). Thus, overall, it would appear that at the genetic level, the greater the caloric intake the less the level of genetic homeostasis and the higher the probability of a loss in the organism's ability to deal with stress.

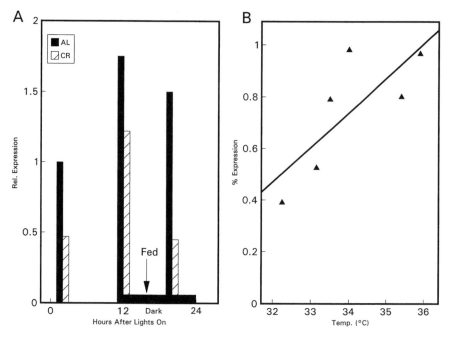

Figure 8.6 Relative expression of c-*myc* oncogene levels as (A) a function of time after lights on and (B) body temperature. Inappropriate expression of c-*myc* is generally higher throughout the day in AL animals than in 40% calorically restricted (CR) ones. 'Fed' indicates when animals (F-344 male rats) are fed; the black bar indicates when lights are off. Activities are in μmol/min/mg protein. Expression also appears to be correlated to body temperature. Figures adapted from Nakamura *et al.* (1989, 1990).

Apoptosis

Apoptosis is a highly regulated and energy-consuming process which effectively removes damaged and preneoplastic cells from the cell population (Steller, 1995). Balanced against factors that regulate proliferation, apoptosis is also essential for keeping cell number constant in tissues. This process is not only important for defence against toxicants, but also for maintaining homeostasis (Kerr *et al.*, 1994; Williams, 1991; Williams and Smith, 1993). Experimental studies in rats have suggested that apoptotic cell death is protective, by removing senescent, DNA-damaged or diseased cells that could potentially interfere with normal function or lead to neoplastic transformation (Ledda-Columbano and Columbano, 1991). Recently, studies by Muskhelishvili *et al.* (1995) have demonstrated that the spontaneous rate of apoptotic cell death is increased either as the level of caloric intake is decreased (Figure 8.7) or with age. The efficacy of increased apoptosis with decreased caloric consumption may be further enhanced due to the induction of a decrease in the rate of cellular proliferation with a decrease in caloric intake.

Table 8.7 Oncogene expression and methylation in animals fed *ad libitum* (AL) or 40% calorically restricted (CR) diets

Cell/Tissue[a]	Oncogene/ Protein	Effect on Expression		DNA Methylation		Reference
		AL	CR	AL	CR	
PA (rat)	c-HA-ras	++++	+	⇓	⇑	Lyn-Cook *et al.* (1995)
PA (rat)	c-Ki-*ras*	+++	+	⇑	⇑	Lyn-Cook *et al.* (1995)
LT (mouse)	c-*myc*			⇑	⇑	Nakamura *et al.* (1989, 1990)
LT (mouse)	c-*myc*					
	(p1, p2, p3)			⇑	⇑	Miyamura *et al.*
	(p4)			⇓	⇑	(1993)
	(p9, p10)			⇑	⇓	
LT (rat)	c-Ha-*ras*	++	+			Himeno *et al.* (1992)
	c-Ki-*ras*	+++	++			
	c-*myc*	++	+++			
	c-*fos*	++++	+			
	TGFα	−	−			
	TGFβ	−	−			
	c-*jun*	−	−			
	c-*erb*A	−	−			
	c-*erb*B	−	−			
	c-*sis*	−	−			
P (rat)	$p21_{mut}$ ――― p21	+++	+			Hass *et al.* (1993)
PA (rat)	$p53_{mut}$ ――― P53	++++	+			Hass *et al.* (1993)

[a]PA, pancreatic acinar cells in culture; LT, Liver tissue.

Table 8.8 Changes in DNA methylation and gene expression in pancreatic acinar cells from Brown–Norway rat[a]

Diet	DNA methylation[b]		DNA expression[c]
	C-H-*ras*	c-K-*ras*	c-H-*ras*
AL	Hypo	Hyper	4X
CR	Hyper	Hyper	1X

[a]Animals at 29 months of age, AL is *ad libitum* feeding, CR is a 40% caloric restriction. Adapted from Haas *et al.* (1993)
[b]HpaII digestion of high-molecular weight DNA (Southern blot).
[c]Slot-analyses of poly (A)[+] mRNA.

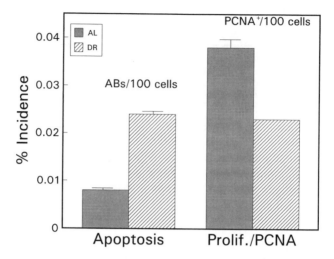

Figure 8.7 Changes in the rates of apoptosis in liver with diet. Apoptotic bodies (AB) per 100 nuclei, measured in male B6C3F1 male mice, at different ages with either *ad libitum* (AL) or restricted (CR) feeding. Grey bars are AL-fed animals; hatched bars are 40% CR mice. Error bars are standard deviation. Data from Muskhelishvili *et al.* (1995).

Conclusions

Over 50 years of work continues to confirm the belief that, while individual dietary components may be of importance in specific age-related changes in tumour occurrence, total caloric intake, as opposed to any one macro- or micro-nutrient, has the greatest overall impact. Since caloric intake modulates nearly every biochemical, molecular, cellular and physiological function associated with cancer it is not surprising that a strong correlation exists between body weight and tumour occurrence (Turturro *et al.*, 1993, 1995). It is also not surprising that, based upon human epidemiological studies, dietary factors are the leading cause of many, if not all, forms of cancer. Now that an extensive body of data has been developed relative to the impact of caloric intake on animal physiology, intermediary metabolism, drug, metabolism, induction of DNA damage, DNA repair, fidelity of DNA replications, apoptosis, neuroendocrine function and immune competency, it is time that these data be applied to the clinical environment. This is now occurring in a collaborative study between the National Center for Toxicological Research and the University of Tennessee at Memphis. This type of work will further improve the use of caloric restriction as a tool in the armamentarium to improve human health and slow the onset of cancer and other diseases.

References

Allaben W, Chou M, Pegram R, Leakey J, Feuers R, Dufy P, Turturro A and Hart R (1990) Modulation of toxicity and carcinogenicity by caloric restriction. *Korean Journal of Toxicology*, **6**, 167–182.

Baron J, Voigt J, Whitter T, Kawabata T, Knapp S, Guengerich F and Jakoby W (1986) Identification of intra tissue sites for xenobiotic activation and detoxication. *Advances in Experimental Medicine and Biology*, **197**, 119–144.

Brash D and Hart R (1977) Molecular biology of aging. In *The Biology of Aging*, Bemke J (ed), Plenum Press Publishing Corp., New York, pp. 57–81.

Busbee D, Miller S, Schroeder M, Srivastava V, Guntupalli G, Merriam E, Holt S, Wilson V and Hart R (1995) DNA polymerase α function and fidelity: dietary restriction as it affects age-related enzyme changes. In *Dietary Restriction: Implications for the Design and Interpretation of Toxicity and Carcinogenicity Studies*, Hart R, Neumann D and Robertson R (eds), ILSI Press, Washington, DC, pp. 245–270.

Chang M, Koestner A and Hart R (1981) Interrelationships between cellular proliferation, DNA alkylation, and age as determinants of ethylnitrosourea-induced neoplasia. *Cancer Letters*, **13**, 39–45.

Chou M, Kong J, Chung K-T and Hart R (1993) Effects of caloric restriction on the metabolic activation of xenobiotics. *Mutation Research*, **295**, 223–235.

Djuric Z, Lu M, Lewis S, Luongo D, Chen X, Heilbrun L, Reading B, Duffy P and Hart R (1992) Oxidative DNA damage levels in rats fed low-fat, high-fat, or caloric-restricted diets. *Toxicology and Applied Pharmacology*, **115**, 156–160.

Djuric Z, Lu MH, Lewis S, Luongo D, Chen X, Heilbrun L, Reading B, Duffy P and Hart R (1995) Effects of dietary calories and fat on levels of oxidative DNA damage. In *Dietary Restriction: Implications for the Design and Interpretation of Toxicity and Carcinogenicity Studies*, Hart R, Neumann D and Robertson R (eds), ILSI Press, Washington, DC, pp. 167–180.

Feuers R, Duffy P, Leakey J, Turturro A, Mittelstaedt R and Hart R (1989) Effect of chronic caloric restriction on hepatic enzymes of intermediary metabolism in the male Fischer 344 rat. *Mechanisms of Ageing and Development*, **48**, 179–189.

Feuers R, Duffy P, Chen F, Desai V, Oriaku E, Shaddock J, Pipkin J, Weindruch R and Hart R (1995) Intermediary metabolism and antioxidant systems. In *Dietary Restriction: Implications for the Design and Interpretation of Toxicity and Carcinogenicity Studies*, Hart R, Neumann D and Robertson R (eds), ILSI Press, Washington, DC, pp. 181–195.

Hart R and Setlow R (1974) Correlation between DNA excision-repair and lifespan in a number of mammalian species. *Proceedings of the National Academy of Sciences, USA*, **71**, 2169–2173.

Hart R and Stephens R (1980) The comparative biology of longevity assurance mechanisms. In *Aging – Its Chemistry*, Proceedings of the 3rd AP Beckman Conference in Clinical Chemistry, Dietz AA (ed), AACC Publications, Winston-Salem, North Carolina, pp. 259–276.

Hart RW and Turturro A (1998) Evolution and dietary restriction. *Experimental Gerontology*, **33**, 53–60.

Hart R, Setlow R and Woodhead A (1977) Evidence that pyrimidine dimers in DNA can give rise to tumors. *Proceedings of the National Academy of Sciences, USA*, **74**, 5574–5578.

Hart R, Sacher G and Hoskins T (1979) DNA repair in a short- and long-lived rodent species. *Journal of Gerontology*, **34**, 808–817.

Hart R, Neumann D and Robertson R (eds) (1995a) *Dietary Restriction: Implications for the Design and Interpretation of Toxicity and Carcinogenicity Studies*, ILSI Press, Washington, DC.

Hart R, Keenan K, Turturro A, Abdo K, Leakey J and Lyn-Cook B (1995b) Symposium overview. Caloric restriction and toxicity. *Fundamental and Applied Toxicology*, **25**, 184–195.

Hart R, Leakey J, Duffy P, Feuers R and Turturro A (1996) The effects of dietary restriction on drug testing and toxicity. *Experimental and Toxicologic Pathology*, **48**, 121–127.

Hass B, Hart R, Lu MH and Lyn-Cook B (1993) Effects of caloric restriction in animals on cellular function, oncogene expression, and DNA methylation *in vitro*. *Mutation Reearch*, **295**, 281–289.

Himeno Y, Engelman R and Good R (1992) Influence of caloric restriction on oncogene expression and DNA synthesis during liver regeneration. *Proceedings of the National Academy of Sciences, USA*, **89**, 5497–5505.

James-Gaylor J, Muskhelishvili L, Gaylor D, Turturro A and Hart R (1998) Upregulation of apoptosis with dietary restriction: Implications for carcinogenesis and aging. *Environmental Health Perspectives*, in press.

Joeschke H (1995) Mechanisms of oxidant stress-induced acute tissue injury. *Proceedings of the Society of Experimental Biology and Medicine*, **209**, 104–111.

Kerr J, Winterford C and Harmon B (1994) Apoptosis. Its significance in cancer and cancer therapy. *Cancer*, **73**, 2013–2026.

Ledda-Columbano G and Columbano A (1991) Apoptosis and hepatocarcinogenesis. In *Apoptosis: the Molecular Basis of Cell Death*, Tomer L and Cope F (eds), Cold Spring Harbor Laboratory Press, New York, pp. 101–119.

Leakey J, Seng J, Manjgaladze M, Kozlovskaya N, Xia S, Lee M-Y, Frame L, Chen S, Rhodes C, Duffy P and Hart R (1995) Influence of caloric intake on drug-metabolizing enzyme expression: relevance to tumorigenesis and toxicity testing. *Dietary Restriction: Implications for the Design and Interpretation of Toxicity and Carcinogenicity Studies*, Hart R, Neumann D, and Robertson R (eds) ILSI Press, Washington, DC, p. 167–180.

Licastro F, Weindruch R, Davis L and Walford R (1988) Effect of dietary restriction upon the age-associated decline of lymphocyte DNA-repair activity in mice. *Age*, **11**, 48–52.

Lipman J, Turturro A and Hart R (1989) The influence of dietary restriction on DNA repair in rodents: a preliminary study. *Mechanisms of Ageing and Development*, **48**, 135–143.

Lyn-Cook B, Blann E, Hass B and Hart R (1995) Oncogene expression and cellular transformation: the effects of dietary restriction. In *Dietary Restriction: Implications for the Design and Interpretation of Toxicity and Carcinogenicity Studies*, Hart R, Neumann D and Robertson R (eds), ILSI Press, Washington, DC, pp. 271–278.

Manjgaladze M, Chen S, Frame L, Seng J, Duffy P, Feuers R, Hart R and Leakey J (1993) Effects of caloric restriction on rodent drug and carcinogen metabolizing enzymes: implications for mutagenesis and cancer. *Mutation Research*, **195**, 201–222.

McCord J (1995) Superoxide radical: controversies, contradictions, and paradoxes. *Proceedings of the Society of Experimental Biology and Medicine*, **109**, 112–117.

Miyamura Y, Tawa R, Koizumi A, Uehara Y, Kurishita H, Kamiyama S and Ono T (1993) Effects of energy restriction on age-associated changes of DNA methylation in mouse liver. *Mutation Research*, **295**, 63–69.

Muskhelishvili L, Hart R, Turturro A and James J (1995) Age-related changes in the intrinsic rate of apoptosis in livers of diet and restricted and *ad libitum*-fed B6C3F1 mice. *American Journal of Pathology*, **147**, 20–24.

Nakamura K, Duffy P, Turturro A and Hart R (1989) The effect of dietary restriction on MYC protooncogene expression in mice: a preliminary study. *Mechanisms of Ageing and Development*, **48**, 199–205.

Nakamura K, Duffy P, Lu MH and Hart R (1990) Dietary fasting reduces hepatic MYC protooncogene expression in *Peromyscus leucopus* mice. *Age*, **13**, 27–31.

Ogawa K, Solt D and Farber E (1980) Phenotypic diversity as an early property of putative preneoplastic hepatocyte populations in liver carcinogenesis. *Cancer Research*, **40**, 725–733.

Poeggeler B, Reiter RJ, Tang D, Chen L and Manchester L (1993) Melatonin, hydroxyl radical-mediated oxidative damage and ageing: a hypothesis. *Journal of Pineal Research*, **14**, 151–168.

Poirier M and Beland F (1994) DNA adduct measurements and tumor incidence during chronic carcinogen exposure in rodents. *Environmental Health Perspectives*, **102**, (Suppl. 6), 161–165.

Spitzer JA (1995) Active oxygen intermediates – beneficial or deleterious? An intro-duction. *Proceedings of the Society of Experimental Biology and Medicine*, **209**, 102–123.

Srivastava VK, Miller S, Schroeder M, Hart R and Busbee D (1993) Age-related changes in expression and activity of DNA polymerase α: some effects of dietary restriction. *Mutation Research*, **295**, 265–280.

Steller H (1995) Mechanisms of genes of cellular suicide. *Science*, **267**, 1445–1449.

Surgeon-General (1988) *The Surgeon-General's Report on Nutrition and Health*, US DHHS, Pub. #88-50210, US DHHS, Washington, DC, pp. 21–82.

Tice R and Setlow R (1985) DNA repair and replication in aging organisms. In *Handbook of the Biology of Aging*, Finch C and Schneider E (eds), Van Nostrand, New York, pp. 173–224.

Turturro A and Hart R (1984) DNA repair mechanism in aging. In *Comparative Pathobiology of major age-related diseases: Current status and research frontiers*, Scarpelli D and Migaki G (eds), A.R. Liss, New York, pp. 19–45.

Turturro A and Hart R (1991) Longevity-assurance mechanisms and caloric restriction. *Annals of the New York Academy of Sciences*, **621**, 363–372.

Turturro A and Hart R (1992) Dietary alteration in the rate of cancer and aging. *Experimental Gerontology*, **27**, 583–592.

Turturro A, Duffy P and Hart R (1993) Modulation of toxicity by diet and dietary macro-nutrient restriction. *Mutation Reseach*, **295**, 151–164.

Turturro A, Blank K, Murasko D and Hart R (1994) Mechanisms of caloric restriction affecting aging and disease. *Annals of the New York Academy of Sciences*, **719**, 159–170.

Turturro A, Duffy P and Hart R (1995) The effect of caloric modulation on toxicity studies. In *Dietary Restriction: Implications for the Design and Interpretation of Toxicity and Carcinogenicity Studies*, Hart R, Neumann D and Robertson R (eds), ILSI Press, Washington, DC, p. 79–98.

Weindruch R and Walford R (1988). *The Retardation of Ageing and Disease by Dietary Restriction*, Charles C. Thomas, Springfield, IL.

Weraarchakull N, Strong R, Wood WE and Richardson A (1989) The effect of aging and dietary restriction on DNA repair. *Experimental Cell Research*, **181**, 197–204.

Williams G (1991) Programmed cell death: apoptosis and oncogenesis. *Cell*, **65**, 1097–1098.

Williams G and Smith C (1993) Molecular regulation of apoptosis: genetic controls on cell death. *Cell*, **74**, 777–779.

9 Lipotropes and Chemical Carcinogenesis

Emmanuel Farber[1] and Amiya K Ghoshal[2]

[1]Department of Pathology, Anatomy and Cell Biology, Jefferson Medical College, Thomas Jefferson University, Philadelphia, PA 19107-6799, USA
[2]Department of Pathology, University of Toronto, Toronto, Ontario, Canada M5S 1A8

Introduction

In the field of nutrition and cancer/cancer development (carcinogenesis), the relationship of lipotropes to chemical carcinogenesis is both an exciting, positive topic and yet is also a very confused one.

The exciting aspect is due to our present realisation that choline deficiency is so far the only model in cancer aetiology and pathogenesis in which a discrete, well-established single nutritional modulation is a direct cause of cancer, without any known or suspected need for added xenobiotics, including carcinogens. Although the literature is replete with suggestions concerning the importance of various lipids, minerals and other dietary components in cancer aetiology and pathogenesis, these remain currently in the realm of popular speculation, with the probable exception of zinc. The genesis of hepatocellular carcinoma in the rat on a choline-devoid diet is well established and appears to be beyond question.

The confusing aspect relates to the chemical and metabolic properties of individual lipotropes and lipotropes as a group, and the metabolic relation between these compounds and choline. Unfortunately, until recently, almost all the studies used 'lipotropes' and 'choline' interchangeably, a practice that has led to great confusion both phenomenologically and mechanistically.

Nutrition and Chemical Toxicity. Edited by Costas Ioannides. © John Wiley & Sons Ltd. ISBN 0 471 97453 6

A brief historical perspective

This topic in physiology, biochemistry and pathology was initiated quite by accident in 1932 when Best and Hunstman (1932) found that dietary raw pancreas was quite effective in preventing fat accumulation and facilitating fat removal from the liver of dogs that were made diabetic experimentally by pancreatectomy. They soon discovered that lecithin and its contained choline were the effective ingredients in the pancreas. Subsequent studies in Best's group (Best et al., 1935) and others later showed that dietary methionine was also effective. The later discoveries of the roles of folic acid and vitamin B_{12} and other less potent nutritional components in the removal of 'fat' from the liver led to the general concept of 'lipotropism and lipotropes' and to the possible role of methylation in this general physiological activity (Best et al., 1953–54).

Studies in several laboratories also observed that the continual chronic exposure of rats and mice to a lipotrope-deficient diet led to the development of fatty cysts (lipodiastemata) and to the progressive development of liver cirrhosis (György and Goldblatt, 1939; Lillie et al., 1942; Hartroft, 1950a,b, 1954; Buckley and Hartroft, 1955; Ashworth et al., 1961; Newberne et al., 1982; Shinozuka and Katyal, 1985).

Also both animal species were shown to develop liver cell cancer on chronic exposure to lipotrope-deficient ('choline-deficient') diets. This was reported first by Copeland and Salmon and their associates (1946; Engel et al., 1947) for the rat, and subsequently by Buckley and Hartroft (1955) for the mouse.

The later discovery of aflatoxins as contaminants of the peanut meal or peanut proteins used in the preparation of the deficient diets threw major doubt on the role of lipotrope-choline-deficiency in the genesis of liver cancer (Salmon and Newberne, 1963; Newberne et al., 1964, 1982; Busby and Wogan, 1984). Peanut meal is a common source of protein in the preparation of lipotrope-deficient diets becaue it is low in methionine. Further research on lipotropes and choline deficiency in respect to carcinogenesis was thrown into disarray – a situation which lasted some 15 years.

The study of choline deficiency in carcinogenesis was revived mainly due to the work of Shinozuka and Lombardi and their colleagues (Shinozuka et al., 1978; Sells et al., 1979; Giambaressi et al., 1982; Newberne et al., 1982). They reported the promoting effect of feeding a choline-devoid, but not a lipotrope-deficient, diet in animals initiated with different chemical carcinogens. Soon thereafter, unequivocal hepatocellular carcinoma was found in rats fed a choline-devoid diet in three different laboratories (Mikol et al., 1983; Ghoshal and Farber, 1984; Yokoyama et al., 1985). There has not as yet been any report that a lipotrope-deficient diet per se with low, but adequate levels of choline, free of aflatoxins or other carcinogens, can induce liver cancer in the rat or mouse (Newberne et al., 1982, Newberne, 1986; Newberne and Rogers, 1986).

The impression derived from the many studies of lipotropes and lipotropism indicated clearly that the lipotropic effect of several dietary constituents appears to be related to their ability to methylate. Presumably, one of the chemical targets for the methylation is phosphatidyl ethanolamine as a precursor for choline in lecithin. Thus, lipotropism is closely related conceptually to methylation. Virtually all experimental and human studies have considered choline deficiency and lipotrope deficiency as being essentially the same with disturbances in methylation, including the genesis of methyl groups and transmethylations, as the fundamental biochemical basis for the pathological changes seen.

Recent studies of Ghoshal, Rushmore, Ghazarian and others in our laboratory have clearly indicated that the 'lumping' of choline deficiency with lipotrope deficiency is very likely unjustified (see Ghoshal and Farber, 1993; Ghoshal, 1995). 'Pure' choline-deficiency in the rat, with a diet devoid of choline, but with adequate but not excessive levels of methionine, folic acid and vitamin B_{12} induces a clinical and pathological picture that is quite different from that seen with lipotrope deficiency. The fundamental biochemical basis for these different syndromes are probably also different mechanistically.

Comparison of effects of choline-deficiency and lipotrope-deficiency in the rat

Before concentrating on the major focus in this discussion, chemical carcinogenesis and lipotropes, it is important to have a clear perspective on how choline deficiency differs from lipotrope deficiency. This brief comparison will enable a more sharply focused view of how choline is closely related to the development of cancer and whether non-choline lipotropes also relate to carcinogenesis (Newberne, 1986; Ghoshal and Farber, 1993; Ghoshal, 1995).

The differences between the response patterns of the rat to a choline-devoid diet (CD) and to a lipotrope-deficient diet (LD) are quite striking and clear-cut (Table 9.1). The CD diets used were made either with pure amino acids (Mikol et al., 1983) or with alcohol-extracted peanut meal, soy protein and casein (Ridout et al., 1954; Young et al., 1956) as the sources of amino acids. The choline content of the control diet was either 0.8% (Ghoshal and Farber, 1984) or 0.2% (Mikol et al., 1983), while the folic acid and vitamin B_{12} contents of both control and CD diets ranged from 2 to 5 mg/kg and 50 μg/kg to 10 mg/kg respectively. The methionine content in both control and CD diets with protein was 1800 mg/kg. The protein diet had no detectable aflatoxin B_1, volatile nitrosamines and nitrosamides, nitrates plus nitrites, malondialdehyde or mutagenic activity with or without activation (Ghoshal and Farber, 1984). The LD diets were quite variable in content, but were generally low or deficient in methionine and choline and low or deficient in folic acid and vitamin B_{12}.

The animals on the LD diets show poor or no weight gain in the different studies (e.g. Hartroft, 1950a,b, 1954; Newberne et al., 1982; Newberne, 1986;

Table 9.1 Comparison of major differences between pathological consequences in the rat with choline-devoid and lipotrope-deficient diets

Consequences	Choline-devoid	Lipotrope-deficient
Body weight	Good weight gain	Poor or no weight gain
Fatty liver	Very rapid periportal (zone 1)	Rapid central (zone 3)
Necrosis	Early (4.5 to 5 days) focal and widespread; at least 50% of hepatocytes within 2 weeks	None; only some ill-defined hepatocyte injury associated with fatty cysts at a late period
'Fatty cysts' (lipodiastemata)	Not seen	Regularly seen after many weeks of LD diet
Cirrhosis	Very infrequent, even after 2 years	Very frequent, almost every rat
Hepatocellular carcinoma	Frequent – at least 50–70% of male rats by 2 years	Uncertain

Zeisel, 1990). This is in contrast to the animals on the CD diets, who showed continual gain in body weight over the many months equal to that of animals fed the control diet with adequate choline levels (0.2 to 0.8 g/100 g) (Mikol *et al.*, 1983; Ghoshal and Farber, 1984). The accumulation of triglycerides (TG) (triacylglycerols) in the liver was equally rapid with CD and LD. However, the LD groups showed the first accumulation in zone 3 ('central') while those in the CD group showed zone 1 ('periportal') fatty liver. Every report on the effects of LD diets in rats that include histological examination stresses the 'central' nature of the fatty liver (e.g. Hartroft 1950a,b, 1954; Shinozuka and Katyal, 1985; Newberne, 1986).

The response of greatest import in the acute phase of the CD deficiency is the highly reproducible liver cell death. This is seen in every male rat, as assessed by three different criteria: (i) histology; (ii) serum enzyme analysis; and (iii) loss of prelabelled DNA (Giambarresi *et al.*, 1982; Ghoshal *et al.*, 1983; Rushmore *et al.*, 1987; Chandar *et al.*, 1987; Chandar and Lombardi, 1988). The degree of cell death is quite considerable, with loss of at least 50% of the hepatocytes within two weeks and lasting many weeks thereafter (Ghoshal *et al.*, 1983). With the LD diets, even minimal or questionable cell death is absent from the liver until many weeks after initiating the diet. Hartroft (1950a,b, 1954), one of the most careful pathogologists to study liver changes in lipotrope deficiency, has stated repeatedly that, 'I have never found clear-cut morphological evidence of acute cell death'. He noted cell death only in association with lipodiastemeta (fatty cysts) at a later time.

Despite the persistence of liver cell death for several months, cirrhosis of the liver is seen in only very few rats, even when fed the CD diet for two years

(Ghoshal and Farber, 1984). This is in sharp contrast to the animals on the LD diets that show a high incidence of liver cirrhosis.

A major difference between the responses to CD and LD relates to the genesis of lipodiastemata (Hartroft, 1950a,b, 1954). These have not been seen in any of the animals fed CD diets, even for long periods of time (Ghoshal and Farber, 1984) and are considered to be a major, if not exclusive, site of origin for the liver fibrosis and cirrhosis in animals fed LD diets.

Unlike the current uncertainties in respect of the carcinogenicity of long-term feeding of LD diet in rats (e.g. Newberne et al., 1982), male Fisher 344 rats develop unequivocal hepatocellular carcinoma, many with metastasis, within two years on a 'pure' CD diet (Mikol et al., 1983; Ghoshal and Farber, 1984; Yokoyama et al., 1985; Chandar and Lombardi, 1988). Exposure to the CD diet for periods as short as 3 and 6 months is sufficient to induce 13 to 27% of liver cancer by 16 months (Chandar and Lombardi, 1988). In all the reports to date, the rats fed the control choline-supplemented diet did not develop liver cancer. Therefore, hepatocellular carcinoma in the rat is unequivocally induced by a pure CD diet with no added or detectable carcinogens. Whether an LD diet, free of aflatoxins or other carcinogens, can also induce hepatocellular carcinoma or other cancers in the rat remains to be established (Newberne et al., 1982).

Pathogenesis of hepatocellular carcinoma with a choline-devoid diet

The topic of 'lipotropes and chemical carcinogenesis' encompasses at last two major areas. The first is the role of lipotropes in the aetiology and pathogenesis of carcinogenesis, and the second is the modulation of chemical carcinogenesis by lipotropes. Although the second may seem to be of greater interest in the context of 'nutrition and chemical toxicity', it cannot be discussed intelligently without a clear view of the first. For example, it has been proposed by Newberne and his colleagues, and by Lombardi and Shinozuka and their colleagues that a major influence of choline deficiency and lipotrope deficiency is in promoting chemical carcinogenesis with known cacinogens. Unfortunately, the assays used were not definitive, since one cannot differentiate between 'true' promotion and the additive effect ('syncarcinogenic effect') (Williams et al., 1987) of two or more carcinogenic processes occurring simultaneously. The studies on the supposed promotion were carried out before it was realised that CD is carcinogenic in its own right and needs no additional carcinogens, of whatever nature, to induce cancer.

The majority, if not all, cancers in humans as well as in animals, both natural and experimental, develop over a relatively long period of time, often involving one-third to one-half or three-quarters of the lifespan. The major segment of this time sequence involves several steps that are not neoplastic, neither benign nor malignant, but focal and seemingly adaptive (Farber, 1996) (Figure 9.1). Several of the steps are reversible in that they show spontaneous remodelling to normal-appearing tissue. There appear to be several different phenotypes before malignancy is seen. The best characterised phenotypes have been described for the liver, especially in rats. The first phenotype occurs during initiation and consists of the appearance of a new biochemical and physiological pattern, the resistance phenotype that appears constitutively. There is a large decrease in the enzymes, such as cytochromes P450, involved in the metabolic activation of many xenobiotics and an increase in their conjugation for excretion (Roomi et al., 1985; Farber, 1996).

This new resistance phenotype occurs in isolated hepatocytes scattered throughout the liver (Gindi et al., 1994) and is constitutive. This phenotype is induced rapidly by a wide variety of genotoxic carcinogens, every one of over 50 so far studied, that either by themselves or after suitable metabolic activation interact with DNA, RNA and protein (Farber, 1996). Also, this phenotype has been found to be induced more slowly by a non-genotoxic carcinogen, clofibrate (Nagai et al., 1993) and by exposure to a CD diet (Ghoshal et al., 1987). For the latter two, the hepatocytes with the resistance phenotype appear between 10 and 24 weeks.

The rare altered hepatocytes that appear during initiation do not show any spontaneous cell proliferation in vivo in the intact organism. Thus, this next major step, clonal expansion occurs actively by selection by providing a stimulus for cell proliferation and, at the same time, inhibiting cell proliferation in the majority of the hepatocytes, but not in the resistant ones (Figure 9.1). This differential inhibition is so far the only established mechanism for clonal expansion during promotion. Diferential stimulation and differential recovery are two other possible mechanisms that so far have not been established (see Farber, 1982).

The pattern of biochemical components in the resistane phenotype does not appear to be 'abnormal' but rather physiological, since it can be induced transiently by exposure to one of several xenobiotics. For example, intravenous lead nitrate (Columbano et al., 1983, 1984; Roomi et al, 1986; Ledda-Columbano et al., 1989) and the antioxidants BHA (butyl hydroxyanisole) and BHT (butyl hydroxy toluene) (Cha and Bueding, 1979; Cha and Heine, 1982) are quite effective.

The genesis of this new constitutive resistance phenotype is a two-step process. The set of biochemical changes is induced by the active form of the carcinogen. The constitutive form of the new phenotype appears after a round of cell proliferation within 96 h thereafter. This resistance phenotype is the basic mechanism for the next step, the clonal expansion to generate hepatocyte nodules. These nodules have two major options: (i) remodelling for the majority; and (ii) persistence. The majority remodel to normal-appearing liver. Presumably, they no longer participate in cancer development. The small minority persist and undergo a series of phenotypic changes, as outlined in Table

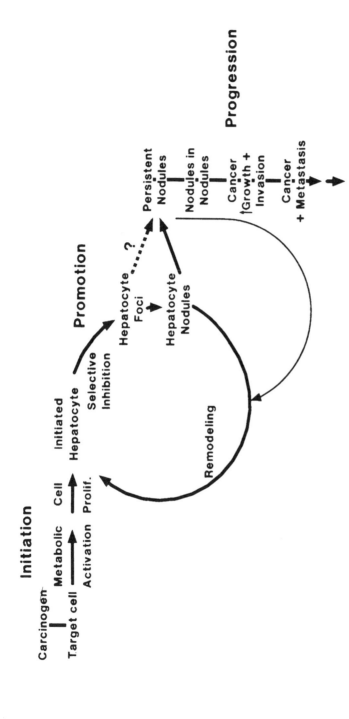

Figure 9.1 Schematic representation of several key steps in the sequence between exposure to a chemical carcinogen and the appearance of hepatocellular carcinoma. Modified from Farber E (1984) with permission.

9.2. The phenotypic outline for nodules generated with chemical carcinogesis, as detailed in Table 9.2 and Figure 9.1 is well established. The nodules in the animals on CD diet have a remarkably similar overall behaviour and set of properties. Although the details of the sequence have not yet been documented, the overall similarity is such as to make it quite certain that the sequences with chemical carcinogens and with the CD diet are similar, if not identical. Thus, one aspect of 'lipotropes and chemical carcinogenesis', that relating to choline deficiency, mirrors chemical carcinogenesis.

The other aspect, namely the effects on the process of carcinogenesis with chemicals is much less clear. As already noted, the experiments on the possible promoting action of choline deficiency are not adequate, since they have not separated 'promotion' and 'syncarcinogenesis'. This can be done, but requires special care. With respect to the possible promoting effects of 'lipotrope deficiency', as LD and CD have been lumped together, it is impossible to arrive at any conclusion, even tentative, in this area. Also, a major complication in this area is the striking effect of LD diet on body weight. As outlined many years ago (Sidransky and Farber, 1958), weight loss or no gain in weight can radically change how the body reacts to many nutritional modulations, even to the point of preventing a response. This may very well have occurred in virtually all of the experiments on 'lipotropes and chemical carcinogenesis'. This is not seen with 'pure' choline deficiency with adequate methionine, folic acid and vitamin B_{12}. Thus, the possible role of 'pure' lipotrope deficiency with adequate, but not excess, choline in promotion of chemical carcinogenesis remains to be analysed, in a rigorous rational manner.

With regard to the initiation of chemical carcinogenesis, there is only one mechanistically controlled study with CD-LD diets (Ghoshal and Farber, 1983). This study showed that feeding a CD diet for a short period of time, sufficient to induce cell death, followed by cell proliferation, can substitute for partial

Table 9.2 Phenotypic properties of persistent nodules leading to cancer

1.	Persistence of resistance phenotype
2.	Spontaneous hepatocyte proliferation
3.	Balance between cell proliferation and cell loss until malignant neoplasia appears
4.	A low progressive remodelling of increasing number of nodules
5.	'Ground-glass hepatocytes' as a common hepatocyte appearance before cancer
6.	Normal diurnal rhythm
7.	Normal response to phenobarbital
8.	New pattern of growth on transplantation to spleen with slow evolution to cancer
9.	Appearance of nodules in nodules
10.	Appearance of hepatocellular carcinoma with nodules with metastasis
11.	Imbalance between cell proliferation and cell loss
12.	'Full-blown' hepatocellular carcinoma
13.	Metastases

hepatectomy or the administration of necrogenic agent such as CCl_4 in inducing the cell proliferation required for initiation. Unfortunately, the several
other studies have not disclosed whether exposure to CD or LD affects the
first step in initiation, activation of the carcinogens (see Rogers, 1975;
Newberne, 1986; Sawada et al., 1990; Schrager et al., 1990; Rogers et al.,
1993; Zeisel and Blusztain, 1994). An attempt to study this was made using
the genesis of bacterial mutagenic derivatives of some chemical carcinogens
(Reddy et al., 1983). Unfortunately, the assay is not reliable in the extrapolation
from in vitro to in vivo. The only reasonably reliable assay so far available is the
extent of interaction of the carcinogens with DNA, RNA and protein under very
carefully controlled in vivo conditions (e.g. Farber et al., 1976).

Of the several studies of the possible effects of CD-LD diets on early steps
in chemical carcinogens, no conclusion is yet possible concerning an effect
on the first step, the activation of chemical carcinogens. The suggestion
concerning an effect on metabolic activation has not yet distinguished
between CD and LD and on whether some of the effects are due to altered
body weights. Also, the possible influence of exposures to CD and to LD on
enzyme activities are conflicting. In one study (Ghoshal et al., 1988), no
change in cytochromes P450, cytochrome b_5, glutathione S-transferase, DT-
diaphorase (quinone reductase), glutathione peroxidase, glutathione reductase, superoxide dismutase (cytosolic and mitochrondrial) and total catalase
activation over an 8-day period were seen. Glutathione concentration
increased over the same period. These results seem to be in conflict with
those of other studies, less well controlled, in which CD-LD diets induced
decreases in cytochromes oxidase or cytochromes P450 (Rogers and
Newberne, 1971; Greim et al., 1975; Poirier et al., 1977; Campbell et al.,
1978; Reddy et al., 1983). These studies unfortunately did not regularly control body weight and did not compensate for changes in liver weight such as
those due to triglyceride accumulation.

Following the two initiation steps and the early clonal expansion to generate foci, the hepatic nodules undergo a series of phenotypic changes as
documented in Table 9.2. As yet, these phenotypes have not been carefully
related to particular steps in the sequence leading to unequivocal malignant
neoplasia. This type of study will no doubt provide much more insight into
how cancer develops. However, it appears that the changes seen with chemical carcinogens seem to be reproduced, at least in principle, in those seen
with cancer development following exposure to a CD diet. The overall similarity between the proposed sequence of changes from the initial exposure to
cancer for chemical carcinogens (genotoxic), non-genotoxic carcinogens such
as clofibrate and carcinogenesis with exposure to a CD diet ('pure choline
deficiency') is outlined in Figure 9.2. At this juncture in our understanding, it
appears that there is an unusual degree of correspondence in all three types
of systems.

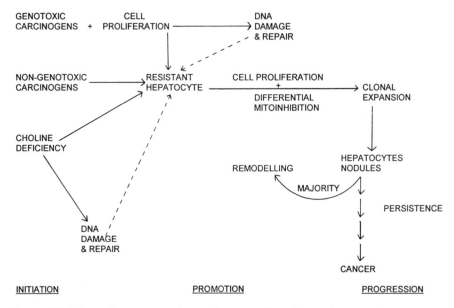

Figure 9.2 Schematic representation of the several similarities between liver carcinogenesis induced by genotoxic chemical carcinogens, non-genotoxic chemical carcinogens and choline deficiency.

Biochemical mechanisms

The exposure of a male rat to a CD diet induced a highly reproducible series of biochemical and biological changes in the liver, which are outlined in Table 9.3. These changes, together with some more general considerations relating to our current views on carcinogenesis, offer a few possibilities for biochemical mechanisms.

There is a widespread feeling that structural gene changes, such as mutations, are the basis for the development of cancer, including the many early phenotypic changes that are regularly seen before the appearance of malignant neoplasia, and that constitute the process of carcinogenesis. They are remarkably similar in principle in many different organs and tissues and with different aetiologic agents including genotoxic carcinogens, some viruses, some forms of radiation and choline deficiency. Although the associations between a whole variety of mutations and cancer are well known, it is not known whether these associations are 'cause or effect'. As discussed lucidly by Prehn (1994), we do not know whether 'cancers beget mutations' or 'mutations beget cancers'. It is possible that many, if not the majority of, phenotypic changes in cancer development are epigenetic rather than genetic, and are the consequence of constitutive changes in gene expression (Prehn, 1994). On this basis, the long period of carcinogenesis before unequivocal malignant neoplasia supervenes

Table 9.3 Sequence of known liver changes with dietary choline deficiency

Time	Biochemical pathology
6–8 hours	Fatty liver, periportal (not central) progressively involving all the liver cells by days 4 to 5
24 hours	Lipid peroxidation in nuclei
48 hours	Alkali-sensitive alteration in DNA (DNA damage and repair)
72 hours	Increase in activity of phospholipase A_2 in microsomes (but not in nuclei)
$4\frac{1}{2}$ to 5 days	Onset of progressive liver cell death with at least 50% by day 14
5 days	Lipid peroxidation in mitochondria
10 weeks	Initiation of liver carcinogenesis with appearance of rare resistant hepatocytes with resistance biochemical phenotype
1 year	First appearance of hepatocellular carcinoma with metastasis

may well be fundamentally a form of adaptation, termed 'clonal adaptation' which has survival value for the reacting organism (Nicholson, 1950; Farber, 1996).

A common form of structural gene change that is a focus for both carcinogens and lipotropes concerns the methylation of DNA. There is considerable evidence that a major form of modulation of gene expression is methylation of cytosine leading mainly to gene suppression, but also sometimes to gene activation (Doerfler, 1983; Taylor, 1984; Razin *et al.*, 1984). This realisation has fostered a large interest in the possibility that alteration in DNA methylation may be a key or at least an important basis for some of the altered behaviour of many different cancers (Halliday, 1979; Nyce *et al.*, 1983; Riggs and Jones, 1983; Locker *et al.*, 1986; Shivapurkur *et al.*, 1986; Hsieh *et al.*, 1989; Wainfan *et al.*, 1989; Jones and Buckley, 1990; Dizik *et al.*, 1991; Wainfan and Poirier, 1992). The majority, if not all, of these studies on cancer suffer from both technical and conceptual deficiencies.

Technically, it is well established that the methylation of cytosine, the only known methylation site in mammalian DNA, occurs post-synthetically. The methylated cytosine in the parent DNA is reproduced as cytosine and is then methylated when double stranded. Obviously, proliferating cells all have a period, albeit quite short, of being under-methylated before the methylation occurs. This is even evident in a more or less reasonably synchronous system, such as after partial hepatectomy (Kanduc *et al.*, 1988, 1991). It is particularly evident in any neoplastic process in which the cell population is almost completely asynchronous. Also, the presence of cell death makes the assay almost uninterpretable with the assay of DNA alterations. Thus, the complexities in the analysis of levels of methylation in cancer and in precancerous changes make any reasonable interpretation virtually impossible. Clearly, the many studies of DNA methylation in cancer are quite technically unreliable. They have to be repeated under much more controlled conditions before any conclusions are acceptable.

This area has a further conceptual problem which applies to all studies of the biochemistry–molecular biology of mechanisms of carcinogenesis. All the studies in mutations and DNA methylation in cancer relate to one or more genes, such as p53, Rb H-K- and N-*ras, myc*, etc. associated with disturbances in cell and the cell cycle. These are either stimulatory or inhibitory for cell proliferation. Yet, no *real* carcinogenic process known in animals and man, other than *in vitro* cell culture, has any disturbance in growth until very late in the process when malignant neoplasia appears. Thus, no gene suggested to be involved in the long period of carcinogenesis has any phenotypic validation. There is not a signal phenotypic validation for any of the studies on methylation of DNA or mutations of DNA until perhaps very late in the carcinogenic process when unequivocal malignant behaviour is present. This pertains equally well to all the carcinogenic systems, including not only chemical carcinogenesis, but also cancer induced by choline deficiency and the possible hypothetical modulations with lipotrope deficiencies.

Another common misconception relates to cell proliferation. It is often stated that cell proliferation, by iteself, can lead to cancer. With choline deficiency, and possibly the several forms of lipotrope deficiencies, cell proliferation is often seen fairly early. As detailed fairly recently (Farber, 1995), there is no evidence that cell proliferation *per se* can lead to cancer. This also pertains to the chronic cell proliferation seen in rats exposed to a CD diet.

A prominent feature in the biochemical pathology of choline deficiency is lipid peroxidation and the genesis of free radicals (Table 9.4). As outlined in Table 9.4, aldehydes as well as other indices of free radical generation are seen in choline deficiency. It has been proposed that the free radicals may play a role in generating the DNA damage seen in the liver with choline deficiency and this may relate to the initiation process (Figure 9.2) as well as to later steps in the carcinogenic process (Ghoshal and Farber, 1993). This speculation suffers from the same severe limitation as do the other considerations relating to DNA and gene alterations, namely the absence of phenotypic validation.

Some brief general considerations

The role of choline in the genesis of cancer is truly an exciting development in the field of nutrition and cancer. However, the possible larger role of lipotropes in carcinogenesis, either by themselves or as modulators of cancer with chemical carcinogens, offers a real challenge. Clearly, the dietary alterations must be much better controlled with the study of single variables, as is already evident with choline deficiency in the presence of methionine, folic acid, vitamin B_{12} and other nutrients related to lipotropism. Such studies could

Table 9.4 Evidence for free radical activity in liver with choline deficiency

1.	Lipid peroxidation in nuclei by 24 hours
2.	Radicophile AD_5 (N-p-methoxphenylacetyldehydroso-alanine) prevents lipid peroxidation
3.	Free radical trapping agents, such as α-phenyl-tert-butylnitrone (PBN) and tert-nitrosobutane (tNB) prevent lipid peroxidation
4.	Calcium and strontium prevent lipid peroxidation
5.	Lipid peroxidation is followed in time by DNA alteration and hepatocyte cell death, and all of these effects are prevented by the above agents
6.	Inhibition of phospholipase A_2 (PLA_2) increases lipid peroxidation, which now appears also in microsomes
7.	Aldehydes appear in liver cells following lipid peroxidation as with other instances of lipid peroxidation in the liver and these are prevented by PLA_2 as well as by inhibiting lipid peroxidation
8.	Radicophiles AD_5, PBN and tNB prevent not only lipid peroxidation, but also DNA alterations and cell death, even when administered after lipid peroxidation appears in the nuclei

add in a major way to our understanding of how diet relates to carcinogenesis and to suggestions for the prevention of cancer development in humans.

Also, an important area that requires major new approaches is the development of ways to show phenotypic validations to nutritional studies. Without reasonable and testable hypotheses with phenotypic properties as end-points, the area will cointinue in the realm of speculation, an unfortunate prospect for the prevention of cancer. Since cancer and all the many steps that precede cancer during carcinogenesis have as the key manifestations phenotypic changes, any rational hypothesis for pathogenesis must have a phenotype as an end-point. As with any multi-step process, the challenge becomes the development of rational hypotheses for each major step, hypotheses that can be tested and that offer mechanistic possibilities for the next step in the process. The slower rates of development of cancer with choline, and other important nutrients offer new possible approaches that could lead to new ways to prevent some cancers.

References

Ashworth CT, Sanders E and Arnold N (1961) Hepatic lipids: fine structural changes in liver cell after high fat, high cholesterol and choline-deficient diets in rats. *Archives of Pathology*, **72**, 33–44.

Best CH and Huntsman ME (1932) The effects of the components of lecithin upon deposition of fat in the liver. *Journal of Physiology*, **75**, 405–412.

Best CH, Huntsman ME and Ridout JH (1935) The lipotropic effect of proteins. *Nature*, **735**, 821–822.

Best CH, Lucas GC and Ridout JH (1953–54) The lipotropic factors. *Annals of the New York Academy of Science*, **57**, 646–653.

Buckley GF and Hartroft WS (1955) Pathology of choline deficiency in the mouse. *Archives of Pathology*, **59**, 185–197.

Busby WF and Wogan GN (1984) Aflatoxins. In *Chemical Carcinogens*, Searle CE (ed), ACS Monograph 182, Washington, vol 2, pp. 945–1136.

Campbell C, Hays JR and Newberne PM (1978) Dietary lipotropes, hepatic mixed function oxidase activities and *in vivo* covalent binding of aflatoxin-B$_1$ in rats. *Cancer Research*, **38**, 4569–4573.

Cha Y-N and Bueding E (1979) Effects of 2(3)-tert-butyl-4-hydroxyanisole administration on the activities of several hepatic microsomal and cytoplasmic enzymes in mice. *Biochemical Pharmacology*, **28**, 1917–1921.

Cha Y-N and Heine HS (1982) Comparative effects of dietary administration of 2(3)-tert-butyl-4-hydroxyanisole and 3, 5-di-tert-4-hydroxytoluene on several hepatic enzyme activities in mice and rats. *Cancer Research*, **42**, 2609–2615.

Chandar N and Lombardi B (1988) Liver cell proliferation and incidence of hepatocellular carcinomas in rats fed consecutively a choline-devoid and choline-supplemented diet. *Carcinogenesis*, **9**, 259–263.

Chandar N, Amenta J, Kandala C and Lombardi B (1987) Liver cell turnover in rats fed a choline-devoid diet. *Carcinogenesis*, **8**, 669–673.

Columbano A, Ledda GM, Sirigu P, Perra T and Pani P (1983) Liver cell proliferation induced by a single dose of lead nitrate. *American Journal of Pathology*, **116**, 83–88.

Columbano A, Ledda-Columbano GM, Coni P, Vargiu M, Faa G and Pani P (1984) Liver hyperplasia and regression after lead nitrate administration. *Toxicologic Pathology*, **12**, 89–95.

Copeland DH and Salmon WD (1946) The occurrence of neoplasms in the liver, lungs and other tissues of rats as a result of prolonged choline deficiency. *American Journal of Pathology*, **22**, 1059–1081.

Dizik M, Christman JK and Wainfan E (1991) Alterations in expression and methylation of specific genes in livers of rats fed a cancer-promoting methyl-deficient diet. *Carcinogenesis*, **12**, 1307–1312.

Doerfler W (1983) DNA methylation and gene activity. *Annual Review of Biochemistry*, **52**, 93–124.

Engel RW, Copeland DH and Salmon WD (1947) Carcinogenic effects associated with diets deficient in choline and related nutrients. *Annals of the New York Academy of Science*, **49**, 49–67.

Farber E (1982) Sequential events in chemical carcinogenesis. In *Cancer: A Comprehensive Treatise*, Becker FF (ed), Vol. 1, 2nd edn, Plenum Publishing Co., New York, pp. 485–506.

Farber E (1984) Cellular biochemistry of the stepwise development of cancer with chemicals: GHA Clowes memorial lecture. *Cancer Research*, **44**, 5463–5474.

Farber E (1995) Cell proliferation as a major risk factor for cancer; a concept of doubtful validity. *Cancer Research*, **55**, 3759–3762.

Farber E (1996) The step-by-step development of epithelial cancer: from phenotype to genotype. *Advances in Cancer Research*, **70**, 21–48.

Farber E, Parker S and Gruenstein M (1976) The resistance of putative premalignant liver cell populations, hyperplastic nodules, to the acute cytotoxic effects of some hepatocarcinogens. *Cancer Research*, **36**, 3879–3887.

Ghoshal AK (1995) New insight into the biochemical pathology of liver in choline deficiency. *Critical Reviews in Biochemisry and Molecular Biology*, **30**, 263–273.

Ghoshal AK and Farber E (1983) The induction of resistant hepatocytes during initiation of liver carcinogenesis with chemicals in rats fed a choline deficient methionine low diet. *Carcinogenesis*, **4**, 801–804.

Ghoshal AK and Farber E (1984) The induction of liver cancer by a dietary deficiency of choline and methionine without added carcinogens. *Carcinogenesis*, **5**, 1367–1370.

Ghoshal AK and Farber E (1993) Biology of Disease; choline deficiency, lipotrope deficiency and the development of liver disease including liver cancer: a new perspective. *Laboratory Investigation*, **68**, 255–260.

Ghoshal AK, Ahluwalia M and Farber E (1983) The rapid induction of liver cell death in rats fed a choline-deficient methionine low diet. *American Journal of Pathology*, **113**, 309–314.

Ghoshal AK, Rushmore TH and Farber E (1987) Initiation of carcinogenesis by a dietary deficiency of choline in the absence of added carcinogens. *Cancer Letters*, **36**, 289–296.

Ghoshal A, Roomi MW, Ahluwalia M, Simmonds W, Rushmore TH, Farber E and Ghoshal AK (1988) Glutathione and enzymes related to free radical metabolism in liver of rats fed a choline-devoid low methionine diet. *Cancer Letters*, **41**, 53–62.

Giambarresi LK, Katyal SL and Lombardi B (1982) Promotion of liver carcinogenesis in the rat by a choline-devoid diet: role of liver cell necrosis and regeneration. *British Journal of Cancer*, **46**, 825–829.

Gindi T, Ghazarian DMD, Deitch D and Farber E (1994) An origin of presumptive preneoplastic foci and nodules from hepatocytes in chemical carcinogenesis in rat liver. *Cancer Letters*, **83**, 75–80.

Greim H, Czyban P, Garro AJ, Hutterer F, Schaffner F and Popper H (1975) Cytochrome P-450 in the activation and inactivation of carcinogens. *Advances in Experimental Medicine and Biology*, **58**, 103–105.

György P and Goldblatt H (1939) Hepatic injury on a nutritional basis in rats. *Journal of Experimental Medicine*, **76**, 185–192.

Halliday R (1979) A new theory of carcinogenesis. *British Journal of Cancer*, **40**, 513–522.

Hartroft WS (1950a) Accumulation of fat in liver cells and in lipodiastemata preceding experimental dietary cirrhosis. *Anatomical Record*, **106**, 61–87.

Hartroft WS (1950b) The locus of the beginning of dietary cirrhosis. *Transactions of the 8th Conference on Liver Injury*, pp. 126–164.

Hartroft WS (1954) The sequence of pathological events in the development of experimental fatty liver and cirrhosis. *Annals of the New York Academy of Science*, **57**, 633–645.

Hsieh LL, Wainfan E, Hoshina S, Dizik M and Weinstein B (1989) Altered expression of retrovirus-like sequences and cellular oncogenes in mice fed methyl-deficient diets. *Cancer Research*, **49**, 3795–3799.

Jones PA and Buckley JD (1990) The role of DNA methylation in cancer. *Advances in Cancer Research*, **54**, 1–23.

Kanduc D, Ghoshal A, Quagliariello E and Farber E (1988) DNA hypomethylation in ethionine-induced rat preneoplastic hepatocyte nodules. *Biochemical Biophysical Research Communications*, **50**, 739–744.

Kanduc D, Rossiello MR, Aresta A, Cavazza C, Quagliariello E and Farber E (1991) Transitory DNA hypomethylation during liver cell proliferation induced by a single dose of lead nitrate. *Archives of Biochemistry and Biophysics*, **286**, 212–216.

Ledda-Columbano GM, Columbano A, Curto M, Ennas MEG, Coni P, Sarma DSR and Pani P (1989) Further evidence that mitogen-induced cell proliferation does not support the formation of enzyme-altered islands in rat liver by carcinogens. *Carcinogenesis*, **120**, 847–850.

Lillie RD, Ashburn LL, Sebrell WH, Daft FS and Lowry JV (1942) Histogenesis and repair of the hepatic cirrhosis in rats produced by low protein diets and preventable with choline. *US Public Health Reports*, **57**, 502–508.

Locker J, Reddy TV and Lombardi B (1986) DNA methylation and hepatocarcinogenesis in rats fed a choline-devoid diet. *Carcinogenesis*, **7**, 1309–1312.

Mikol YB, Hoover KL, Creasia D and Poirier LA (1983) Hepatocarcinogenesis in rats fed methyl-deficient amino-acid defined diets. *Carcinogenesis*, **4**, 1619–1629.

Nagai MK, Armstrong D and Farber E (1993) Induction of resistant hepatocytes by clofibrate, a non-genotoxic carcinogen. *Proceedings of the American Association for Cancer Research*, **34**, 981.

Newberne PM (1986) Liptotropic factors and oncogenesis. In *Essential Nutrients in Carcinogenesis*, Poirier LA, Newberne PM and Pariza MW (eds), Plenum Publishing Corporation, New York, pp. 223–251.

Newberne PM and Rogers AE (1986) Labile methyl group and the promotion of cancer. *Annual Review of Nutrition*, **6**, 407–432.

Newberne PM, Carlton WW and Wogan GN (1964) Hepatomas in rats and hepatomal injury induced by peanut meal or *Aspergillus flavus* extract. *Pathology Vet*, **1**, 105–132.

Newberne PM, DeCamago LV and Clark AS (1982) Choline deficiency, partial hepatectomy and live tumors in rats and mice. *Toxicologic Pathology*, **10**, 95–109.

Nicholson GW deP (1950) *Studies on Tumor Formation*, Butterworth & Co., London, pp. 249–261.

Nyce J, Weinhouse S and Magee PN (1983) 5-Methylctyosine depletion during tumor development: an extension of the miscoding concept. *British Journal of Cancer*, **48**, 463–475.

Poirier LA, Grantham PH and Rogers AE (1977) The effects of a marginally lipotrope-deficient diet on the hepatic levels of S-adenosyl-methionine and on urinary metabolites of 2-acetylaminofluorene in rats. *Cancer Research*, **37**, 744–748.

Prehn, RT (1994) Cancers beget mutations versus mutations beget cancers. *Cancer Research*, **54**, 5296–5300.

Razin A, Cedar H and Riggs AD (eds) (1984) *DNA Methylation, Biochemistry and Biological Significance*, Springer-Verlag, New York.

Reddy TV, Ramanathan R, Shinozuka H and Lombardi B (1983) Effects of dietary choline deficiency in the mutagenic activation of chemical carcinogens by rat liver fractions. *Cancer Letters*, **18**, 41–48.

Ridout JH, Lucas CC, Patterson JM and Best CH (1954) Changes in chemical composition during the development of cholesterol fatty livers. *Biochemical Journal*, **58**, 297–301.

Riggs AD and Jones PA (1983) 5-Methylcytosine, gene regulation and cancer. *Advances in Cancer Research*, **54**, 1–23.

Rogers AE (1975) Variable effects of a lipotrope deficient, high fat diet on chemical carcinogenesis in rats. *Cancer Research*, **35**, 2469–2474.

Rogers AE and Newberne PM (1971) Nutrition and aflatoxin carcinogenesis. *Nature*, **299**, 62–63.

Rogers AE, Zeisel SH and Groopman J (1993) Commentary. Diet and carcinogenesis. *Carcinogenesis*, **14**, 2205–2217.

Roomi MW, Ho RK, Sarma DSR and Farber E (1985) A common biochemical pattern in hepatocyte nodules generated in four different models in the rat. *Cancer Research*, **45**, 564–571.

Roomi NW. Columbano A, Ledda-Columbana GM and Sarma DSR (1986) Lead nitrate induces certain biochemical properties characteristic of hepatocyte nodules. *Carcinogenesis*, **7**, 1643–1646.

Rushmore TH, Ghazarian DM, Subrahmanyan V, Farber E and Ghoshal AK (1987) Probable free radical effects on rat liver nuclei during early hepatocarcinogenesis with a choline-devoid low methionine diet. *Cancer Research*, **47**, 6731–6740.

Salmon WD and Newberne PM (1963) Occurrence of hepatomas in rats fed diets containing peanut meal as a major source of protein. *Cancer Research*, **23**, 571–575.

Sawada N, Poirier L, Moran S, Xu Y-H and Pitot HC (1990) The effect of choline and methionine deficiencies on the number and volume percentage of altered hepatic foci in the presence or absence of diethylnutrosamine initiation in rat liver. *Carcinogenesis*, **11**, 273–281.

Schrager TF, Newberne PM, Pikul AG and Groopman JD (1990) Aflatoxin DNA adduct formation in chronically dosed rats fed a choline-deficient diet. *Carcinogenesis*, **11**, 177–180.

Sells MA, Katyal SL, Sell S, Shinozuka H and Lombardi B (1979) Induction of foci of altered gamma-glutamyl-transpeptidase positive hepatocytes in carcinogen-treated rats fed a diet devoid of choline. *British Journal of Cancer*, **40**, 274–283.

Shinozuka H and Katyal SL (1985) Pathology of choline deficiency. In *Nutritional Pathology*, Sidransky H (ed) Marcel Dekker, New York, pp. 279–320.

Shinozuka H, Lombardi B, Sell S and Yammarino RM (1978) Early histological and functional alterations of ethionine liver carcinogenesis in rats fed a choline-deficient diet. *Cancer Research*, **38**, 1092–1098.

Shivapurkur N, Wilson MJ, Hoover KL, Mikol YB, Creasia D and Poirier LA (1986) Hepatic DNA methylation and liver tumor formation in male C3H mice fed methionine-and-choline-deficient diets. *Journal of the National Cancer Institute*, **77**, 213–217.

Sidransky H and Farber E (1958) Chemical pathology of acute amino acid deficiencies. I-Morphologic changes in immature rats fed threonine-, methionine- and histidine-devoid diets. *AMA-Archives of Pathology*, **66**, 119–134.

Taylor JH (1984) *DNA Methylation and Cellular Differentiation*, Springer-Verlag, New York.

Wainfan E and Poirier L (1992) Methyl group in carcinogenesis: effects on DNA methylation and gene expression. *Cancer Research*, **54**, 2071S–2077S.

Wainfan E, Dizik M, Stender M and Christman JK (1989) Rapid appearance of hypomethylated DNA in livers of rats fed cancer-promoting, methyl-deficient diets. *Cancer Research*, **49**, 4094–4097.

Williams GM, Maruyama H and Tanaka T (1987) Lack of rapid initiating, promoting or sequential syncarcinogenic effects of di (2 ethylhexyl) phthalate in rat liver carcinogenesis. *Carcinogenesis*, **8**, 875–880.

Yokoyama S, Sells MA, Reddy TV and Lombardi B (1985) Hepatocarcinogenesis and promoting action of a choline-devoid diet in the rat. *Cancer Research*, **45**, 2834–2842.

Young RJ, Lucas CC, Patterson JM and Best CH (1956) Lipotropic dose-response studies in rats: comparisons of choline, betaine and methionine. *Canadian Journal of Biochemistry and Physiology*, **34**, 713–720.

Zeisel SH (1990) Choline deficiency. *Journal of Nutritional Biochemistry*, **1**, 332–349.

Zeisel SH and Blusztain JK (1994) Choline and human nutrition. *Annual Review of Nutrition*, **14**, 269–296.

10 Expression of Chemical Toxicity in Vitamin Deficiency and Supplementation

Gary Williamson

Biochemistry Department, Institute of Food Research, Norwich Research Park, Colney, Norwich, NR4 7UA, UK

Introduction

This chapter examines free radicals as chemical toxins which can lead to a manifestation of toxicity as carcinogenesis. Free radicals, especially reactive oxygen species (ROS), are generated by both endogenous metabolism and by external insults such as UV light, chemical toxins, cigarette smoke, diesel exhaust fumes, burnt food, infection, inflammation, etc. By a series of events, production of ROS leads to modified cellular components, especially lipids, proteins and DNA. Modification of these cellular targets leads to altered gene expression and cellular growth effects, including carcinogenesis. Protection against the ROS insult is provided by dietary antioxidants such as vitamins E and C, flavonoids and selenium, and by endogenous defences such as glutathione and glutathione-linked enzymes. Many dietary antioxidants also influence antioxidant defences. Epidemiological studies show that diets rich in fruit and vegetables, and therefore antioxidants, reduce the risk of many cancers. Animal studies show cancer protective (chemopreventive) effects of dietary antioxidants, and studies on humans using biomarkers to indicate cancer susceptibility often indicate a protective effect of antioxidants. The evidence overall is strongly indicative that antioxidants reduce cancer risk in humans, but conclusive proof of this effect continues to be elusive. The coverage of the chapter is shown in Figure 10.1. The potential information available in this area is huge, and only certain aspects of the field are covered. The chapter should be read with frequent reference to Figure 10.1, since this illustrates how the components of the whole chapter fit together. There is not enough space to

Nutrition and Chemical Toxicity. Edited by Costas Ioannides. © John Wiley & Sons Ltd. ISBN 0 471 97453 6

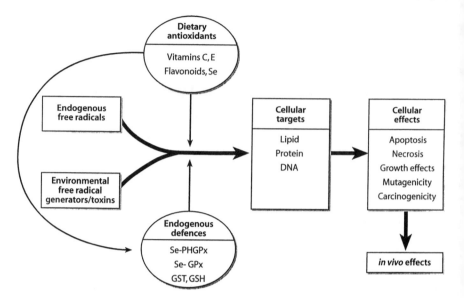

Figure 10.1 Interactions between toxicity of reactive oxygen species, antioxidants, cellular effects and consequences for the organism. Se-PHGPx, selenium-dependent phospholipid glutathione peroxidase; Se-GPx, selenium-dependent glutathione peroxidase; GST, glutathione-S-transferase; GSH, glutathione.

cover any aspect in detail, but at least one review or book is included in each of the sections, to enable the reader to examine each further.

Sources of free radicals

ENDOGENOUS SOURCES OF FREE RADICALS

Normal metabolic processes involving the transfer of electrons are tightly coupled. However, a small amount of 'leakage' occurs, and 1–3% of the oxygen which is inhaled generates superoxide (Halliwell and Aruoma, 1997). These reactive oxygen species (such as superoxide, hydroxyl radical, hydrogen peroxide and singlet oxygen) can react with DNA, lipid and protein and modify structure and function. Several small biological molecules, such as adrenaline, dopamine and tetrahydrofolates, generate superoxide and hydrogen peroxide on direct oxidation by O_2. Phagocytes produce ROS to kill invading organisms, and inflammation increases the production of ROS, partly owing to increased phagocytic activity. Several enzymes are also particularly likely to lead to the production of ROS, and some of these are indicated below.

Lipoxygenases

Lipoxygenases catalyse a pro-oxidant reaction and convert unsaturated lipids to lipid hydroperoxides (see p. 240). These are intermediates in eicosanoid synthesis, which are involved in the inflammatory response. Lipid hydroperoxides are products of oxidative damage to lipids and uncontrolled production can lead to disruption of membrane permeability and modification of DNA by reactive aldehydic products. Lipoxygenases have been reviewed (Nelson and Seitz, 1994; Gaffney, 1996).

Cytochrome P450

Cytochromes P450 are a large family of enzymes which catalyse a variety of oxygenation, demethylation and hydroxylation reactions. Some families of cytochromes P450 are involved in the metabolism of xenobiotics, and are inducible by a wide range of dietary and environmental compounds. Increased cellular membrane levels of cytochromes P450 leads to increased susceptibility of the membranes to lipid peroxidation (Minotti, 1989; Lambert *et al.*, 1996). Several reviews are available on the cytochromes P450 (Hasemann *et al.*, 1995; Poulos, 1995; Guengerich, 1995).

Cytokines

Cytokines are proteins which are produced by a wide variety of cells and influence the behaviour of other cells. Typical cytokines are tumour necrosis factors, (transforming) growth factors, interleukins and interferons. These proteins activate signal transduction mechanisms in cells, which leads to altered gene expression. Tumour necrosis factors and interleukins give rise to the inflammatory response, which involves intracellular production of free radicals, via activation of phospholipases. ROS are involved in mediation of the response of cytokines. This complex area is the subject of several books and reviews (Arai *et al.*, 1990; Clemens, 1991; Damas, 1991; Grimble, 1996).

ENVIRONMENTAL SOURCES OF FREE RADICALS

Free radicals and ROS can arise from a variety of external sources. UV irradiation is significant for initiation of skin carcinogenesis and for cataractogenesis (Spector *et al.*, 1993). Environmental ozone, cigarette smoke and diesel exhausts all generate free radicals (Halliwell and Cross, 1995). Dietary quinolines from burnt meat and fish may be mutagenic and pro-oxidant (Parke and Ioannides, 1994). Dioxin from some industrial bleaching processes is also strongly pro-oxidant via induction of Phase I enzymes (Schrenk *et al.*, 1995). Undoubtedly, the greatest source of free radicals is cigarette smoke, and this increases the risk of lung cancer in smokers compared with non-smokers.

Mechanisms by which free radicals interact with biological systems

INTERACTIONS WITH LIPIDS

Lipids containing unsaturated fatty acids rapidly break down in the presence of transition metals by a process of lipid peroxidation to produce lipid hydroperoxides. Once initiated, the process is autocatalytic, which means that a few initiating events can lead to total membrane destruction in the absence of antioxidants. The process is highly dependent on the presence of transition metals, especially iron, and on oxygen. Most iron is very efficiently sequestered by ferritin and transferrin, but oxidative stress can cause the mobilisation of iron from these iron stores. For example, superoxide can cause release of iron from ferritin (Buettner *et al.*, 1987). Iron and hydrogen peroxide form hydroxyl radicals by Fenton chemistry, which damage biological molecules, including lipids. The products of lipid peroxidation are a complex mixture, but include alkenals, which react with biological targets including DNA (Eisenbrand *et al.*, 1995). There is a vast literature on lipid peroxidation, and the interested reader is referred to several reviews on the subject (Horton and Fairhurst, 1987; Gutteridge and Halliwell, 1990; Esterbauer, 1991; Halliwell *et al.*, 1992).

INTERACTIONS WITH PROTEIN

Proteins are targets for free radical attack, but the mechanism of the reactions involved is not as well studied as lipid peroxidation. Like lipids, proteins form hydroperoxides on reaction with ROS, but each amino acid shows different reactivity (Figure 10.2; Gebicki and Gebicki, 1993). Protein hydroperoxides break down to give a variety of products, especially carbonyls. Carbonyl groups can be readily measured using 2,4-dinitrophenylhydrazine, and so have been used as an estimate of protein damage, but the method also measures proteins that have reacted with products of lipid peroxidation (Halliwell and Aruoma, 1997).

INTERACTIONS WITH DNA

There are a large number of oxidative 'hits' on DNA per cell, since DNA damage occurs continously *in vivo*. A low level of DNA damage products can be measured in human cells and tissues, and this reflects a steady-state level of balance between repair and damage. This baseline level is affected by many factors, including ROS, genotoxins, mutagens, carcinogens and radiation. Several ROS-modified forms of DNA bases have been described. The most frequently oxidised DNA base products are thymine glycol, 8-hydroxyguanine and 8-oxoguanine (Halliwell and Aruoma, 1997). DNA single-strand breaks can arise from oxidation of the sugar phosphate backbone. Some structures of the products of DNA damage are shown in Figure 10.3. There are several

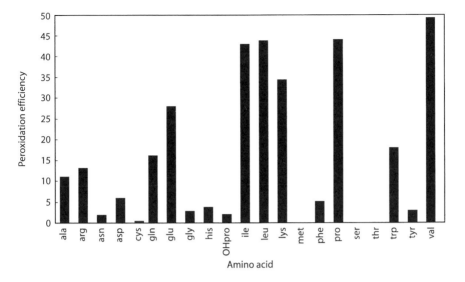

Figure 10.2 Relative susceptibility of amino acids to oxidative damage by γ rays. The peroxidation efficiency is the number of peroxide groups per hydroxyl radical generated ($\times 100$). From Gebicki and Gebicki (1993).

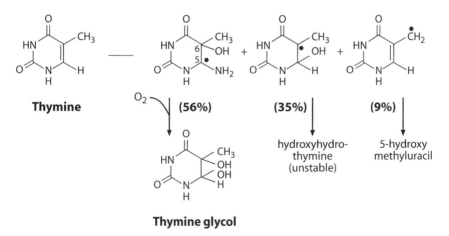

Figure 10.3 Products of free radical-mediated oxidative damage to one of the bases of DNA, thymine.

mechanisms of DNA repair, which include repairing strand breaks and replacing modified bases.

Diet has a considerable impact on the rate of oxidative damage. Several studies have shown that products of DNA damage in humans decrease on consumption of antioxidants. Consumption of Brussels sprouts decreased 8-hydroxyguanine, an oxidative DNA damage marker, in the urine (Verhagen *et al.*, 1995) and consumption of antioxidant-rich fruit and vegetables decreased steady state levels of urinary thymidine glycol (Table 10.1).

CELL PROGRESSION DURING CARCINOGENESIS AS A RESULT OF FREE RADICAL-MEDIATED DAMAGE

Cancer arises as a result of genetic alterations, either inherited or from the mutation of somatic cells. The malignant phenotype requires more than one genetic error, which arises during cell replication. For these errors to become permanent, the defect must occur in a population of stem cells. The risk of this series of events is increased by damaged DNA, or by increasing the rate of replication. Thus DNA damage occurring at important sites greatly increases the risk of a cell entering the progression stage of carcinogenesis. Several important genes have been identified, and modification of these genes has consequences for the progression of the cell. This is a large area of active research, and the reader is referred to papers on the p53 gene (Harris, 1993) and the proto-oncogenes *fos* and *jun* (Patel *et al.*, 1994; Karin, 1995; Rahmsdorf, 1996).

Interaction of antioxidants with free radicals

This section is in many ways the most important since it links the previous two sections and also is focused on mechanisms which explain the epidemiological observations. Dietary antioxidants can act either directly, via free radical scavenging mechanisms, or by stimulation of endogenous defences via signal transduction pathways. The net result is a decrease in the amount of ROS generated, a decrease in the species likely to give ROS and an increase in repair of damage caused by ROS.

Table 10.1 Yield of human urinary thymidine glycol for isocaloric (2400 kcal/day) and isocompositional (carbohydrates, lipids, proteins) diets with or without fruit and vegetables

Urinary marker	Fruit and vegetables in the diet	Absence of fruit or vegetables in the diet
Thymidine glycol (nmol/kg·day)	0.21 ± 0.05	0.60 ± 0.05

Adapted from Simic (1994).

CHEMICAL MECHANISMS OF INTERACTION

The most important direct-acting antioxidants in the diet are α-tocopherol (vitamin E), ascorbic acid (vitamin C), flavonoids and hydroxycinnamates.

General mechanism of free radical scavenging

The mechanism of lipid peroxidation involves formation of a lipid radical as an initiation step:

$$LH + R\cdot \rightarrow L\cdot + RH$$

The initiating radical may be a hydroxyl ion, generated by reaction of hydrogen peroxide with iron. The lipid radical rapidly reacts with oxygen to give a lipid hydroperoxide.

$$L\cdot + O_2 \rightarrow LOO\cdot$$

$$LOO\cdot + LH \rightarrow LOOH + L\cdot$$

This new lipid radical can then react with oxygen to continue these propagation reactions. The reaction can be terminated by the reaction of two radicals:

$$L\cdot + L\cdot \rightarrow L{-}L$$

The statistical likelihood of this reaction occurring depends on the half-life of the lipid radical. A shorter half-life leads to greater chance of propagation and less chance of termination reactions. A free radical scavenger, X, can substitute for LH in the above equation.

$$LOO\cdot + XH \rightarrow LOOH + X\cdot$$

This implies that the ability of X to be efficient at terminating the chain reactions is defined by the half-life of $X\cdot$. A longer half-life increases the chance of the two X radicals meeting:

$$X\cdot + X\cdot \rightarrow X{-}X$$

Thus, a compound that forms a very stable $X\cdot$ intermediate will be an effective antioxidant in this system (Halliwell et al., 1992).

α-Tocopherol

Vitamin E is a naturally occuring mixture of tocol (6-hydroxy-2-methyl-(4,8,12-trimethyltridecyl)chromane) derivatives, and α-tocopherol is the most biologically active. Vitamin E is active in a number of tests for antimutagenicity (Odin, 1997). It is highly lipid soluble and protects cellular membranes and circulating lipoproteins from oxidation. Oxidation of α-tocopherol by a radical leads to the relatively stable radical intermediate tocopheroxyl radical, which yields tocopherylquinone as the ultimate metabolite. The tocopherylquinone is also efficiently recycled back to α-tocopherol by several cellular reductants, especially NAD(P)H, and the action of NAD(P)H is increased by the presence of reduced glutathione (GSH) (Morrissey *et al.*, 1994). The tocopheroxyl radical may be reduced by ascorbic acid (see below).

Ascorbic acid

Ascorbic acid (vitamin C) is a widely distributed water-soluble compound and is an important antioxidant in plasma (Weber *et al.*, 1996) and aqueous humour (McLauchlan *et al.*, 1998). Ascorbate reacts rapidly with many ROS, and the resulting ascorbyl radical (semidehydroascorbate) is relatively unreactive. The radical is enzymically converted back to ascorbate by NADH- or glutathione-dependent enzymes. In extracellular fluids, these reactions do not occur and so ascorbate is rapidly depleted by oxidative stress. Ascorbate is highly pro-oxidant in the presence of iron, but normally iron is sequestered. In tissue damage or disease, iron is released which may cause the formation of damaging ROS in the presence of ascorbate. Ascorbic acid has been the subject of several reviews (Cohen and Bhagavan, 1995; Buettner and Jurkiewicz, 1996).

Flavonoids

Flavonoids are a large group of compounds which occur in large amounts in many plant foods. The most relevant in terms of dietary antioxidants are the flavones, flavonols and anthocyanins. The flavones are catechin, epicatechin, galloyl esters of epicatechin, and polymerised forms of all of these molecules, and are found in high levels in tea. Flavonols are found at high levels in onions, apples, tea, wine and broccoli, and almost always occur as glycosides; antho-cyanins occur at high levels as the main pigment in berries such as black-currants. The structure of these classes are shown in Figure 10.4. There is a

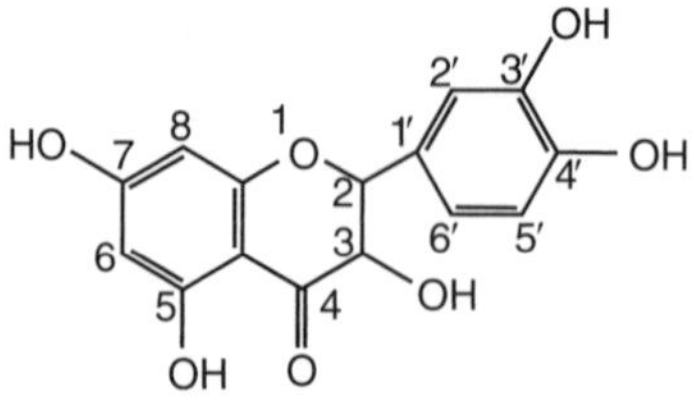

Q-3-glucoside (isoquercitrin) - high in apple and pear
Q-3,4'-diglucoside - high in onions
Q-4'-glucoside - high in onions
Q-3-rutinoside (rutin) - high in tea

Figure 10.4 Structures of commonly occurring quercetin glycosides and their occurrence in plant material.

large amount of literature on the biological effects of quercetin aglycone (i.e. with no sugar attached) (Gandhi and Khanduja, 1993; Stavric, 1994; Cook and Samman, 1996; Cao et al., 1997), since quercetin is commercially available. However, there is very little free quercetin in the diet. Onions contain two flavonol glycosides, the 4′-monoglucoside and the 3,4′-diglucoside (Rhodes and Price, 1996). Broccoli contains quercetin 3-sophoroside and kaempferol 3-sophoroside (Plumb et al., 1997) and tea contains quercetin 3-rutinoside (Biedrich et al., 1989). All of these compounds are antioxidants, but the substitution position and, to a lesser extent, the nature of the sugar, strongly influence these properties (Williamson et al., 1996).

Catechins and (+)-epicatechin are found at high levels in tea, often as a gallate or galloyl ester (Cao et al., 1997; Mitscher et al., 1997). Green tea contains high levels of these compounds. During fermentation to black tea, many of these polyphenolics become polymerised. This class of compounds are generally good antioxidants (Cao et al., 1997) and are absorbed by humans (Lee et al., 1995).

Hydroxycinnamates

Hydroxycinnamates include ferulic, caffeic, p-coumaric and sinapic acids. Many of these phenolics are present at an extremely high level in many diets (Herrmann, 1989). They are found almost entirely linked to another component, and are often ester-linked to sugars or acids. Chlorogenic acid is caffeic acid ester linked to quinic acid, is found at very high levels in coffee and apple juice and is a good antioxidant (Miller et al., 1995). Broccoli contains several esters of sinapic acid, which are antioxidants (Plumb et al., 1997). Cereal brans contain high levels of ester-linked ferulic acid which affects antioxidant activity in the colon (Kroon et al., 1997). Cereal brans also contain relatively large amounts of diferulates, which are also antioxidants (Garcia-Conesa et al., 1997).

ENDOGENOUS DEFENCES

Glutathione S-transferases (GST) are a large group of enzymes which have been divided into several classes: α, μ, π and θ. These enzymes play several roles in protection of cells from oxidative damage (Sun et al., 1996). GSTs conjugate electrophilic chemicals with glutathione, which facilitates excretion of these molecules and may protect from chemically induced carcinogenesis. Some of the GSTs also reduce hydroperoxides, which are products of biomolecules with ROS. The protection of membranes and of DNA are likely to be important functions of GSTs.

Selenium-dependent phospholipid glutathione peroxidase (Se-PHGPx) is a selenium-dependent enzyme which is highly active on membrane phospholipid hydroperoxides, and, in the presence of glutathione, inhibits lipid peroxidation (Roveri *et al.*, 1994). It is found at high levels in the testes, which is a site of extensive cellular replication. Further, selenium deficiency in experimental animals leads to a almost complete loss of 'classical' glutathione peroxidase, but retention of Se-PHGPx (Guan *et al.*, 1995). The activity of Se-PHGPx on phospholipid hydroperoxides is several orders of magnitude higher than the best GST. This leads to interesting differences in the defence profiles of individual organs. For example, the liver contains high levels of GST α, which is the most efficient form of GST for phospholipid hydroperoxides, and only moderate levels of Se-PHGPx. In testes, levels of GST are relatively low, but Se-PHGPx is very high, which means that the latter is a much more important defence against membrane peroxidation than GSTs. Interestingly, Se-PHGPx has a remarkably high activity on thymine hydroperoxides (Bao *et al.*, 1997; Figure 10.5), which is a model compound representing early DNA oxidative damage products. Further, Se-PHGPx specially binds to chromatin (Godeas *et al.*, 1996), and is found in tissues with high levels of DNA replication (Cockell *et al.*, 1996), which implies a very important role for this enzyme in protection against DNA oxidative damage.

NAD(P)H quinone reductase is a flavoprotein which reduces phenolics by a mechanism which involves two electrons (Belinsky and Jaiswal, 1993; Cadenas, 1995). This is in contrast to certain cytochromes P450, which reduce phenolics by one-electron steps, generating a free radical intermediate which may 'leak' from the cytochrome P450 (Lambert *et al.*, 1996). However, some drugs are metabolised by NAD(P)H:quinone reductase to a form which is more toxic (Walton *et al.*, 1992). On balance, however, it is generally considered that this enzyme is an antioxidant defence. There are also a limited number of substrates which are more toxic after conjugation with glutathione by glutathione S-transferases, but on balance the GSTs are definitely a defensive system.

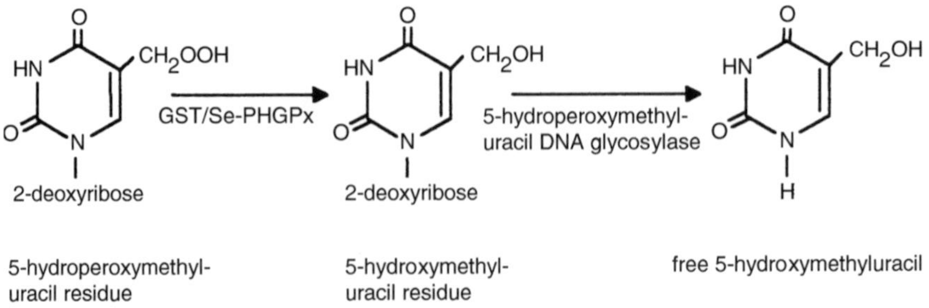
CH2OOH
HN
O
N
2-deoxyribose
GST/Se-PHGPx
CH2OH
2-deoxyribose
5-hydroperoxymethyl-
uracil DNA glycosylase
H
5-hydroperoxymethyl-
uracil residue
5-hydroxymethyl-
uracil residue
free 5-hydroxymethyluracil

Figure 10.5 Action of selenium-dependent phospholipid glutathione peroxidase (Se-PHGPx) on thymine hydroperoxides, a model compound representing oxidatively-damaged DNA; GST, glutathione-S-transferase.

'Classical' intracellular glutathione peroxidase is a selenium-dependent enzyme which catalyses the reduction of hydrogen peroxide to water, and the reduction of lipid and other organic hydroperoxides to alcohols, at the expense of oxidation of glutathione to glutathione disulphide (Ursini et al., 1995; Tappel, 1984). The glutathione disulphide is in turn reduced back to glutathione by the action of the NADPH-dependent enzyme, glutathione reductase. This illustrates that maintenance of a suitable intracellular reducing environment is energy-dependent. Intracellular glutathione peroxidase is not active on membrane hydroperoxides, and furthermore, mice which have no glutathione peroxidase do not exhibit increased sensitivity to hyperoxia (Ho et al., 1997). This demonstrates that Se-PHGPx is probably more important in protection of the cellular components against oxidative stress, and that glutathione peroxidase may act primarily as a reductant of hydrogen peroxide and as a selenium store.

Superoxide dismutase is dependent on cations for activity. Mn-SOD requires dietary manganese, whereas Cu/Zn-SOD requires dietary copper and zinc. SOD reduces superoxide to hydrogen peroxide, and is an important defence mechanism provided that hydrogen peroxide is rapidly removed by glutathione peroxidase or catalase. Catalase is found almost exclusively in peroxisomes and catalyses the disproportionation of hydrogen peroxide to water and oxygen. The relative importance of each antioxidant enzyme is impossible to measure, but estimates in specific cases have been made (Michiels et al., 1994).

EFFECT OF DIETARY ANTIOXIDANTS ON CELLULAR ENDOGENOUS DEFENCES

Many of the most important endogenous defences against ROS are induced or repressed by diet. In this way, dietary vitamins and phytochemicals modulate defence mechanisms and so play an important role in maintaining the redox status of a cell, in addition to acting as free radical scavengers as already discussed. Diet affects many enzymes which affect the production or scavenging of ROS. Enzymic antioxidants include glutathione S-transferases (mainly α and θ classes), SePHGPx, glutathione peroxidase and superoxide dismutase. In addition, drug-metabolising enzymes such as glutathione S-transferases, quinone reductase and glucuronosyl transferases remove the compounds that can give rise to ROS and so act as a further antioxidant defence.

Many enzymes which are involved in cellular defence are controlled at the transcriptional level by the antioxidant responsive element (ARE) (Table 10.2). The consensus sequence for the ARE is TMAnnRTGAYnnnGCR (Wasserman and Fahl, 1997). The ARE binds to various transcription factors, which includes a p160 protein (Wang and Williamson, 1994; Wasserman and Fahl, 1995), and the transcription factors nrf1, nrf2 and maf (Kataoka et al., 1996; Itoh et al., 1997). There is also the 12-O-tetradecanoyl-phorbol-13-acetate responsive

Table 10.2 Proteins whose expression may be controlled by the antioxidant responsive element identified by screening of DNA databanks for the sequence TMAnnRTGAYnnnGCR in promoter regions

Primate enzymes	Rodent enzymes
NAD(P)H:quinone reductase	Glutathione S-transferase Ya
β-Globin	Glutathione S-transferase P
Myoglobin	Ferritin L
Alzheimer gene STM2	β-Globin
Collagenase	GSH transporter
P450 aromatase	Interleukin 6
	Tyrosinase

Other enzymes which may be regulated by the ARE are UDP-glucuronosyl transferase and haem oxygenase. Adapted from Wasserman and Fahl (1997).

element (TRE), which is found in the promoter region of many genes and controls expression resulting from a variety of stresses including hydrogen peroxide. The ARE and TRE are found as overlapping sequences in some genes, such as NAD(P)H:quinone reductase from human and rat (Favreau and Pickett, 1995). Some genes have a 'pure' ARE without the TRE consensus sequence (TGAG/CTCA), such as the rat GST Ya gene (Bergelson *et al.*, 1994). Signal transduction mechanisms in response to oxidative stress and to dietary sulphur compounds and some phenolics activate defence mechanisms via the ARE and TRE, but the mechanism is not yet understood (Figure 10.6).

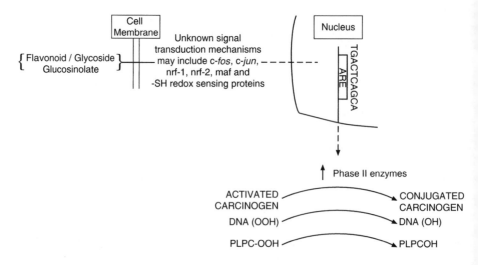

Figure 10.6 Simplified schematic diagram showing the interaction of phytochemicals with signal transduction pathways. PLPC, phospholipid hydroperoxide.

Selenium regulates expression of Se-PHGPx and of GPx by a post-transcriptional mechanism, which involves mRNA stabilisation (Imai *et al.*, 1995; Bermano *et al.*, 1996).

WHICH DIETARY COMPOUNDS AFFECT EXPRESSION VIA ANTIOXIDANT RESPONSIVE ELEMENTS?

Vitamin A, C and E regulate expression of NAD(P)H:quinone reductase but not glutathione S-transferase in a human colon epithelial cell line (Wang and Higuchi, 1995). However, glucosinolate breakdown products are probably the most effective regulators of antioxidant enzymes (Zhang *et al.*, 1992). Glucosinolates are a class of sulphur-containing compounds which break down on disruption of the plant tissues containing them, to produce a range of highly biologically active products (Fenwick *et al.*, 1983). High levels of glucosinolates are found almost exclusively in *Brassica* vegetables such as broccoli, Brussels sprouts, cauliflower and cabbage, and are responsible for the spicy flavour of watercress, mustard and horseradish (Rosa *et al.*, 1996). Typical breakdown products of the glucosinolates are isothiocyanates, nitriles and thiocyanates, depending on the conditions of processing of the vegetable. In the past, certain glucosinolates were studied for their potential goitrogenic properties. These properties arise from the glucosinolate progoitrin, which is found at high levels only in rape seed. However, this glucosinolate is low in human food, and *Brassica* vegetables normally consumed contain high levels of other glucosinolates, such as aliphatic and indole glucosinolates (Fenwick *et al.*, 1983). For induction of antioxidant and detoxifying enzymes, the most effective glucosinolates are the methylsulphinyl derivatives, which give rise to methylsulphinylpropyl- and methylsulphinylbutyl-isothiocyanates. In cultured cells, a concentration of only 0.2 μM is required to double the activity of NAD(P)H:quinone oxidoreductase (Zhang *et al.*, 1992). Glucosinolate breakdown products reduce cancer risk in a number of experimental models (Jongen, 1996; Voerhoeven *et al.*, 1997).

Cysteine sulphoxides are found in alliums, such as onions, garlic and leeks. Breakdown products such as allyl sulphide and allyl disulphide are effective inducers of antioxidant defences such as glutathione S-transferase and NAD(P)H:quinone reductase, at least in animal models (Sparnins *et al.*, 1988). Less information is available on humans.

Quercetin and 4′-substituted derivatives are the only representatives among the flavonoids which show an induction of antioxidant enzymes such as NAD(P)H:quinone reductase (Plumb *et al.*, 1997). It is not known if the induction by these phenolics is relevant in humans.

Effects of dietary nutrient antioxidants on progression of chemically induced carcinogenesis *in vivo*

EPIDEMIOLOGY

Epidemiological studies based on observing populations have shown a strong relationship between a high intake of fruit and vegetables and a decrease in the risk of cancer at certain sites (Table 10.3). However, epidemiology can provide much less convincing evidence about particular foods or food components and health. The epidemiological evidence on flavonoids, for example, is mixed, and it cannot be proven whether or not flavonoids are anticarcinogenic by epidemiology alone. These types of studies provide hypotheses which can be tested by experimental science. A full review on the epidemiological evidence on the relationship between food and cancer can be found in the book by Hill *et al.* (1994).

ANIMAL STUDIES

A large number of experiments have been performed using animal models to show that administration of certain compounds before a carcinogen can decrease the number of tumours which subsequently develop by up to 100% (Table 10.4). To reduce the time for tumour growth in this type of study, high doses of both carcinogen and anticarcinogen are administered. These experiments are useful as part of a battery of tests to determine the efficacy and develop hypotheses for the mechanism of action of putative anticarcinogens, but only provide indicators for human anticarcinogens. The approach was pioneered by Wattenberg and co-workers (Wattenberg, 1983, 1985; Wattenberg *et al.*, 1980).

Table 10.3 Epidemiological evidence for protection against carcinogenesis by fruit and vegetables. Relative risk of various cancers in three tertiles of consumption of fruit and vegetables (low intake normalised to unity)

Cancer site	Food	High intake	Middle intake	Low intake
Pancreas	Vegetables	0.4	0.7	1.0
Pancreas	Fruit	0.5	0.7	1.0
Prostate	Vegetables	0.3	0.8	1.0
Prostate	Fruit	0.4	0.8	1.0
Bladder	Vegetables	0.4	1.0	1.0
Bladder	Fruit	0.4	1.0	1.0
Liver	Vegetables	0.2	0.8	1.0
Liver	Fruit	0.6	1.3	1.0

Adapted from Hill *et al.* (1994).

Table 10.4 Reduction in tumour yield in animals after chemically induced carcinogenesis by treatments with antioxidants

Compound	Tumour inducer	Species	Target organ	Δ yield (%)[a]
Ascorbic acid	UV	Mouse	Skin	90
Ascorbic acid	Diethylstilbestrol	Hamster	Kidney	50
Ascorbic acid	Dimethylhydrazine/ oestradiol diproprionate	Mouse	Uterus	44
Quercetin	Azoxymethane	Mouse	Colon	75
Quercetin	N-methyl-N- nitrosourea	Mouse	Skin	55
Rutin	Azoxymethane	Mouse	Colon	63
Vitamin E	DMBA/TBA[b]	Mouse	Skin	35
Vitamin E	UV	Mouse	Skin	48
Vitamin E	DMBA	Hamster	Buccal pouch	43
EGC[c]	DMBA	Mouse	Skin	64

[a]Decrease in yield of tumours, expressed as a percentage of the control.
[b]DMBA, 7,12-dimethylbenz[a]anthracene; TPA, 12-O-tetradecanoyl phorbol-13-acetate.
[c]EGC, (+)-epigallocatechin.
Adapted from Dragsted et al. (1993).

HUMAN STUDIES: CANCER INCIDENCE AND BIOMARKERS

Several compounds have been tested in large human trials for lower cancer incidence in at-risk populations, and some are listed below (Greenwald, 1996). At the time of writing, several other studies were also ongoing.

The α-tocopherol, β-carotene lung cancer prevention study (ATBC) tested if daily oral doses of vitamin E and/or β-carotene could reduce rates of lung and other cancers in 29 133 male smokers over five to eight years. Vitamin E supplementation produced a 34% decrease in the incidence of prostate cancer, and a small but insignificant decrease (16%) in colorectal cancer. β-Carotene, however, produced an 18% increase in the incidence of lung cancer. The isotretinoin efficacy trial showed that daily oral doses of this retinoid reduced rates of secondary tumours by 83% in 100 high-risk people who had initially been treated for head and neck cancer. The Linxian general population trial showed that there was a 21% decrease in stomach cancer deaths among 29 584 people taking beta-carotene, vitamin E and selenium over a six-year period in China.

Conclusions

There is now very strong evidence from epidemiology, animal models, cellular studies, molecular models and human studies that fruit and vegetables reduce the risk of certain cancers, especially those of the gastrointestinal tract. Two of the major mechanisms which bring about this protection are: (i) a decrease in reactive oxygen species by dietary antioxidants; and (ii) the induction of cellular defence enzymes. A link between individual dietary components and health is unlikely, as a variety of dietary components act, possibly synergistically, to maintain health and protect against chronic disease. Nevertheless, in order to build a mechanistic picture of the role of dietary vitamins and phytochemicals in protecting against the toxicity of reactive oxygen species, it is important first to consider the action of single components and then how they might interact.

References

Arai K, Lee F, Miyajima A, Miyatake S, Arai N and Yokota T (1990) Cytokines: coordinators of immune and inflammatory responses. *Annual Review of Biochemistry*, **59**, 783–836.

Bao, Y-P, Jemth P, Mannervik B and Williamson G (1997) Reduction of thymine hydroperoxide by phospholipid hydroperoxide glutathione peroxidase and glutathione transferase. *FEBS Letters*, **410**, 210–212.

Belinsky M and Jaiswal AK (1993) QR expression in normal and tumour tissues. *Cancer Metastasis Review*, **12**, 103–117.

Bergelson S, Pinkus R and Daniel V (1994) Intracellular glutathione levels regulate fos/jun induction and activation of glutathione S-transferase gene expression. *Cancer Research*, **54**, 36–40.

Bermano G, Arthur JR and Hesketh JE (1996) Selective control of cytosolic glutathione peroxidase and phospholipid hydroperoxide glutathione peroxidase mRNA stability by selenium supply. *FEBS Letters*, **387**, 157–160.

Biedrich P, Engelhardt UH and Herzig B (1989) Determination of quercetin 3-O-rutinoside (rutin) in black tea by HPLC. *Zeitschrift fuer Lebensmittel Untersuchung und Forschung*, **189**, 149–150.

Buettner GR and Jurkiewicz BA (1996) Catalytic metals, ascorbate and free radicals: combinations to avoid. *Radiation Research*, **145**, 532–541.

Buettner GR, Saran M and Bors W (1987) The kinetics of the reaction of ferritin with superoxide. *Free Radical Research Communications*, **2**, 369–372.

Cadenas E (1995) Antioxidant and prooxidant functions of DT-diaphorase in quinone metabolism. *Biochemical Pharmacology*, **49**, 127–140.

Cao, G, Sofic E and Prior RL (1997) Antioxidant and pro-oxidant behaviour of flavonoids: structure-activity relationships. *Free Radicals in Biology and Medicine*, **22**, 749–760.

Clemens MJ (1991) *Cytokines, Medical Perspectives Series*, BIOS Scientific Publishers, Oxford, UK.

Cockell KA, Brash AR and Burk RF (1996) Influence of selenum status on activity of phospholipid hydroperoxide glutathione peroxidase in rat liver and testis in comparison with other selenoproteins. *Journal of Nutritional Biochemistry*, **7**, 333–338.

Cohen M and Bhagavan HN (1995) Ascorbic acid and gastrointestinal cancer. *Journal of the American College of Nutrition*, **14**, 565–578.

Cook NC and Samman S (1996) Flavonoids – Chemistry, metabolism, cardioprotective effects, and dietary sources. *Journal of Nutritional Biochemistry*, **7**, 66–76.

Damas P (1991) The cytokines: a possible role in sepsis. *Current Opinions in Anaesthesiology*, **4**, 241–246.

Dragsted LO, Strube M and Larsen JC (1993) Cancer-protective factors in fruits and vegetables: biochemical and biological background. *Pharmacology and Toxicology*, **72**, S116–S135.

Eisenbrand G, Schuhmacher J and Golzer P (1995) The influence of glutathione and detoxifying enzymes on DNA damage induced by 2-alkenals in primary rate hepatocytes and human lymphoblastoid cells. *Chemical Research in Toxicology*, **8**, 40–46.

Esterbauer H (1991) Lipid peroxidation products: formation, chemical properties and biological activities. In *Free Radicals in Liver Injury*, Poli G, Cheeseman KH, Dianzani MU and Slater TF (eds), IRL Press, Oxford, pp. 29–47.

Favreau LV and Pickett CB (1995) The rat quinone reductase antioxidant response element – identification of the nucleotide sequence required for basal and inducible activity and detection of antioxidant response element-binding proteins in hepatoma and non-hepatoma cell lines. *Journal of Biological Chemistry*, **270**, 24468–24474.

Fenwick GR, Heaney RK and Mullin WJ (1983) Glucosinolates and their breakdown-products in food and food plants. *CRC Critical Reviews in Food Science and Nutrition*, **18**, 123–201.

Gaffney BJ (1996) Lipoxygenases: structural principles and spectroscopy. *Annual Reviews of Biophysics and Biomolecular Structures*, **25**, 431–459.

Gandhi RK and Khanduja KL (1993) Impact of quercetin composition on phase 1 and phase 2 drug metabolizing enzymes in mice. *Journal of Clinical and Biochemical Nutrition*, **14**, 107–112.

Garcia-Conesa MT, Plumb GW, Kroon PA, Wallace G and Williamson G (1997) Antioxidant properties of ferulic acid dimers. *Redox Report*, **3**, 239–244.

Gebicki S and Gebicki JM (1993) Formation of peroxides in amino acids and proteins exposed to oxygen free radicals. *Biochemical Journal*, **289**, 743–749.

Godeas C, Tramer F, Micali F, Roveri A, Majorino M, Nisii C, Sandri G and Panfili E (1996) Phospholipid hydroperoxide glutathione peroxidase (PHGPx) in rat testis nuclei is bound to chromatin. *Biochemical and Molecular Medicine*, **59**, 118–124.

Greenwald P (1996) Chemoprevention of cancer. *Scientific American*, **September**, 64–67.

Grimble RF (1996) Interaction between nutrients, pro-inflammatory cytokines and inflammation. *Clinical Science*, **91**, 121–130.

Guan JY, Komura S, Ohishi N and Yagi K (1995) Difference in effects of classic and phospholipid hydroperoxide glutathione peroxidases on liver lipid peroxide level in selenium-deficient rats. *Biochemistry and Molecular Biology International*, **37**, 1103–1110.

Guengerich FP (1995) Human cytochrome P450 enzymes. In *Cytochrome P450: Structure, Mechanism, and Biochemistry*, 2nd edn, Ortiz de Montellano PR (ed), Plenum Press, New York, pp. 473–535.

Gutteridge JMC and Halliwell B (1990) The measurement and mechanism of lipid peroxidation in biological systems. *Trends in Biochemical Sciences*, **15**, 129–135.

Halliwell B and Aruoma OI (1997) Free radicals and antioxidants: the need for *in vivo* markers of oxidative stress. In *Antioxidant Methodology:* in vivo *and* in vitro *concepts*, Aruoma OI and Cuppett SL (eds), AOCS Press, Champaign, IL, pp. 1–22.

Halliwell B and Cross CE (1995) Oxygen derived species: their relationship to human disease and environmental stress. *Environmental Health Perspectives*, **102**, S5–S12.

Halliwell B, Gutteridge JMC and Cross CE (1992) Free radicals, antioxidants and human disease: where are we now? *Journal of Laboratory and Clinical Medicine*, **119**, 598–620.

Harris CC (1993) p53: at the crossroads of molecular carcinogenesis and risk assessment. *Science*, **262**, 1980–1981.

Hasemann CA, Kurumbail RG, Boddupalli SS, Peterson JA and Deisenhofer J (1995) Structure and function of cytochromes P450: a comparative analysis of three crystal structures. *Structure*, **3**, 41–62.

Herrmann K (1989) Occurrence and content of hydroxycinnamic and hydroxybenzoic acid compounds in foods. *Critical Reviews in Science of Nutrition*, **28**, 315–347.

Hill MJ, Giacosa A and Caygill CPJ (1994) *Epidemiology of Diet and Cancer*, Ellis Horwood Series in Food Science and Technology, Chichester, UK.

Ho YS, Magnenat JL, Bronson RT, Cao J, Gargano M, Sugawara M and Funk CD (1997) Mice deficient in cellular glutathione peroxidase develop normally and show no increased sensitivity to hyperoxia. *Journal of Biological Chemistry*, **272**, 16644–16651.

Horton AA and Fairhurst S (1987) Lipid peroxidation and mechanisms of toxicity. *CRC Critical Reviews in Toxicology*, **18**, 27–79.

Imai H, Sumi D, Hanamoto A, Arai M, Sugiyama A, Chiba N, Kuchino Y and Nakagawa Y (1995) Molecular cloning and functional expression of a cDNA for rat phospholipid hydroperoxide glutathione peroxidase: 3′-untranslated region of the gene is necessary for functional expression. *Journal of Biochemistry Tokyo*, **118**, 1061–1067.

Itoh K, Chiba T, Takahashi S, Ishii T, Igarashi K, Katoh Y, Oyake T, Hayashi N, Satoh K, Hatayama I, Yamamoto M and Nabeshima Y (1997) An Nrf2/small maf heterodimer mediates the induction of phase II detoxifying enzyme genes through antioxidant elements. *Biochemical and Biophysical Research Communications*, **236**, 313–322.

Jongen WMF (1996) Glucosinolates in *Brassica*: occurrence and significance as cancer-modulating agents. *Proceedings of the Nutrition Society*, **55**, 433–446.

Karin M (1995) The regulation of AP-1 activity by mitogen-activated protein kinases. *Journal of Biological Chemistry*, **270**, 16483–16486.

Kataoka K, Noda M and Nishizawa M (1996) Transactivation activity of maf nuclear oncoprotein is modulated by jun, fos and small maf proteins. *Oncogene*, **12**, 53–62.

Kroon PA, Faulds CB, Ryden P, Robertson JA and Williamson G (1997) Release of bound ferulic acid from fibre and its potential as an antioxidant in the human colon. *Journal of Agriculture and Food Science*, **45**, 661–667.

Lambert N, Chambers SJ, Plumb GW and Williamson G (1996) Human cytochrome P-450s are pro-oxidants in iron ascorbate-initiated microsomal lipid peroxidation. *Free Radical Research*, **24**, 177–185.

Lee M, Wang Z, Li H, Chen L, Sun Y, Gobbo S, Balentine DA and Yang CS (1995) Analysis of plasma and urinary tea polyphenols in human subjects. *Cancer Epidemiology*, **4**, 393–399.

McLauchlan WR, Sanderson J, Quinlan M and Williamson G (1998) Measurement of the total antioxidant activity of human aqueous humour. *Clinical Chemistry*, **44**, 888–889.

Michiels C, Raes M, Toussaint O and Remacle J (1994) Importance of Se-glutathione peroxidase, catalase, and Cu/Zn-SOD for cell survival against oxidative stress. *Free Radicals in Biology and Medicine*, **17**, 235–248.

Miller NJ, Diplock AT and Rice-Evans CA (1995) Evaluation of the total antioxidant activity as a marker of the deterioration of apple juice oil storage. *Journal of Agricultural and Food Chemistry*, **43**, 1794–1801.

Minotti G (1989) *tert*-Butyl hydroperoxide dependent microsomal release of iron and lipid peroxidation. *Archives of Biochemistry and Biophysics*, **273**, 144–147.

Mitscher LA, Jung M, Shankel D, Dou JH, Steele L and Pillai SP (1997) Chemoprotection: a review of the potential therapeutic antioxidant properties of green tea (*Camellia sinensis*) and certain of its constituents. *Medical Research Reviews*, **17**, 327–365.

Morrissey PA, Quinn PB and Sheehy PJA (1994) Newer aspects of micronutrients in chronic disease: vitamin E. *Proceedings of the Nutrition Society*, **53**, 571–582.

Nelson MJ and Seitz SP (1994) The structure and function of lipoxygenase. *Current Opinions in Structural Biology*, **4**, 878–884.

Odin AP (1997) Vitamins as antimutagens: advantages and some possible mechanisms of antimutagenic action. *Mutation Research Reviews*, **386**, 39–67.

Parke DV and Ioannides C (1994) The effects of nutrition on chemical toxicity. *Drug Metabolism Reviews*, **26**, 739–765.

Patel LR, Curran T and Kerppola TK (1994) Energy transfer analysis of fos-jun dimerization and DNA binding. *Proceedings of the National Academy of Science USA*, **91**, 7360–7364.

Plumb GW, Price KR, Rhodes MJC and Williamson G (1997) Antioxidant properties of the major polyphenolic compunds in broccoli. *Free Radical Research*, **27**, 429–435.

Poulos TL (1995) Cytochrome P450. *Current Opinions in Structural Biology*, **5**, 767–774.

Rahmsdorf HJ (1996) Jun: transcription factor and oncoprotein. *Journal of Molecular Medicine*, **74**, 725–747.

Rhodes MJC and Price KR (1996) Analytical problems in the study of flavonoid compounds in onions. *Food Chemistry*, **56**, 1–5.

Rosa EAS, Heaney RK, Fenwick GR and Portas CAM (1996) Glucosinolates in crop plants. *Horticultural Reviews*, **19**, 99–215.

Roveri A, Maiorino M, Nisii C and Ursini F (1994) Purification and characterisation of phospholipid hydroperoxide glutathione peroxidase from rat testis mitochondrial membranes. *Biochimica et Biophysica Acta*, **1208**, 211–221.

Schrenk D, Stuven T, Gohl G, Viebahn R and Bock KW (1995) Induction of CYPIA and glutathione S-transferase activities by 2,3,7,8-tetrachlorodibenzo-*p*-dioxin in human hepatocyte cultures. *Carcinogenesis*, **16**, 943–946.

Simic MG (1994) DNA markers of oxidative processes *in vivo* – relevance to carcinogenesis and anticarcinogenesis. *Cancer Research*, **54**, S1918–S1923.

Sparnins VL, Barany G and Wattenberg LW (1988) Effects of organosulfur compounds from garlic and onions on benzo[a]pyrene-induced neoplasia and glutathione S-transferase activity in mouse. *Carcinogenesis*, **9**, 131–134.

Spector A, Wang G-M, Wang R-R, Garner WH and Moll H (1993) The prevention of cataract caused by oxidative stress in cultured rat lenses. I. H_2O_2 and photochemically induced cataract. *Current Eye Research*, **12**, 163–179.

Stavric B (1994) Quercetin in our diet: from potent mutagen to probable anticarcinogen. *Clinical Biochemistry*, **27**, 245–248.

Sun QA, Komura S, Ohishi N and Yagi K (1996) Alpha-class isozymes of glutathione S-transferase in rat liver cytosol possess glutathione peroxidase activity toward phospholipid hydroperoxide. *Biochemistry and Molecular Biology International*, **39**, 343–352.

Tappel AL (1984) Selenium glutathione peroxidase and synthesis. *Current Topics in Cellular Regulation*, **24**, 87–97.

Ursini F, Maiorino M, Brigelius-Flohe R, Aumann KD, Roveri A, Schomburg D and Flohe L (1995) Diversity of glutathione peroxidases. *Methods in Enzymology*, **252**, 38–53.

Verhagen H, Poulsen HE, Loft S, Van Poppel G, Willems MI and van Bladeren PJ (1995) Reduction of oxidative DNA damage in humans by Brussels sprouts. *Carcinogenesis*, **16**, 969–970.

Verhoeven DTH, Verhagen H, Goldbohm RA, Van den Brandt PA and Van Poppel G (1997) A review of mechanisms underlying anticarcinogenicity by *Brassica* vegetables. *Chemico-Biological Interactactions*, **103**, 79–129.

Walton MI, Bibby MC, Double JA, Plumb JA and Workman, P (1992) DT-Diaphorase activity correlates with sensitivity to the indoloquinone-EO9 in mouse and human colon carcinomas. *European Journal of Cancer*, **28A**, 1597–1600.

Wang B and Williamson G (1994) Detection of a nuclear protein which binds specifically to the antioxidant responsive element (ARE) of the human NAD(P)H:quinone
oxidoreductase gene. *Biochimica et Biophysica Acta*, **1219**, 645–652.

Wang WQ and Higuchi CM (1995) Induction of NAD(P)H:quinone reductase by vitamins A, E and C in colo205 colon cancer cells. *Cancer Letters*, **98**, 63–69.

Wasserman WW and Fahl WE (1995) The antioxidant responsive element. In *The
Oxygen Paradox*, Davies KJA and Ursini F (eds), CLEUP Press, Padova, Italy, pp.
413–424.

Wasserman WW and Fahl WE (1997) Functional antioxidant responsive elements.
Proceedings of the National Academy of Science USA, **94**, 5361–6366.

Wattenberg LW (1983) Inhibition of neoplasia by minor dietary constituents. *Cancer
Research*, **43**, 2448S–2453S.

Wattenberg LW (1985) Chemoprevention of cancer. *Cancer Research*, **45**, 1–8.

Wattenberg LW, Coccia JB and Lam LKT (1980) Inhibitory effects of phenolic compounds on benzo[a]pyrene induced neoplasia. *Cancer Research*, **40**, 2820–2823.

Weber, P, Bendich A and Schalch W (1996) Vitamin C and human health – A review of
recent data relevant to human requirements. *International Journal of Vitamin Nutrition
and Research*, **66**, 19–30.

Williamson G, Plumb GW, Uda Y, Price KR and Rhodes MJC (1996) Dietary quercetin
glycosides: antioxidant activity and induction of the anticarcinogenic phase II marker
enzyme quinone reductase in Hepa1c1c7 cells. *Carcinogenesis*, **17**, 2385–2387.

Zhang Y, Talalay P, Cho C-G and Posner GH (1992) A mjaor inducer of anticarcinogenic protective enzymes from broccoli: isolation and elucidation of structure.
Proceedings of the National Academy of Science, USA, **89**, 2399–2403.

11 Safety Evaluation of Vitamins and Minerals

John N Hathcock

Nutritional and Regulatory Science, Council for Responsible Nutrition, 1300 19th Street, NW, Suite 310, Washington, DC, 20036-1609, USA

Introduction

With the accumulation of evidence that intakes higher than the Recommended Dietary Allowances (RDAs) of certain vitamins and minerals decrease the risk of chronic diseases, there is much interest in the use of dietary supplements and food fortification to increase intakes of specific vitamins and minerals. With these increases in intake, careful evaluation of the scientific evidence related to their safety is crucial.

The United States National Academy of Sciences, Codex Alimentarius Commission, the European Commission, and several countries, including Canada, France, Germany, Greece, Japan, Mexico and the United Kingdom are considering safety limits for vitamins and minerals. Both the RDA-based and several risk assessment methods are being considered as the potential basis for setting nutrient safety limits. The scientific issues related to these different approaches to nutrient safety will be examined and illustrated with some examples.

Identification of an appropriate 'safety limit' for intake of a nutrient requires careful attention to the meanings of the words 'safe' and 'limit'. Safety may be defined as the complete absence of hazard (Coon, 1973), and also as 'reasonable certainty in minds of competent scientists that the substance is not harmful under the intended conditions of use' (Code of Federal Regulations, 1995). Complete safety can never be demonstrated because it would require proof of a negative – that there is no risk whatever to anyone under any condition of use. Although some regulatory authorities have used the term 'safe and adequate' to mean 'safety limit', a more accurate meaning of this term would be 'the recommended intake, an amount that is also safe' (Hathcock, 1996). The

Nutrition and Chemical Toxicity. Edited by Costas Ioannides. © John Wiley & Sons Ltd. ISBN 0 471 97453 6

term 'safe' may be applied to 'an intake to give an adequate margin of safety below the level that causes effect' (Hathcock, 1993, 1996). A 'safety limit' may be properly defined as the highest intake that provides an adequate margin of safety below those that produce adverse effects.

Derivation of safety limits from toxicity data

The approaches that have been used to define and identify safety limits for nutrients include RDA-based limits and risk assessment methods. The risk assessment methods that have been employed include the acceptable daily intake (ADI) (Lehman and Fitzhugh, 1954), reference dose (RfD) (Barnes and Dourson, 1988), nutrient safety limit (NSL) (Hathcock, 1993, 1996), direct use of an appropriate human No Observed Adverse Effect Level (NOAEL) as a limit (Hathcock, 1997a), and an upper limit (UL) (Food and Nutrition Board, 1997).

RDA-BASED LIMITS

The RDAs are defined and designed to meet the known nutrient needs for most healthy persons, that is, to provide for the recognised essential functions of nutrients (Food and Nutrition Board, 1989). The RDAs are not intended to assess the safety of high intakes of vitamins and minerals. Therefore, limits based on the RDAs reflect nutritional policy, and not safety considerations.

The limits proposed by some international organisations, several European countries and Mexico have been based on arbitrary small multiples of the RDAs, with the RDA multiple sometimes depending on the nutrient group and perhaps the retail outlet. The number of multiples of the RDA chosen as a safety limit varies considerably, but 100% of the RDA was incorporated into the final guidelines from Mexico's Health Department (Health Department, 1996), and was listed in the proposed draft guidelines from the Codex Alimentarius Commission's Committee on Nutrition and Foods for Special Dietary Uses (1995, 1996). The Codex Alimentarius Committee, however, is currently considering risk assessment methods as well as the RDA-based approach to limits (Codex Alimentarius Commission, 1996).

Despite the obvious ease, convenience and extensive use of RDA-based methods to identify 'safety limits', this method remains inherently invalid and subject to several specific disadvantages. First, the RDAs are defined and intended to describe certain nutritional benefits and do not describe safety limits. Also, any multiples of RDAs that provide adequate margins of safety for all vitamins and minerals will be excessively restrictive for some. Conversely, any multiples high enough to avoid excessive restriction for any nutrient may not provide sufficient margins of safety for others. Moreover, limits set at or near the RDAs to achieve wide margins of safety will preclude the known health benefits of certain nutrients at intakes higher than the RDAs. For example, a safety limit of 100% of the RDAs for all minerals generates a limit for selenium that is three times lower than the intake with demonstrated benefits and safety (Clarke *et al.*, 1996), and ten times lower than the lowest intakes known to produce adverse effects (Hathcock, 1997b).

RISK ASSESSMENT (RA) APPROACHES TO NUTRIENT SAFETY LIMITS

RA for identification of safety limits for nutrients may appropriately employ most, but not all, of methods and assumptions used to set limits for other substances. The basics of the RA approach are simple: (i) identification of a NOAEL or Lowest Observed Adverse Effect Level (LOAEL); and (ii) division by an appropriate Safety Factor (SF) to identify a 'safety limit'. Customary approaches include the Acceptable Daily Intake (ADI) and the Reference Dose (RfD). The ADI uses the NOAEL or LOAEL and a fixed SF (usually 10 or 100, depending on NOAEL versus LOAEL and the data source – animals or humans). The RfD also uses the NOAEL or LOAEL, but refines the SF into a Modifying Factor (MF) and four different Uncertainty Factors (UFs). The MF and UFs are usually set at 10, 3 or 1. Thus, the composite SF used in calculation of an RfD could possibly vary from 1 to 100 000, although 10 000 is often set as the maximum composite SF (Dourson *et al.*, 1996).

Some progress is being made toward refining the UFs into data-derived, science-based components that reflect more detailed knowledge of pharmacokinetic and pharmacodynamic variations between and within species (Renwick, 1993). These refinements have been accepted and adopted by only a few policymakers (Dragula and Burin, 1994).

Issues in selection of NOAEL or LOAEL values

For all risk assessment methods of calculating safety limits, the first crucial factor is the identification of the NOAEL or LOAEL. In attempts to protect the public health, there is a tendency to select the 'worst case' for human effects from the entire scientific and medical literature as the LOAEL, with the implication that safe levels must be even lower. Policy based on the 'worst case' is frequently not justified for two reasons: (i) the 'worst-case' report is likely to represent either inappropriate methods or unreliable information; and (ii) the 'safety limit' is likely to be so low that it would prevent benefits from certain nutrients at higher intakes. The selection of animal data for calculation of 'safe' human intakes usually involves identification of the pivotal study and critical effect.

For nicotinic acid, the lowest reported daily intake associated with a single case of adverse outcome is 500 mg per day, but most cases are related to intakes of more than 1000 mg (Rader *et al.*, 1992). The case with a reported intake of 500 mg involved slow-release (SR) niacin and perhaps pre-existing liver disease. This reported intake, like many self-reported intakes by patients, is subject to much uncertainty. If the limitations of this 'worst-case' report are ignored, and 500 mg is selected as the LOAEL, the calculated Nutrient Safety Limit (NSL) values are from 50 to 260 mg (Hathcock, 1993). Subsequent data from a randomised clinical trial found no adverse effects from the administration of 500 mg, demonstrating that this intake is not appropriate as the LOAEL (McKenney et al., 1994). The results did show moderate adverse effects from both SR and unmodified nicotinic acid at intakes of 1000 mg, indicating that this intake is an appropriate LOAEL.

Pyridoxine is another example. The worst-case report suggests adverse effects from intakes as low as 50 mg per day (Dalton and Dalton, 1987). If these data are used to identify the LOAEL, the calculated safety limits range from 5 to 26 mg per day (Hathcock, 1993). The research methods behind the report finding adverse effects at 50 mg, however, involved several weaknesses and limitations. The data are given little credence by most pyridoxine experts, and no other report has suggested adverse effects at intakes of 200 mg or less. Nevertheless, this report was recently used in the UK as the basis of a 50 mg LOAEL that was divided by 5 to identify a suggested safety limit of 10 mg for pyridoxine (Committee on Toxicity, 1997). In contrast to this excessively cautious limit, there are no credible reports of adverse effects related to pyridoxine intakes of 200 mg or less. Additionally, there has long been ample clinical data related to intakes of 20–25 mg per day to directly establish the safety of these intakes (Rose, 1978). Clearly, a restriction to 10 mg is not needed to achieve safety safe use of pyridoxine.

For vitamin E, the report of the lowest intake related to adverse effects (increased haemorrhagic stroke) came from a clinical trial involving men given 50 mg of dl-α-tocopherol acetate (equivalent to 50 IU with this form of vitamin E) (ATBC Cancer Prevention Study Group, 1994). This intake is far lower than intakes shown to interfere with platelet adherence and aggregation – a reasonable basis for hypothesising that there could be an increased risk of stroke. Use of these data to select 50 mg as the LOAEL for vitamin E also ignores the statistical expectation of some random occurrence of 'significant' effects in a large clinical trial with multiple endpoints. Nevertheless, it has been used in France as the basis for setting a safety limit for vitamin E (Bernier, 1995). In comparison with other available data, and based on specific design characteristics of the study, it is inappropriate to use these data to identify a LOAEL for vitamin E. The selection of 50 mg as the LOAEL is contrary to public health interests because no identifiable protection against toxicity is provided and much higher intakes (100 to 800 IU) have been shown to reduce the risk of heart disease.

Acceptable daily intakes

For environmental chemicals and for food additives, including vitamins and minerals used to fortify conventional foods, many authorities including JEFCA (the Joint Expert Committee on Food Additives, of the World Health

Organization and the Food and Agriculture Organization of the United Nations), the US FDA, and US EPA have used the acceptable daily intake (ADI) as the basis for regulatory limits (Lehman and Fitzhugh, 1954; Food Safety Council, 1982; Dourson and Stara, 1983). The ADI is identified by dividing a marginally toxic or marginally non-toxic intake by a safety factor (SF), yielding an intake level considered acceptably safe. The toxic or non-toxic intakes are determined experimentally as the NOAEL or the LOAEL. A larger SF is used with the LOAEL than with the NOAEL.

Environmental chemicals and most food additives have technological rather than nutritional uses, and thus the SF used is relatively large. Depending on whether the data come from animal or human experiments and whether the data identify a NOAEL or a LOAEL, the number is usually 10 or 100. The equation is

$$ADI = NOAEL \text{ (or LOAEL)} \div SF.$$

The recent recommendation on pyridoxine from the Committee on Toxicity in the United Kingdom, is an example of the ADI process applied to a vitamin. In that instance, a SF of 5 was applied to a worst-case LOAEL, with a resulting safety limit that is lower than intakes known to be safe for adults. Also, fixed SF values as low as 5 can result in ADIs below the RDAs for several vitamins and minerals (Hathcock, 1993). Also, any one SF applied to all nutrients may produce ADIs that are too low to be rational 'safety limits' for some and too high for others.

Reference Dose

The US Environmental Protection Agency (EPA) has now replaced the ADI with the Reference Dose (RfD), a term that 'considers the systemic toxicity of a chemical and determines a level that probably will not cause deleterious effects over a lifetime of exposure' (Barnes and Dourson, 1988). The RfD was developed for use in setting regulatory limits for environmental contaminants. This term was appropriately intended to avoid implication that any exposure to such chemicals was completely 'safe' or 'acceptable'. Thus, the RfD considers only adverse effects and the level of confidence in the data. This approach to safety limits, however, can present problems when applied to nutrients, because no consideration is given to the beneficial effects of nutrient consumption. This omission leads to many anomalies when the RfD method is applied to essential trace elements.

For calculation of the RfD, the SF has been refined into multiple components described as an uncertainty factor (UF) and a modifying factor (MF). Thus, the RfD is calculated as:

$$RfD = NOAEL \text{ (or LOAEL)} \div (UF \times MF).$$

UF represents one or the product of several factors (generally 10-fold each, but sometimes less). The MF is generally 1.0, but may be as high as 10. Clearly, multiple uncertainties will lead to a very large composite SF and a very low RfD. The specific choices are set through the judgement of experts on a case-by-case basis. When appropriate human data are available, all UF and MF values may be as low as 1.0, which is the equivalent of using the NOAEL directly as the safety limit.

RfD values have been developed for several essential trace elements, but not for any vitamins (IRIS, 1997a). In calculations of the RfDs for essential trace elements, the final composite safety factor selected has varied greatly – from 1000 for trivalent chromium down to 1 for fluoride and manganese (Table 11.1). With the exception of trivalent chromium, the EPA's calculations of RfD values (converted to the basis of a 70-kg man) range only from 1.4 (zinc for adult males, and molybdenum) to 5 (selenium), when expressed as multiples of the RDA.

Applied to zinc, the RfD method and the SF value selected have produced anomalous and illogical results. At first, a composite SF of 10 was selected and applied to the LOAEL of 60 mg (1 mg/kg body weight/day). The resulting RfD of 6 mg was deemed unacceptable because it was far lower than the RDA (Abernathy et al., 1993). A composite SF of 3 was then selected, yielding an RfD of 0.3 mg/kg, or 21 mg for a 70-kg man. The RfD of 0.3 mg/kg is below the zinc RDAs for children through age 10 years and males of age 11–14 years. Although the RfD of 21 mg for a 70-kg man may not seem illogical, it is derived from the RfD of 0.3 mg/kg, a value that is irrational as a general safety limit because it is below the RDAs for many age–sex groups. Moreover, it was developed from data on adult females, but applied to all age–sex groups.

Table 11.1 Safety factors used for EPA's reference doses

Value	B	Cr(3+)	F	Mn	Mo	Se	Zn
NOAEL (mg/kg/day)	8.8[a]	A1468	0.06	0.14	None	0.015	None
LOAEL (mg/kg/day)	29[a]	None	0.12	None	0.14	0.023	1.0
Composite SF (UF × MF)	100	1000	1	1	30	3	3
RfD (per kg)	0.09 mg	1.0 mg	0.06 mg	0.14 mg	5 μg	5 μg	0.3 mg
RfD, daily total (per 70 kg)	6.3 mg	70 mg	4.2 mg	9.8 mg	350 μg	350 μg	21[b] mg
RI = RDA or upper ESADDI	2.0 mg	200 μg	2.0 mg	5.0 mg	250 μg	70 μg	15[b] mg
Ratio = RfD ÷ RI	3.15	350	2.1	1.96	1.4	5	1.4[b]

[a]Data from animal studies.
[b]For adult men; the RfD equals the RDA for pregnant women; the RfD is less than the RDA for children.
NOAEL, No observed Adverse Effect Level; LOAEL, Lowest Observed Adverse Effect Level; SF, Safety Factor; UF, Uncertainty Factor; MF, Modifying Factor; RfD, Reference Dose; RI, Recommended Intake; RDA, Recommended Dietary Allowance; ESADDI, Estimated Safe and Adequate Daily Dietary Intake.

The basis for the selection of specific composite safety factors used in RfD calculations is not always apparent. For example, the database for selenium (Levander and Burk, 1994), seems larger and includes more relevant human studies than that for manganese (Keen and Zidenberg-Cherr, 1996), which should justify selection of a lower SF for selenium than for manganese. For essential trace elements, EPA's range of safety factors, with the NOAELs, and resulting RfD values, are shown in Table 11.1. For fluoride and manganese, EPA has set the composite SF at 1.0 in calculating the RfD; this is equivalent to direct use of the human NOAEL as the safety limit.

If default assumptions are excessively cautious, adjustment of the composite SF value after an initial calculation can automatically produce RfD values that are at or near the RDAs. Thus, the RfD method lends itself to a pattern of misuse that is the practical equivalent of using RDA-based safety limits (Hathcock, 1996).

Nutrient safety limits

A safety limit approach known as the Nutrient Safety Limit (NSL) is a risk assessment method, rather than an RDA-based method, but is defined so that the calculated limit is never below the recommended intake (Hathcock, 1993, 1996). It provides adequate margins of safety below adverse intake levels but avoids identifying 'safety limits' that are below the recommended intakes (RI) by including both the human LOAEL and the RI. The NSL is calculated as an intermediate value between the LOAEL and the RI. The RI used should be the highest intake that provides definite health benefits without causing adverse effects. Depending on the degree of caution desired, the intermediate value calculated can be the arithmetic mean, geometric mean, or any percentile of the range between the LOAEL and the RI.

After the identification of the LOAEL and RI values for a nutrient, the NSL value, in comparison with other types of safety limits, will depend on the specific calculation method. For example, the arithmetic mean or the geometric mean of the LOAEL and RI (Hathcock, 1993, 1996). The NSL calculated as the geometric mean (31 mg) or arithmetic mean NSL (40 mg) are both above the RfD (Hathcock, 1993). For selenium, the geometric mean NSL (244 μg) is below the RfD, and the arithmetic mean NSL (462 μg) is above the RfD (350 μg). The desired level of caution can be set in advance and used consistently for all nutrients or for specific types of adverse effects, but through the arithmetic and geometric means methods, the NSL is calculated with at least a two-fold actual SF below the LOAEL.

Direct use of human NOAELs as safety limits

If a human NOAEL is identified from appropriate data, the safety of that intake is directly established. Comparison with other data is needed, however, to evaluate whether the NOAEL is likely to be a maximum safe level, that is, a 'safety limit', or whether higher intakes may also provide adequate margins of safety. If a LOAEL can be identified, the difference between it and the NOAEL gives evidence of the margin of safety when the NOAEL is selected as the nutrient limit. If a human LOAEL cannot be identified, or if the NOAEL is based on little data, the relative toxicity from animal data may be used to assess the confidence warranted by the NOAEL.

This method is equivalent to using the NOAEL and a SF of 1.0. It is appropriate for nutrients with sufficient data to estimate both the NOAEL and the LOAEL, except when the NOAEL is calculated as a maximum, and is not a direct observation of safety at the specified intake. For example, based on epidemiological evidence from China, the LOAEL for selenium is 910 μg, the NOAEL is 853 μg, and the lower 95 percentile confidence limit of the NOAEL is 600 μg. In comparison, no adverse effects have been observed in association with intakes of more than 700 μg in the US. This combination of epidemiological data does not provide an appropriate basis for the direct identification of a 'safety limit', but does allow calculation of an appropriate total intake safety limit below these values. For the direct identification of a supplemental intake NOAEL, the data from the 10-year clinical trial with 200 μg of supplemental selenium found none of the known clinical or biochemical indicators of selenium toxicity, thus demonstrating the safety of that level of supplementation. Although these data establish the safety of a 200 μg supplement, they do not suggest that this is the maximum safe intake.

For nutrients with no demonstrated oral toxicity at any level tested, NOAEL values represent only the highest intake for which there is adequate evidence of safety. Such data do not suggest that the NOAEL values are the limits of the range of safe intakes. Indeed, the evidence for some nutrients such as vitamin B_{12}, suggests that intakes much higher than the established NOAEL are also likely to be safe.

Tolerable upper intake levels (ULs)

The Food and Nutrition Board of US National Academy of Sciences has recently defined and set for some nutrients ULs that are defined as 'the maximum level of total chronic daily intake of a nutrient judged to be unlikely to pose a risk of adverse health effects to the most sensitive members of the healthy population' (Food and Nutrition Board, 1997). Selection of the ULs involved hazard identification, dose–response assessment, UL estimation, exposure assessment, intake estimation, and risk characterisation. The dose–response assessment criteria included:

- Selection of data
- Identification of NOAEL (or LOAEL) and critical end-points
- Uncertainty assessment

- Selection of UFs for specific nutrients
- Derivation of the ULs

This process differs somewhat in definition from the direct use of the human NOAEL as a safety limit (i.e. SF = 1). In practice for the nutrients mutually addressed, the UL values from the NAS are very consistent with the NOAEL and LOAEL assessment for adults by Hathcock (Hathcock, 1997a) (Table 11.2). Comparison of these approaches reveals that, in general, the CRN values for human NOAEL are conservatively selected and, without an SF, approximate to the FNB UL values that have been derived through use of a small UF.

Evidence on selected vitamins and minerals

VITAMIN A

Consumption of 25 000 to 50 000 IU (7500 to 15 000 µg RE) of preformed retinol equivalents daily for periods of several months or more by women of child-bearing age can produce multiple adverse effects, including liver toxicity and possibly birth defects (Hathcock et al., 1990). The smallest daily supplement of vitamin A reported to be associated with liver cirrhosis in adults is 25 000 IU retinol equivalents (7500 µg RE) during six years (Geubel et al., 1991). The smallest daily supplement generally considered to generate any risk of birth defects is also 25 000 IU (7500 µg RE) (Hathcock et al., 1990). One report, however, concluded there was a significantly increased risk of neural crest birth defects at maternal daily supplemental levels of 'more than 10 000 IU' (more than 3000 µg RE) (Rothman et al., 1995). The average supplemental intake by this range group of women was 21 675 IU (6500 µg RE), but unfortunately the authors did not identify individual supplemental intakes in the seven cases associated with birth defects. Several issues have been raised about the validity of the defect classification scheme used and the resulting likelihood that the study overestimated the risk associated with vitamin A at the

Table 11.2 Comparison of nutrient safety limits for 50 year-old adults

Nutrient	FNB			CRN	
	NOAEL, (LOAEL)	UF	UL	NOAEL	LOAEL
Calcium (g)	(5 g)	2	2.5 g	1.5 g	> 2.5 g
Phosphorus (g)	~10 g	2.5	4 g	1.5 g	> 2.5 g
Magnesium (mg)	360[a]	~1	350	700[b]	Uncertain
Vitamin D (µg)	60	1.2	50	20	50

[a]Identified for 'non-food' magnesium.
[b]Total magnesium intake.
CRN, Council for Responsible Nutrition; FNB, Food and Nutrition Board; LOAEL, Lowest Observed Adverse Effect Level; NOAEL, No Observed Adverse Effect Level; UF, Uncertainty Factor; UL, Upper Intake Level.

levels identified in this study (Oakley and Erickson, 1995; Shaw *et al.*, 1996; Werler *et al.*, 1996). The finding by Rothman *et al.* (1995) was not confirmed in a more recent study (Lammer *et al.*, 1996).

Some reports suggest the possibility that there may be some risk of vitamin A toxicity at supplementation levels below 20 000 IU (6000 µg RE) per day. One report to the US Food and Drug Administration suggested a characteristic birth defect in association with maternal supplementation at 18 000 IU (5400 µg RE) per day (Rosa *et al.*, 1986). Another report found marginal indications in elderly subjects of adverse effects on the liver with chronic supplementation at levels of 5000 to 10 000 IU (1500 to 3000 µg RE) per day (Krasinski *et al.*, 1989). However, this observation has not been confirmed (Stauber *et al.*, 1991) and the same laboratory was unable to repeat this finding in later studies (Johnson *et al.*, 1992). No other reports have indicated adverse effects from vitamin A at these supplemental levels.

NOAEL: 3000 µg RE (10 000 IU). LOAEL: 6500 µg RE (21 600 IU).

β-CAROTENE

β-Carotene is considered to be virtually non-toxic because humans tolerate high dietary dosages without apparent harm, and animal studies also failed to find any toxic effects (Bendich, 1988; Hathcock *et al.*, 1990; Diplock, 1995). Standard toxicological tests, including teratogenic, mutagenic and carcinogenic assays, have been performed on β-carotene without any evidence of harmful effects. There is no evidence that conversion of β-carotene to vitamin A contributes to vitamin A toxicity, even when β-carotene is ingested in large amounts (Olson, 1994).

The only documented biological effect of high β-carotene intake has been coloration of the skin related to hypercarotenaemia, but this occurs only at extremely high intake levels. Intakes as high as 180 mg/day have been given to humans for several months without observed adverse effects other than skin discoloration (Mathews-Roth, 1986).

Because of the extensive safety record of β-carotene, clinical trials were designed with the assumption that the only likely effects would be benefits. Questions about the safety of β-carotene have been raised by the results of the ATBC (ATBC, 1994) and CARET (Omenn *et al.*, 1996) trials which observed significant increases in lung cancer risk in high-risk populations (long-term smokers or asbestos workers) who were given supplements of β-carotene (20 or 30 mg/day). On the other hand, there was evidence in the CARET study that β-carotene may reduce the risk of lung cancer in former smokers. In contrast to the unexpected increases in lung cancer risk in the ATBC and CARET trials, no increased risk was observed in the PHS trial that included more than two thousand smokers and lasted approximately 12 years (Hennekens *et al.*,

1996), compared with the five to seven years in the ATBC and CARET trials, or in three other shorter-term trials (Greenberg et al., 1990, 1994; Blot et al., 1993). Moreover, observational studies have found reduced risk of lung cancer or other disease associated with increased β-carotene intakes (Hennekens, 1986; Menkes et al., 1986; Rimm et al., 1993). The effects of alcohol or high intakes of retinol on the liver have been postulated to explain the adverse outcome with β-carotene in the ATBC and CARET studies (Lachance, 1996).

NOAEL: 25 mg. LOAEL: None established.

VITAMIN D

Excess vitamin D intakes for a prolonged basis lead to hypercalcaemia. Excessive production of the active metabolite (calcitriol, 1α,25-dihydroxy-cholecalciferol) or greatly increased blood concentration of its immediate precursor (25-hydroxy vitamin D) can overstimulate intestinal absorption of calcium and cause excessive calcium mobilisation from bone (Norman, 1996).

The amount of daily vitamin D ingestion needed to produce adverse effects varies widely. In most adults, daily intake in excess of 50 000 IU (1.25 mg) is needed to produce toxicity (Miller and Hayes, 1982), but much less may cause adverse effects in some persons. In certain diseases such as sarcoidosis, Mycobacterium infections such as tuberculosis, or idiopathic hypercalcaemia, toxicity can occur at levels of vitamin D intake only somewhat above normal (> 25 μg, or 1000 IU per day). A causal relationship between excess vitamin D intake and idiopathic hypercalcaemia is unlikely, although persons with idiopathic calcaemia may be subject to adverse effects of vitamin D at lower intakes than those who are normal (Select Committee on GRAS Substances, 1978).

In children of unreported body weight (certainly between 10 and 30 kg), the amount of dietary vitamin D that has led to adverse effects may be as low as 2000 to 4000 IU (50–100 μg) per day. In full-term infants, adverse effects are reported to occur with intakes as low as 1800 IU (45 μg) per day (Chesney, 1989) but no adverse effects occurred in a six-month study of infants given 1600 IU per day (Fomon et al., 1966). No adverse effects were observed in a clinical trial involving 3000 elderly women given 800 IU (20 μg) per day for 18 months (Chapuy et al., 1992).

There are numerous reports that confirm a variety of adverse effects of very high intakes when used as a drug, administration of activated forms, or parenteral administration of vitamin D or its activated forms (Nanji, 1985; Goldman and Wheeler, 1987; Schwartzman and Franck, 1987; Allen and Shah, 1992; Boulard et al., 1994; Oymak et al., 1994; Matsukawa et al., 1995). These circumstances do not relate to the usual intakes of vitamin D from foods or dietary supplements and thus most reports of adverse effects related to vitamin D provide no useful information about the safety of dietary sources of vitamin D.

NOAEL: 20 μg (800 IU). LOAEL: 50 μg (2000 IU).

VITAMIN E

The lack of toxicity of vitamin E has been consistently reported for 20 years in the research literature. The only reported contradiction concerns possibly decreased blood coagulation. Some studies have reported decreased platelet reactivity (and thus possible decreased clotting capacity) in response to vitamin E addition *in vitro*. However, studies with vitamin E supplementation have shown no changes in platelet aggregation or adhesion with daily vitamin E intakes as high as 1200 IU (800 mg α-TE) (Steiner, 1991, 1993). There is a case report of prolonged bleeding time during chronic warfarin therapy in a man taking 1200 IU of vitamin E per day (Corrigan and Ulters, 1981). However, in a recent study, 800 and 1200 IU were not found to influence prothrombin times in patients on warfarin therapy (Kim and White, 1996). Also, it has been reported that a vitamin E intake of 900 IU per day does not affect coagulation activity in persons not taking anticoagulant drugs (Kitagawa and Mino, 1989).

The ATBC study observed an increase in the number of deaths from haemorrhagic stroke (ATBC, 1994), but there has been no corroboration of this observation in any of the many other studies on vitamin E over the past 20 years. The number of haemorrhagic stroke cases associated with vitamin E treatment and control groups were 66 and 44, respectively, a small fraction of the total subjects in the trial (29 133). The authors did not publish any confidence intervals or tests of statistical significance related to these data. However, because this study evaluated associations of many disease states, it would not be surprising if some appeared statistically significant on the basis of random occurrence. The ATBC study was not designed to differentiate between haemorrhagic and ischaemic stroke. Furthermore, a variety of factors which may promote haemorrhagic stroke such as hypertension, occurrence of cerebral metastasis of lung cancer and potential effects of chemotherapy have not yet been accounted for by the investigators. Nevertheless, this result in the ATBC study has been cited (Bernier, 1995) as sufficient cause for restrictive limits on vitamin E intake. The uniqueness of this observation in the ATBC study and the lack of support in other studies involving higher intakes of vitamin E suggest that attribution of such increased risk to the intake of 50 IU of vitamin E (50 mg of dl-α-tocopherol acetate) is not warranted. Such attribution ignores statistical issues related to multiple endpoints and is contradicted by other data that show effects on platelets only at higher intakes.

NOAEL: 800 mg α-TE. LOAEL: None established.

PYRIDOXINE

Both deficiency and excess of pyridoxine produce neurological disturbances (Hathcock and Rader, 1990). The first report of pyridoxine neurotoxicity in humans described a sensory neuropathy of the extremities in women with daily intakes of 2000 to 6000 mg, mostly taken in an attempt to control premenstrual symptoms (Schaumburg et al., 1983). The neuropathy slowly, and perhaps incompletely, regresses after cessation of the elevated dose (Albin et al., 1987; Albin and Albers, 1990; Santoro et al., 1991). Most cases of sensory neuropathy have resulted from intakes greater than 600 mg/day but some evidence suggests that neuropathy may result from doses as low as 300 to 500 mg in some individuals (Parry and Bredesen, 1985; Bendich and Cohen, 1990; Hathcock and Rader, 1990). The total dose over an unspecified time may give a better prediction of the potential for neurotoxic response than either the daily dose or duration of the high intake (Bendich and Cohen, 1990).

There is controversy over the validity of the single report of adverse effects at daily intakes near 100 mg or less (Dalton and Dalton, 1987). Although this report is often cited as evidence that pyridoxine intakes below 100 mg/day can cause sensory neuropathy, the data showed an average intake of 117 mg/day among women with symptoms, and an identical average intake (116 mg/day) in the control group. The group with symptoms had taken pyridoxine longer – an average 2.9 years, compared with 1.6 years for those without symptoms. Some women in each group had intakes of 50 mg or less. Likely inaccuracies in the telephone survey method and a lack of objective neurological assessment could have introduced bias. The symptoms observed had no dose–response relationship to pyridoxine intake but did suggest a time–response relationship.

Some reports have suggested that high intakes of pyridoxine may carry risk of oxalate kidney stones. Such concerns seem unfounded. The reported cases may have been associated with the drug pyridoxilate (a combination of pyridoxine and glyoxalate) (Daudon et al., 1987), and a recent prospective epidemiological study found the relative risk of oxalate renal stones to be decreased for men consuming more than 40 mg of pyridoxine in comparison with those consuming less that 3 mg (Curhan et al., 1996).

Estimation of NOAEL and LOAEL values from the available data may be complicated by the dose–time interaction. A pyridoxine intake of 500 mg/day carries a risk of neurotoxicity and this level is identified as the LOAEL for long-term use.

Severe methodological problems in the report by Dalton and Dalton (1987) on intakes near 100 mg include lack of objective neurological measurements and lack of dose verification by any means other than an interview. They state that neurological examinations were given, but they describe neither the methods nor the results. There is no indication that the withdrawal and rechallenge for a few patients was done in a blinded manner, thus raising the distinct possibility of biased results. These weaknesses are so large that in the absence of any other report of adverse effects at similar intakes during the decade since their publication, together with the absence of adverse effects in other reports from well-controlled studies at much higher intakes (Bendich and Cohen, 1990), indicate that the Dalton and Dalton report may not be used as a reliable indicator of risk.

NOAEL: 200 mg. LOAEL: 500 mg.

The NOAEL and LOAEL values identified from human data are not contradicted by animal data. A well-controlled study in dogs found a strong neuropathy with doses of 250 mg/kg/day, but only a very mild one at 50 mg/kg/day (Phillips et al., 1978). This dose–response relationship suggests that the LOAEL of 50 mg/kg/day is close to being a NOAEL. Thus, extrapolation to humans need not employ a composite safety factor any larger than 30. This factor is derived from 10 for variation among humans, and 3 (and probably less) for conversion to the NOAEL. With a total safety factor of 10, the dog LOAEL would convert to 300 mg/day for a 60-kg person (and 30 would give 100 mg/day). An additional safety factor of 10 is clearly not needed because of the human data that clearly show the resulting 'limit' to be far below the human NOAEL. The former practice of using multiple 10-fold safety factors is now recognised as being unnecessarily restrictive, and sometimes produces an illogical result.

NICOTINIC ACID

The flushing reaction produced by nicotinic acid has been recognised for more than half a century (Bean, 1978). When taken on an empty stomach, crystalline nicotinic acid in doses as small as 10 mg may produce a mild but noticeable flushing reaction. While not desirable, such reactions produce no known adverse consequences, and they are seldom perceptible when small amounts of nicotinic acid are taken in tablet or capsule form, or consumed with food.

Serious side effects of nicotinic acid have occasionally occurred when gram-quantities were taken to lower serum lipids (Rader et al., 1992). Liver toxicity and serious gastrointestinal effect can sometimes occur in persons consuming 1 g or more per day of nicotinic acid. Gastrointestinal side effects may include indigestion, nausea, vomiting and diarrhoea and, in some persons, necessitate discontinuation of nicotinic acid. Liver toxicity is most commonly monitored by increases in serum transaminase enzymes of liver origin released by damage to liver cells. Small increases in serum concentrations of transaminases do not indicate significant liver damage and return to normal after cessation of nicotinic acid intake. More severe reactions may produce jaundice, fatigue, or, in at least one case, fulminate liver failure (Clementz and Holmes, 1989).

There is a strong correspondence between the minimum adverse effect level identified through clinical trials and that suggested by the published anecdotal case reports. Many severe reactions is nicotinic acid, especially liver toxicity, have involved ill-advised or inadvertent switching from unmodified nicotinic acid preparations to slow-release formulations (Rader *et al.*, 1992). Most reported adverse reactions to nicotinic acid have occurred with intakes of 2 to 6 g/day. There are only two anecdotal cases reported where intake levels were below 1000 mg, one for slow-release nicotinic acid at 500 mg/day and one for unmodified nicotinic acid at 750 mg/day (Rader *et al.*, 1992). The clinical trial of McKenney *et al.* (1994) used two groups of adult subjects, one for immediate-release and one for slow-release nicotinic acid, who were observed initially and for six weeks at each dosage level: 500, 1000, 1500, 2000 and 3000 mg/day. The data showed no adverse reactions at 500 mg/day for either form of nicotinic acid, but statistically significant effects beginning at 1000 mg/day (gastrointestinal effects for unmodified nicotinic acid, and mild liver toxicity for slow-release nicotinic acid). Gram quantities of nicotinic acid should not be self-administered as a dietary supplement but may be safely used under the care and monitoring of a physician.

The amount of information on nicotinamide is much smaller than that for nicotinic acid, but there appears to be much less use at high levels than for nicotinic acid. Nicotinamide intakes of 3 g/day or more have resulted in gastrointestinal and liver effects (Rader *et al.*, 1992).

> NOAEL: Nicotinic acid, 500 mg; Nicotinamide, 1500 mg.
> LOAEL: Nicotinic acid, 1000 mg; Nicotinamide, 3000 mg.

FOLIC ACID

Three major concerns have been identified as possible adverse effects from excessive levels of folic acid intake: (i) the masking of pernicious anaemia, thus allowing the neurologic disease of vitamin B_{12} deficiency to progress unchecked; (ii) the disruption of zinc function by folic acid; and (iii) the antagonism of medications, especially antifolate agents. Each of these presents serious concerns and warrants careful consideration of the evidence. The evidence is weak that folic acid has adverse effects by these or any other mechanism (Campbell, 1996).

Masking pernicious anaemia

Administration of high levels of folic acid to pernicious anaemia patients can mask the anaemic manifestations while allowing the neurological disease (posterolateral spinal cord degeneration) to progress (Butterworth and Tamura, 1989). Fortunately, this devastating complication is unlikely to occur with the amounts of folic acid intake achieved through ordinary diets and the vast majority of dietary supplements. The convincing reports of the masking effect involve administration of 5 mg or more folic acid per day. A few early reports showed some response in certain haematological indices in pernicious anaemia patients taking folic acid doses as low as 0.1 mg to 0.8 mg. These effects are sometimes interpreted as indicating possible risk from increased folic acid intakes (Savage and Lindenbaum, 1995). Such possible risk is speculative because more than 25% of vitamin B_{12}-deficient patients who are not taking folic acid display no anaemia (normal haematocrit and normal mean cell volume) but show only neurological signs (Healton et al., 1991). Thus, a report of an individual with neurological signs of vitamin B_{12} deficiency who had also taken folic acid supplements (Brantigan, 1997) cannot be concluded to be evidence of a masking effect. There is no clear evidence that folic acid changes the time course or neurological outcome in vitamin B_{12} deficiency. Although there are a few reports of an incomplete masking effect resulting from amounts of folic acid less than 1 mg, the effect is unusual at that intake and is predictable only at 5 mg or more (Food and Drug Administration, 1993). Many pernicious anaemia patients who respond to folic acid may also be deficient in folic acid (Dudley and Coltman, 1970). Although haemoglobin and haematocrit respond in some patients, particularly with high oral doses or parenteral administration, folic acid does not completely normalise haematological morphology in vitamin B_{12} deficiency (Herbert, 1963).

Folic acid–zinc interactions

Certain folic acid–zinc interactions are well documented. The folate conjugase enzyme must act on food pteroylpolyglutamates for absorption, which does not occur in zinc deficiency (Butterworth and Tamura, 1989). The crucial issue, however, is whether higher intakes of folic acid have adverse consequences through a disruption of zinc bioavailability or function, and, if so, the levels of folic acid associated with such effects. Some reports suggest that as little as 350 μg of supplemental folic acid can adversely affect zinc nutrimental value (Milne et al., 1984; Mukherjee et al., 1984; Simmer et al., 1987), but more recent reports indicate no adverse effects of folic acid on zinc uptake or function (Tamura et al., 1992; Kauwell et al., 1995).

The suggestion that folic acid intakes of less than 400 μg per day cause adverse outcomes of pregnancy through the antagonism of zinc functions (Mukherjee et al., 1984) was not supported by a larger, multi-centre study involving a 10-fold higher intake of folic acid throughout pregnancy (Wald et al., 1991).

It is difficult to resolve differences in the scientific literature regarding a possible adverse effect of folic acid on zinc nutriment. These incompatible results can likely be attributed to the widely different experimental approaches used. In general, methods based on rate of uptake and plasma concentration tend to show effects at lower folic acid intakes, whereas zinc balance methods tend to show effects only at higher intakes. Large, well-conducted clinical trials have found no adverse effects of folic acid on pregnancy through zinc antagonism or any other mechanism, but they have demonstrated a clear benefit in reducing the risk of NTDs (Walt *et al.*, 1991; Czeizel and Dudas, 1992).

Folic acid–drug interactions

At very high levels of intake, folic acid has been reported to interfere with the effectiveness of anticonvulsant drugs such as Dilantin (diphenylhydantoin) used in controlling epilepsy (Food and Drug Administration, 1993, 1996). Folic acid doses of 5 to 30 mg orally have produced some evidence of increased frequency of seizures in epileptics, but there is no evidence of such effects at lower intakes of folic acid. It might be expected that increased folic acid intakes could interfere with actions of folate antagonistic drugs such as methotrexate. In contrast, administration of 1 mg folic acid daily, for six months in patients with rheumatoid arthritis who were treated with low-dose methotrexate, actually decreased methotrexate toxicity without affecting its efficacy for therapy (Morgan *et al.*, 1990). Drug antagonisms by folic acid have been reported, but the effects are varied and the levels at which they occurred are scattered. Effects in categories other than these three are so inconsistent that they do not support any specific LOAEL value.

NOAEL: 1000 μg. LOAEL: Not less than 5000 μg.

CALCIUM

No adverse effects are usually observed in healthy adults consuming up to 2500 mg of calcium per day (Food and Nutrition Board, 1989). Using milk alkali syndrome as the critical end-point, some adverse effects may occur with intakes of 4–5 g/day, but intakes as low as 1–2 g/day may lead to hypercalciuria in persons with renal stones (Food and Nutrition Board, 1997). High intakes may induce constipation and may also put some otherwise healthy hypercalcinuric men at risk of urinary stone formation. However, higher calcium intakes have generally been associated with decreased risk of kidney stones (Curhan *et al.*, 1993). Higher intakes of calcium may also inhibit the intestinal absorption of other essential minerals, notably iron, zinc and manganese (Greger, 1988).

Calcium intakes of up to 2500 mg are safe for normal adults, and this intake may be identified as the NOAEL. Adverse effects in normal adults have been observed only with chronic intakes considerably above 2500 mg/day. Thus, the LOAEL is distinctly greater than 2500 mg/day, but the exact value cannot be identified.

NOAEL: 2500 mg; LOAEL: Uncertain but in the range of 4–5 g or higher.

BORON

Boron has a low potential for causing obvious adverse effects in humans, as indicated by the widespread use of boric acid between 1870 and 1920 as a food preservative. This use of boric acid led to intakes of up to 500 mg per day without adverse effects other than nausea and loss of appetite (Nielsen, 1996). In pregnant rats, dietary boric acid can cause foetal development defects and growth deficits (Price et al., 1996). In studies with dogs, high intakes of boric acid have caused testicular atrophy and decreased sperm production (Weir and Fisher, 1972). Intakes of 500 mg boric acid (72 mg boron) per day for 50 days by adults led to disturbed appetite and digestion (Nielsen, 1996).

In a study in dogs, Weir and Fisher (1972) found adverse effects with an intake of 29 mg/kg/day over 38 weeks of treatment, and this level became the LOAEL. The next lower dose of 8.8 mg/kg/day produced no adverse effects and therefore this intake became the NOAEL. The foetal development NOAEL in rats is higher that the NOAEL in male dogs. The US Environmental Protection Agency applied a 100-fold margin of safety to the NOAEL in dogs to calculate a 'safe' intake (i.e. a Reference Dose) of 0.09 mg per day, or 6.3 mg per day in a 70-kg man (IRIS, 1997b).

The clinical trials with an upper intake of 3 mg per day produced no adverse effect, but this intake may be too low to be a meaningful NOAEL for humans because few intake levels have been studied. The EPA Reference Dose (equivalent to 6.3 mg/day in a 70-kg man) that was extrapolated from animals with a 100-fold safety factor, may be considered a safe level of human intake. This intake level could be suggested as a NOAEL, except that it would be a misnomer because it is based on calculation rather than observation. For boron intakes by adults, the Reference Dose of 6.3 mg per day does not require application of any additional safety factor (i.e. the safety factor is 1.0). It is not a direct human NOAEL, but it may be considered safe.

CHROMIUM (III)

No credible data or reports have shown adverse effects of chromium III (valence 3^+) in humans, and animal data also suggest that orally administered chromium is extremely innocuous (Dourson, 1994; Nielsen, 1994a,b; Hathcock, 1996). In addition, the Medline database lists no published cases of adverse reactions in humans.

In contrast, chromium VI (chromate, valence 6^+) is clearly established as the work-related aetiologic agent in lung disease, including lung cancer in chromate and stainless steel workers (Gad, 1989). One report described chromosome breakage in vitro by high concentrations of chromium (III) picolinate added directly to cells (Stearns et al., 1995). These data showed that even at the high concentrations used in vitro, the only evidence for DNA damage resulted from picolinic acid, not chromium. Overall, the data of Stearns and co-workers do not provide appropriate evidence that chromium III in food or dietary supplements carries any risk of causing DNA damage or cancer.

The US EPA has reviewed all relevant data on chromium toxicity and calculated an RfD, a safety limit involving a margin of safety below the levels with evidence of adverse effects, for chromium III and also for chromium VI (IRIS, 1997c). Application of a composite safety factor of 1000 to the animal data gives an RfD of 1.47 mg/kg (Dourson, 1994), which with rounding converts to 70 mg/day in the adult male. The RfD for chromium III (70 000 μg) is 350 times the upper value of the nutritional range (the Estimated Safe and Adequate Daily Dietary Intake) of 50–200 μg for adults (Food and Nutrition Board, 1989). Thus, chromium III has an extraordinarily wide margin of safety. In contrast, hexavalent chromium (Cr^{6+}), a form not found in the diet, has significant toxic potential, and thus the RfD for chromium VI, calculated by EPA for a 70 kg man, is only 335 μg/day (Dourson, 1994).

In summary, there is no evidence of toxicity in humans from orally ingested trivalent chromium (Cr^{3+}), and extrapolation from animal data indicates that it is extraordinarily safe. The benign character of chromium III should not be confused with the established toxicity of chromium VI.

There are no data on which to base a LOAEL for chromium III in humans. The highest intake reported for a group of people under good observation is 1000 μg/day (Anderson *et al.*, 1996), therefore this value is identified as the NOAEL. Because of the extremely high RfD calculated from animal data (70 000 μg/day) through application of a large safety factor (1000), it is likely that the NOAEL is limited by experience with high intakes and not by any known potential for adverse effects.

SELENIUM

Excess selenium intake due to consumption of seleniferous plants by animals produces a wide range of adverse effects (National Research Council, 1983). Chronic toxicity signs in livestock include cirrhosis, lameness, hoof malformations, hair loss and emaciation. In laboratory animals, the signs most commonly include cirrhosis. The minimum dietary level of selenium recognised to produce adverse effects in farm animals is 4–5 μg/g dry weight of diet.

An episode of human poisoning by selenium involved a manufacturing error that resulted in a dietary supplement product which actually contained 182 times the amount of selenium declared on the label (Jensen *et al.*, 1984; Helzlsouer *et al.*, 1985). Adverse effects occurred within a few weeks and included effects on hair, nails and liver. Human selenium poisoning in a high-selenium area of China also produced adverse effects on nails, skin, the nervous system and teeth (Yang *et al.*, 1983). The adverse effects occurred in susceptible persons with intakes of 910 μg/day or more. No adverse effects have been associated with lower levels, but the ratio of plasma selenium to erythrocyte selenium have been found to increase with dietary intakes of

750 μg/day or more (Yang et al., 1989b). Human surveys in seleniferous areas of the United States have failed to find any signs of selenium intoxication with intakes up to slightly more than 700 μg/day (Longnecker et al., 1991). Because the chemical forms of selenium in foods grown in seleniferous areas are not known, the human data on adverse effects from chronically high intakes apply only to total dietary selenium and not to any specific form. No adverse effects were observed in the 8- to 10-year clinical trial by Clark et al. (1996; Combs and Clark, 1997) at daily supplemental intakes of 200 μg selenium in yeast.

With adverse effects established in a few individuals at chronic dietary intakes of 910 μg/day, this value may be identified as the LOAEL for skin, hair, nails and liver effect. The data of Yang et al. (1989b) did not show any overt adverse effects but identified an increase in the ratio of plasma selenium to erythrocyte selenium at intakes of 750 μg/day. Therefore, this intake level is not selected as a NOAEL. Although this change in ratio is not itself an adverse effect, it may indicate that the ability to eliminate excess selenium is nearly saturated. Application of regression methods to the data of Yang et al. (1989a, b) supports a NOAEL of 853 μg/day for the Chinese adult of 55 kg weight (Combs, 1994; Poirier, 1994). The US EPA has set the NOAEL at 0.015 mg/kg/day (Poirier, 1994; IRIS, 1997d), a value that corresponds to a NOAEL of 1050 μg for a 70-kg man, or 822 μg for a 55-kg adult. In the Chines population with an average LOAEL of 910 μg selenium intake, the lower 95% confidence limit was 600 μg per day (Yang and Zhou, 1994).

Considering these factors, a NOAEL is set at 200 μg supplemental selenium per day, based on the absence of adverse effects at this supplemental level in the clinical trial of Clark and co-workers, and on the substantial margin of safety it provides below the levels that are associated with adverse effects.

NOAEL: 200 μg. LOAEL: 910 μg.

References

Abernathy CO, Cantilli R, Du JT and Levander OA (1993) Essentiality versus toxicity: some considerations in the risk assessment of essential trace elements. In *Hazard Assessment of Chemicals*, Saxena J (ed), Hemisphere Publishing, New York, pp. 81–113.

Albin RL and Albers JW (1990) Long-term follow-up of pyridoxine-induced acute sensory neuropathy-neuronopathy. *Neurology*, **40**, 1319.

Albin RL, Albers JW, Greenberg HS, Townsend JB, Lynn RB, Burke JM and Alessi AG (1987) Acute sensory neuropathy-neuronopathy from pyridoxine overdose. *Neurology*, **37**, 1729–1732.

Allen SH and Shah JH (1992) Calcinosis and metastatic calcification due to vitamin D intoxication. *Hormone Research*, **37**, 68–77.

Anderson R, Cheng N, Bryden N, Polansky M, Cheng N, Chi J and Feng J (1996) Beneficial effects of chromium for people with type II diabetes (abstract). American Diabetes Association Annual Science Sessions.

ATBC: The Alpha-Tocopherol, Beta Carotene (ATBC) Cancer Prevention Study Group (1994). The effect of vitamin E and beta carotene on the incidence of lung cancer and other cancers in male smokers. *New England Journal of Medicine*, **330**, 1029–1035.

Barnes DG and Dourson M (1988) Reference dose (RfD): description and use in health risk assessments. *Regulatory Toxicology and Pharmacology*, **8**, 471–486.

Bean WB (1978) Some aspects of pharmacologic use and abuse of water-soluble vitamins. In *Nutrition and Drug Interactions*, Hathcock JN and Coon J (eds), Academic Press, New York, pp. 667–685.

Bendich A (1988) The safety of beta carotene. *Nutrition and Cancer*, **11**, 207–214.

Bendich A and Cohen M (1990) Vitamin B$_6$ safety issues. *Annals of the New York Academy of Sciences*, **585**, 321–323.

Bernier JJ (1995) *Rapport sur les limites de sécurité dans les consommations alimentaires des vitamines et minéraux*, Ministère de l'Économie et des Finances, Ministère du Travail et des Affaires Sociales, Ministère de l'Agriculture, de la Pêche et de l'Alimentation, Paris.

Blot WJ, Lie J-Y, Taylor PR, Guo W, Dawsey S, Wang G-Q, Yang CS, Zheng S-F, Gail M, Li G-Y, Yu Y, Liu B-Q, Tangrea J, Sun Y-H, Liu F, Fraumeni JF Jr., Zhang Y-H and Li B (1993) Nutrition intervention trials in Linxian, China: supplementation with specific vitamin/mineral combinations, cancer incidence, and disease-specific mortality in the general population. *Journal of the National Cancer Institute*, **85**, 1483–1492.

Boulard JC, Hanslik T, Alterescu R and Baglin A (1994) Hypercalcémie symptomatique après association vitamine D diurétiques thiazidiques: 2 observations chez des femmes dosés (letter). *La Presse Medicale*, **22**, 96.

Brantigan CO (1997) Folate supplementation and the risk of masking vitamin B$_{12}$ deficiency. *Journal of the American Medical Association*, **277**, 884.

Butterworth CE Jr and Tamura T (1989) Folic acid safety and toxicity: a brief review. *American Journal of Clinical Nutrition*, **50**, 353–358.

Campbell NR (1996) How safe are folic acid supplements? *Archives of Internal Medicine*, **156**, 1638–1644.

Chapuy MC, Arlot ME, Duboeuf F, Brun J, Crouzet B, Arnaud S, Delmas PD and Meunier PJ (1992) Vitamin D$_3$ and calcium to prevent hip fractures in elderly women. *New England Journal of Medicine*, **327**, 1637–1642.

Chesney RW (1989) Vitamin D: Can an upper limit be defined? *Journal of Nutrition*, **119**, 1825–1828.

Clark LC, Combs GF, Turnbull BW, Slate EH, Chalker DK, Chau J, Davis LS, Glover DA, Graham GF, Gross EG, Krongrad A, Lesher JL Jr, Park HF, Sanders BB, Smith CL and Taylor JR (1996) Effect of selenium supplementation for cancer prevention in patients with carcinoma of the skin. A randomized controlled trial. *Journal of the American Medical Associations*, **276**, 1957–1963.

Clementz GL and Holmes AW (1989) Nicotinic acid-induced fulminant hepatic failure. *Journal of Clinical Gastroenterology*, **9**, 582–584.

Code of Federal Regulations (CRF) (1995) Title 21, part 170.22, Government Printing Office, Washington, DC.

Codex Alimentarius Commission (1995) *Draft guidelines for dietary supplements (vitamins and minerals)*, Committee on Nutrition and Foods for Special Dietary Uses. ALINORM 95/26. Food and Agriculture Organization of the United Nations/World Health Organization, Joint Office, Rome.

Codex Alimentarius Commission (1996) *Report of the twentieth session of the Codex Committee on Nutrition and Foods for Special Dietary Uses, ALINORM 97/26*. Food and Agriculture Organization of the United Nations/World Health Organization, Joint Office, Rome.

Combs GF Jr (1994) Essentiality and toxicity of selenium: a critique of the recommended dietary allowance and the reference dose. In *Risk Assessment of Essential Elements*, Mertz W, Abernathy CO and Olin SS (eds), ILSI Press, Washington, DC, pp. 167–183.

Combs GF Jr and Clark LC (1997) Selenium. In *Antioxidants Disease Prevention*, Garewal HS (ed), CRC Press, New York, pp. 97–113.

Committee on Toxicity (1997) Department of Health, London, UK. *World Food Chemistry News*, January 22, p. 5.

Coon JM (1973) Toxicology of natural food chemicals: a perspective. In *Toxicants Occurring Naturally in Foods*, 2nd edn, National Academy of Sciences, Washington DC, pp. 573–591.

Corrigan JJ Jr and Ulfers LL (1981) Effect of vitamin E on prothrombin levels in warfarin-induced vitamin K deficiency. *American Journal of Clinical Nutrition*, **34**, 1701–1705.

Curhan GC, Willett WC, Rimm EB and Stampfer MJ (1993) A prospective study of dietary calcium and other nutrients and the risk of symptomatic kidney stones. *New England Journal of Medicine*, **328**, 833–838.

Curhan GC, Willett WC, Rimm EB and Stampfer MJ (1996) A prospective study of the intake of vitamins C and B_6, and the risk of kidney stones in men. *Journal of Urology*, **155**, 1847–1851.

Czeizel A and Dudas I (1992) Prevention of the first occurrence of neural-tube defects by preconceptual vitamin supplementation. *New England Journal of Medicine*, **327**, 1832–1835.

Dalton K and Dalton MJT (1987) Characteristics of pyridoxine overdose neuropathy syndrome. *Acta Neurologica Scandinavica*, **76**, 8–11.

Daudon M, Revillaud RJ, Normand M, Petit C and Jungers P (1987) Pyridoxilate-induced calicium oxalate calculi: a new drug-induced metabolic nephrolithiasis. *Journal of Urology*, **138**, 258–261.

Diplock AT (1995) Safety of antioxidant vitamins and beta-carotene. *American Journal of Clinical Nutrition*, **62**, 1510S–1516S.

Dourson ML (1994) The chromium reference dose. In *Risk Assessment of Essential Elements*, Mertz W, Abernathy CO and Olin SS (eds), ILSI Press, Washington DC, pp. 207–212.

Dourson M and Stara JF (1983) Regulatory history and experimental support of uncertainty (safety) factors. *Regulatory Toxicology and Pharmacology*, **3**, 224–238.

Dourson ML, Fleter SP and Robinson D (1996) Evolution of science-based uncertainty factors in noncancer risk assessment. *Regulatory Toxicology Pharmacology*, **24**, 108–120.

Dragula C and Burin G (1994) International harmonization for the risk assessment of pesticides: results of an IPCS survey. *Regulatory Toxicology and Pharmacology*, **20**, 337–353.

Dudley GM and Coltman CA (1970) Resolution of ineffective erythropoiesis of pernicious anemia and 'strongly suggestive' folate lack in response to folic acid. *American Journal of Clinical Nutrition*, **23**, 147–155.

Fomon SJ, Younoszal MK and Thomas LN (1966) Influence of vitamin D on linear growth of normal full-term infants. *Journal of Nutrition*, **88**, 345–350.

Food and Drug Administration (1993) Food labeling: health claims and label statements; folate and neural tube defects; proposed rules. *Federal Register*, **58**, 53254–53288.

Food and Drug Administration (1996) Food labeling: health claims and label statements; folate and neural tube defects. *Federal Register*, **61**, 8752–8781.

Food and Nutrition Board (1989) *Recommended Dietary Allowances*, 10th edn, National Academy of Sciences Press, Washington, DC.

Food and Nutrition Board, Standing Committee on the Scientific Evaluation of Dietary Reference Intakes (1997) *Dietary reference intakes for calcium, phosphorus, magnesium, vitamin D, and fluoride*, National Academy Press, Washington, DC.

Food Safety Council (1982) *A proposed food safety evaluation process*, Nutrition Foundation, Washington, DC.

Gad SC (1989) Acute and chronic systemic chromium toxicity. *Science of the Total Environment*, **86**, 149–157.

Geubel AP, De Galocsy C, Alves N, Rahier J and Dive C (1991) Liver damage caused by therapeutic vitamin A administration: estimate of dose-related toxicity in 41 cases. *Gastroenterology*, **100**, 1701–1709.

Goldman JM and Wheeler MF (1987) Vitamin D-induced hypercalcemia (letter). *American Journal of Medicine*, **82**, 1277.

Greenberg ER, Baron JA, Stukel TA, Stevens MM, Mandel JS, Spencer SK, Elias PM, Lowe N, Nierenberg DW, Bayrd G, Vance JC, Freeman DH Jr, Clendenning WF and Kwan T (1990) A clinical trial of beta carotene to prevent basal-cell and squamous-cell cancers of the skin. *New England Journal of Medicine*, **323**, 789–795.

Greenberg ER, Baron JA, Tosteson TD, Freeman DH Jr, Beck GJ, Bond JH, Colaccio TA, Coller JA, Frankl HD, Haile RW, Mandel JS, Nierenberg DW, Rothstein R, Snover DC, Stevens MM, Summers RW and van Stoek U (1994) A clinical trial of antioxidant vitamins to prevent colorectal adenoma. *New England Journal of Medicine*, **331**, 141–147.

Greger JL (1988) Effect of variations in dietary protein, phosphorus, electrolytes and vitamin D on calcium and zinc metabolism. In *Nutrient Interactions*, Bodwell CD and Erdman JW Jr (eds), Marcel Dekker, New York, pp. 205–227.

Hathcock JN (1993) Safety limits for nutrient intakes: concepts and data requirements. *Nutrition Reviews*, **51**, 278–285.

Hathcock JN (1996) Safety limits for nutrients. *Journal of Nutrition*, **126**, 2386S–2389S.

Hathcock JN (1997a) *Vitamin and mineral safety*, Council for Responsible Nutrition, Washington, DC.

Hathcock JN (1997b) Vitamins and minerals: efficacy and safety. *American Journal of Clinical Nutrition*, **66**, 427–437.

Hathcock JN and Rader JI (1990) Micronutrient safety. *Annals of the New York Academy of Science*, **587**, 257–266.

Hathcock JN, Hattan DG, Jenkins MY, McDonald JT, Sundaresan PR and Wilkening VL (1990) Evaluation of vitamin A toxicity. *American Journal of Clinical Nutrition*, **52**, 183–202.

Health Department (1996) *Guidelines to the Regulations to General Health Law in Matters of the Sanitary Control of Goods and Services*. Under-Ministry of Regulation and Sanitary Development, Mexico.

Healton EB, Savage DG, Brust JCM, Garrett TJ and Lindenbaum J (1991) Neurologic aspects of cobalamin deficiency. *Medicine*, **70**, 229–245.

Helzlsouer K, Jacobs R and Morris S (1985) Acute selenium intoxication in the United States. *Federation Proceedings*, **44**, 1670.

Hennekens CH (1986) Micronutrients and cancer prevention. *New England Journal of Medicine*, **315**, 1288–1289.

Hennekens CH, Buring JE, Manson JE, Stampfer M, Rosner B, Cook NR, Belanger C, LaMotte F, Gaziano JM, Ridker PM, Willet W and Peto R (1996) Lack of effect of long-term supplementation with beta carotene on the incidence of malignant neoplasms and cardiovascular disease. *New England Journal of Medicine*, **334**, 1145–1190.

Herbert V (1963) Current concepts in therapy: megaloblastic anemia. *New England Journal of Medicine*, **268**, 201–203.

IRIS (1997a) *Integrated Risk Information System Database IRIS-NCAR (non-carcinogenic)*, US Environmental Protection Agency. Available from the US National Library of Medicine through Toxline.

IRIS (1997b) *Boron. Integrated Risk Information System Database IRIS-NCAR (non-carcinogenic)*, US Environmental Protection Agency. US National Library of Medicine through Toxline.

IRIS (1997c) *Chromium. Integrated Risk Information System Database IRIS-NCAR (non-carcinogenic)*, US Environmental Protection Agency. US National Library of Medicine through Toxline.

IRIS (1997d) *Selenium. Integrated Risk Information System Database IRIS-NCAR (non-carcinogenic)*, US Environmental Protection Agency. US National Library of Medicine through Toxline.

Jensen R, Clossen W and Rothenberg R (1984) Selenium intoxication – New York. *Morbidity and Mortality Weekly Report*, **33**, 157–158.

Johnson EJ, Krall EA, Dawson-Hughes B, Dallal GE and Russell RM (1992) Lack of an effect of multivitamins containing vitamin A on serum retinyl esters and liver function tests in healthy women. *Journal of American College of Nutrition*, **11**, 682–686.

Kauwell GP, Bailey LB, Gregory JF III, Bowling DW and Cousins RJ (1998) Zinc status is not adversely affected by folic acid supplementation and zinc intake does not impair folate utilization in human subjects. *Journal of Nutrition*, **125**, 66–72.

Keen CL and Zidenberg-Cherr S (1996) Manganese. In *Present Knowledge of Nutrition*, 7th edn, Ziegler EE and Filer LJ (eds), ILSI Press, Washington, DC, pp. 334–343.

Kim JM and White RH (1996) Effect of vitamin E on the anticoagulant response to warfarin. *American Journal of Cardiology*, **77**, 545–546.

Kitagawa M and Mino M (1989) Effects of elevated d-alpha(RRR)-tocopherol dosages in man. *Journal of Nutritional Science and Vitaminology (Tokyo)*, **35**, 133–142.

Krasinski SD, Russell RM, Otradovec CL, Sadowski JA, Hartz SC, Jacob RA and McGandy RB (1989) Relationship of vitamin A and vitamin E intake to fasting plasma retinol, retinol-binding protein, retinyl esters, carotene, α-tocopherol, and cholesterol among elderly and young adults: increased plasma retinyl esters among vitamin A supplement users. *American Journal of Clinical Nutrition*, **49**, 112–120.

Lachance PA (1996) 'Natural' cancer prevention. *Science*, **272**, 1860–1861.

Lammer EJ, Shaw GM, Wasserman CR and Block G (1996) High vitamin A intake and risk for major anomalies involving structures with an embryological cranial neural cerse cell component. *Teratology*, **53**, 91–92.

Lehman AJ and Fitzhugh OG (1954) 100-Fold margin of safety. *Association of Food Drug Officials: US Quarterly Bulletin*, **18**, 33–35.

Levander OA and Burk RF (1994) Selenium. In *Modern Nutrition in Health and Disease*, 8th edn, Shils ME, Olson JA and Shike M (eds), Lea & Febiger, Philadelphia, pp. 242–251.

Longnecker MP, Taylor PR, Levander OA, Howe M, Veillon C, McAdam PA, Patterson, KY, Holden JM, Stampfer MJ, Morris JS and Willett WC (1991) Selenium in diet, blood, and toenails in relation to human health in a seleniferous area. *American Journal of Clinical Nutrition*, **53**, 1288–1294.

Matsukawa Y, Ikeda E, Hayama T, Nishinanita S, Sawada S and Horie T (1995) Ectopic calcinosis possibly due to 1 alpha (OH) vitamin D_3 in a patient with systemic lupus erythematosus. *Clinical and Experimental Rheumatology*, **13**, 91–94.

Mathews-Roth MM (1986) Beta-carotene therapy for erythropoietic protoporphyria and other photosensitivity diseases. *Biochimie*, **68**, 875–884.

McKenney JM, Proctor JD, Hamis S and Chinchilli VM (1994) A comparison of the efficacy and toxic effects of sustained vs immediate-release niacin in hypercholesterolemic patients. *Journal of the American Medical Association*, **271**, 672–677.

Menkes MS, Comstock GW, Vuilleumier JP, Helsing KJ, Rider AA and Brookmeyer R (1986) Serum beta-carotene, vitamins C and E, selenium, and the risk of lung cancer. *New England Journal of Medicine*, **315**, 1250–1254.

Miller DR and Hayes KC (1982) Vitamin excess and toxicity. In *Nutritional Toxicology*, vol. 1, Hathcock, JN (ed), Academic Press, New York, pp. 81–133.

Milne DB, Canfield WK, Mahalko JR and Sandstead HH (1984) Effect of oral folic acid supplements on zinc, copper, and iron absorption and excretion. *American Journal of Clinical Nutrition*, **39**, 535–539.

Morgan SL, Baggott JE, Vaughn WH, Young PK, Austin JV, Krumdieck CL and Alarcon GS (1990) The effect of folic acid supplementation on the toxicity of low-dose methotrexate in patients with rheumatoid arthritis. *Arthritis and Rheumatism*, **33**, 9–18.

Mukherjee MD, Sandstead HH, Ratnaparkhl MV, Johnson, LK, Milne DB and Stelling HP (1984) Maternal zinc, iron, folic acid, and protein nutriture and outcome of human pregnancy. *American Journal of Clinical Nutrition*, **40**, 496–507.

Nanji AA (1985) Symptomatic hypercalcaemia precipitated by magnesium therapy. *Postgraduate Medical Journal*, **61**, 47–48.

National Research Council (1983) *Selenium in Nutrition, revised*. National Academy Press, Washington, DC.

Nielsen FH (1994a) Ultratrace minerals. In *Modern Nutrition in Health and Disease*, 8th edn, Shils ME, Olson JA and Shike EM (eds), Lea & Febiger, Philadelphia, pp. 269–286.

Nielsen, FH (1994b) Chromium. In *Modern Nutrition in Health and Disease*, 8th edn, Shils ME, Olson JA and Shike M (eds), Lea & Febiger, Philadelphia, pp. 264–268.

Nielsen FH (1996) Other trace elements. In *Present Knowledge of Nutrition*, 7th edn, Ziegler EE and Filer LJ (eds), ILSI Press, Washington, DC, pp. 353–377.

Norman AW (1996) Vitamin D. In *Present Knowledge of Nutrition*, 7th edn, ILSI Press, Washington, DC, pp. 120–129.

Oakley GP and Erickson JD (1995) Vitamin A and birth defects. *New England Journal of Medicine*, **333**, 1414–1415.

Olson JA (1994) Vitamin A, retinoids and carotenoids. In *Modern Nutrition in Health and Disease*, 8th edn, Shils ME, Olson JA and Shike M (eds), Lea & Febiger, Philadelphia, pp. 287–307.

Omenn GS, Goodman GE, Thomquist MD, Balmes J, Cullen MR, Glass A, Keogh JP, Meyskens FL, Valanis B, Williams JH, Barnhart S and Hammar S (1996) Effects of a combination of beta-carotene and vitamin A on lung cancer and cardiovascular disease. *New England Journal of Medicine*, **334**, 1150–1155.

Oymak O, Ak-polat T, Arik N, Yasavul C, Turgan Q and Caglar S (1994) Hyperammonemic encephalopathy due to vitamin D induced hypercalcemia in a uremic patient (letter). *Nephron*, **66**, 369.

Parry GJ and Bredesen DE (1985) Sensory neuropathy with low-dose pyridoxine. *Neurology*, **35**, 1466–1468.

Phillips WEJ, Mills JHL, Charbonneau SM, Tryphonas L, Hatina GV, Zawidzka Z, Bryce FR and Munro IC (1978) Subacute toxicity of pyridoxine hydrochloride in the beagle dog. *Toxicology and Applied Pharmacology*, **44**, 323–333.

Poirier KA (1994) Summary of the derivation of the reference dose for selenium. In *Risk Assessment of Essential Elements*, Mertz W, Abernathy CO and Olin SS (eds), ILSI Press, Washington, DC, pp. 157–166.

Price CJ, Strong PL, Marr MC, Myers CB and Murray FJ (1996) Developmental toxicity NOAEL and postnatal recovery in rats fed boric acid during gestation. *Fundamental and Applied Toxicology*, **32**, 179–193.

Rader JI, Calvert RJ and Hathcock JN (1992) Hepatic toxicity of un-modified and time-release preparations of niacin. *American Journal of Medicine*, **92**, 77–81.

Renwick AG (1993) Data-derived safety factors for the evaluation of food additives and environmental contaminants. *Food Additives and Contaminants*, **10**, 275–305.

Rimm EB, Stampfer MJ, Ascherio A, Giovannucci E, Colditz GA and Willett WC (1993) Vitamin E consumption and the risk of coronary heart disease in men. *New England Journal of Medicine*, **328**, 1450–1456.

Rosa FW, Wilk AL and Kelsey FO (1986) Teratogen update: vitamin A congeners. *Teratology*, **33**, 355–364.

Rose DP (1978) Effects of oral contraceptives on nutrient utilization. In *Nutrition and Drug Interrelations*, Hathcock JN and Coon J (eds), Academic Press, New York, pp. 161–187.

Rothman KJ, Moore LL, Singer MR, Nguyen UDT, Mannino S and Milunsky A (1995) Teratogenicity of high level vitamin A intake. *New England Journal of Medicine*, **333**, 1369–1373.

Santoro L, Ragno M, Nucciotti, Barbieri F and Caruso G (1991) Pyridoxine neuropathy: a four year electrophysiological and clinical follow-up of a severe case. *Acta Neurologica*, **13**, 13–18.

Savage DG and Lindenbaum J (1995) Folate-cobalamin interactions. In *Folate in Health and Disease*, Bailey L (ed), Dekker, New York, pp. 237–285.

Schaumburg H, Kaplan J, Windebank A, Vick N, Rasmus S, Pleasure D and Brown MJ (1983) Sensory neuropathy from pyridoxine abuse. *New England Journal of Medicine*, **309**, 445–448.

Schwartzman MS and Franck WA (1987) Vitamin D toxicity complicating the treatment of senile, postmenopausal, and glucocorticoid-induced osteoporosis. *American Journal of Medicine*, **82**, 224–230.

Select Committee on GRAS Substances (SCOGS) Life Sciences Research Office (LSRO) (1978) *Evaluation of the health aspects of vitamin D_2 and vitamin D_3 as food ingredients*, Federation of American Societies for Experimental Biology, Washington, DC.

Shaw GM, Wasserman CR, Block G and Lammer EJ (1996) High maternal vitamin A intake and risk of anomalies of structures with a cranial neural crest cell contribution. *Lancet*, **347**, 899–900.

Simmer K, James C and Thompson RPH (1987) Are iron-folate supplements harmful? *American Journal of Clinical Nutrition*, **45**, 122–125.

Stauber PM, Sherry B, VanderJagt DJ, Baghavan HN and Garry PJ (1991) A longitudinal study of the relationship between vitamin A supplementation and plasma retinol, retinyl esters, and liver enzyme activities in a healthy elder population. *American Journal of Clinical Nutrition*, **54**, 878–883.

Stearns DM, Wise JP Sr, Patierno SR and Wetterhahn KE (1995) Chromium (III) picolinate produces chromosome damage in Chinese hamster ovary cells. *FASEB Journal*, **9**, 1643–1648.

Steiner M (1991) Influence of vitamin E on platelet function in humans. *Journal of the American College of Nutrition*, **10**, 466–473.

Steiner M (1993) Vitamin E: more than an antioxidant. *Clinical Cardiology*, **16**, 16–18.

Tamura T, Goldberg RL, Freeberg LE, Cliver SP, Cutter GR and Hoffman HJ (1992) Maternal serum folate and zinc concentrations and their relationships to pregnancy outcome. *American Journal of Clinical Nutrition*, **56**, 365–370.

Wald N, Sneddon J, Densem J, Frost C and Stone R (1991) The MRC Vitamin Study Research Group. Prevention of neural tube defects: results of the Medical Research Council Vitamin Study. *Lancet*, **338**, 131–137.

Weir RJ and Fisher RS (1972) Toxicological studies on borax and boric acid. *Toxicology and Applied Pharmacology*, **23**, 351–364.

Werler MM, Lammer EJ and Mitchell AA (1996) Teratology of high vitamin A intake (letter). *New England Journal of Medicine*, **334**, 1195–1196.

Yang G and Zhou R (1994) Further observations on the human maximum safe dietary selenium intake in a seleniferous area of China. *Journal of Electrolytes and Trace Elements in Health and Disease*, **8**, 159–165.

Yang G, Wang S, Zhou R and Sun S (1983) Endemic selenium intoxication of humans in China. *American Journal of Clinical Nutrition*, **37**, 872–881.

Yang G, Zhou R, Yin S, Gu L, Yan B, Liu Y, Liu Y and Li X (1989a) Studies of safe maximal daily dietary selenium intake in a seleniferous area in China, 1: selenium intake and tissue levels of the inhabitants. *Journal of Electrolytes and Trace Elements in Health and Disease*, **3**, 77–87.

Yang G, Yin S, Zhou R, Gu L, Yan B, Liu Y and Liu Y (1989b) Studies of safe maximal daily dietary selenium intake in a seleniferous area in China, 2: relation between selenium intake and the manifestation of clinical signs and certain biochemical alterations in blood and urine. *Journal of Electrolytes and Trace Elements in Health and Disease*, **3**, 123–130.

12 Naturally Occurring Organosulphur Compounds as Potential Anticarcinogens

Hideki Mori[1] and Akiyoshi Nishikawa[2]

[1]Department of Pathology, Gifu University School of Medicine, 40 Tsukasa-machi, Gifu 500–8705, Japan
[2]Division of Pathology, National Institute of Public Health Sciences, 1-18-1, Kamiyoga, Setagaya-ku, Tokyo, 158–0098, Japan

Introduction

Dietary factors are believed to have a profound impact on the occurrence of human cancers. Minor dietary constituents have been found to exert chemopreventive effects, supporting the data from epidemiological studies that frequent consumption of fruits and vegetables is linked to reduce cancer risk. Recent attention has been focused on identifying dietary phytochemicals having the capability to prevent mutagenesis and carcinogenesis. Chemoprevention embraces the concept that non-carcinogenic naturally occurring products or synthetic compounds can inhibit the process of carcinogenesis. Such an ideal strategy would be possible if the initiating and promoting processes were understood and countervailing agents were shown to be efficaceous with no or low toxicity and side effects. A number of agents have proved effective against chemical mutagenesis and carcinogenesis, i.e. blocking agents and suppressive agents (Wattenberg, 1985). Epidemiological and laboratory studies have suggested that plant-derived dietary chemicals are a major source of chemopreventive agents (Committee on Diet, Nutrition and Cancer, 1982; Wattenberg, 1992a,b).

Naturally occurring organosulphur compounds are a candidate class of such chemopreventive agents. One of the representative groups of the naturally occurring organosulphur compounds are allyl sulphur compounds, most of which have been identified in garlic or onions (Wargovich, 1992). The other

Nutrition and Chemical Toxicity. Edited by Costas Ioannides. © John Wiley & Sons Ltd. ISBN 0 471 97453 6

group is organic isothiocyanates and glucosinolates which are biosynthetic precursors of the isothiocyanates. Both agents are present in substantial amounts in cruciferous vegetables (Zhang and Talalay, 1994; Hecht, 1995). Animal studies have revealed the anticarcinogenic efficacy of these organosulphur compounds in multiple organs such as the lung, oesophagus, forestomach, liver and colon (Wattenberg, 1985, 1992a,b; Wargovich, 1992). As possible mechanisms of the chemoprevention by these organosulphur compounds or plant extracts containing them, effects on the activities of Phase I (cytochrome P450) and Phase II [quinone reductase and glutathione S-transferase (GST)] enzymes have been considered to be most important (Wargovich, 1992; Zhang and Talalay, 1994; Hecht, 1995). However, recent studies have revealed alternative mechanisms such as effects on the arachidonate cascade, antioxidant properties (Imai et al., 1994; Mori et al., 1996a), effects on the immune system (Morioka et al., 1993) and on cell proliferation (Mori et al., 1996b; Sundaram and Milner, 1996a).

In this review, the properties, significance and mode of action of these naturally occurring anticarcinogenic organosulphur compounds, including allyl sulphur compounds, isothiocyanates and others will be discussed.

Allyl sulphur compounds

The antibiotic and fungicidal properties of garlic (*Allium sativum* L.) were known historically, and attention focused on its medical properties in the treatment of a wide range of human diseases. Epidemiological studies have suggested that garlic and related allium foods may have protective effects against tumour formation (Mei et al., 1982; Steinmetz et al., 1994). Animal investigations have also provided evidence that garlic and associated organosulphur compounds inhibit the development of neoplasms in the colon, lung, oesophagus, forestomach, mammary gland and skin (Wargovich, 1992). Recently, the efficacy of cancer prevention by high-selenium garlic has been reported (Ip and Lisk, 1995). Garlic contains a complex mixture of allyl sulphur compounds which have been shown to afford protection in carcinogenesis. Diallyl sulphide (DAS) and diallyl disulphide (DADS), which are representative lipid-soluble allyl sulphur compounds present in garlic, have been extensively studied for their chemopreventive function. DAS has been reported to inhibit dimethylhydrazine (DMH)-induced cancer of the colon in mice (Wargovich, 1987; Sumiyoshi and Wargovich, 1990), N-nitrosomethylbenzylamine (NMBA)-induced oesophageal cancer in rats (Wargovich et al., 1988), and benzo[a] pyrene (BP)-induced forestomach tumorigenesis in mice (Sparnins et al., 1988). DADS has also been reported to prevent N-methyl-N-nitrosourea (MNU)-induced mammary carcinogenesis in rats (Schaffer et al., 1996). Recently, our group has demonstrated that DADS has also anticarcinogenic activity against 2-amino-1-methyl-6–phenylimidazo[4,5-b]pyridine (PhIP)-induced mammary carcinogenesis in rats (Suzui et al., 1997). Both DAS and

DADS are also known to inhibit aflatoxin B_1- or diethylnitrosamine (DEN)-induced development of liver preneoplastic foci in rats (Jang et al., 1989; Habermignard et al., 1996). Furthermore, DAS reduces DMH-induced colonic nuclear aberrations in mice (Sumiyoshi and Wargovich, 1990), and DADS inhibits the growth of both canine and human tumour cells in vitro (Sundaram and Milner, 1993, 1996a). Takahashi et al. (1992) have reported potential inhibitory effects of DADS on colon and renal carcinogenesis in the system for multi-organ carcinogenesis in rats. Conversely, the same workers demonstrated an enhancing effect of DAS on hepatocarcinogenesis in the same model (Takahashi et al., 1992). Allyl methyl disulphide (AMD), allyl methyl trisulphide (AMT), allyl mercaptan (AM), diallyl trisulphide (DAT), dipropyl trisulphide (DPT), propyl methyl disulphide (PMD) and propyl methyl trisulphide (PMT) are other types of lipophilic allyl sulphur compounds present in garlic and related foods (Sparnins et al., 1988; Wattenberg et al., 1989). Of these, DAT, DPT, AMD and AMT were found to possess chemopreventive effects against BP-induced forestomach carcinogenesis in mice (Sparnins et al., 1986), and AMD was also shown to inhibit BP-induced pulmonary carcinogenesis in mice (Sparnins et al., 1988). Furthermore, both AM and AMD were demonstrated to have similar effects in the mouse model using DEN as the model carcinogen (Wattenberg et al., 1989).

Water-soluble allyl sulphur compounds are also present in garlic, such as S-allyl cysteine (SAC), S-methyl cysteine (SMC), L-cysteine and L-methionine (Wargovich, 1992). SAC inhibited DMH-induced cancer of the colon in mice (Sumiyoshi and Wargovich, 1990) and aberrant crypt foci formation in rats (Hatano et al., 1996). Moreover, SAC was reported also to reduce DMBA-induced DNA adducts in mammary tissue (Amagase and Milner, 1993) and to suppress MNU-induced mammary carcinogenesis in rats (Schaffer et al., 1996). Recently, SMC and cysteine were shown to prevent the induction of glutathione S-transferase placental form (GST-P)-positive foci, during the initiation and promotion phases of hepatocarcinogenesis in rats (Takada et al., 1997). However, such organosulphur compounds from garlic and onions were also shown to increase the formation of GST-P positive foci (Takada et al., 1994a,b) (Table 12.1).

The chemopreventive effects of allyl sulphur compounds are believed to be closely related to modulation Phase I or Phase II enzymes. CYP2E1 is an isoform of the cytochromes P450 superfamily which is responsible for metabolic activation of various types of chemical carcinogens of relatively small molecular size. DAS was reported to inhibit hepatic monooxygenase activity, which catalyzes the oxidation of azoxymethane to methylazoxymethanol (Brady et al., 1988). DAS, DADS and allyl methyl sulphide (AMS) are known to suppress P450 activity in rat liver (Reicks and Crankshaw, 1996), and DAS and diallyl sulphone, a metabolite of DAS, are potent inhibitors of hepatic CYP2E1 activity (Brady et al., 1991a,b). In contrast, DAS induces CYP2B1 activity as demonstrated by Brady et al. (1988).

Table 12.1 Anticarcinogenic effects of naturally occurring organosulphur compounds

Compounds	Animal models	References
Allyl sulphur compounds		
DAS	DMH (colon; mouse), NMBA (oesophagus; rat), BP (forestomach; mouse), aflatoxin B_1 (liver foci; rat), DEN (liver foci; rat)	Habermignard et al. (1996); Sparnins et al. (1988); Wargovich et al. (1988); Jang et al. (1989); Sumiyoshi and Wargovich (1990)
DADS	MNU (mammary gland; rat), aflatoxin B_1 (liver foci; rat), DEN (liver foci; rat)	Jang et al. (1989); Habermignard et al. (1996); Schaffer et al. (1996)
DAT	BP (forestomach; mouse)	Sparnins et al. (1988)
DPT	BP (forestomach; mouse)	Sparnins et al. (1988)
AMD	BP (forestomach, lung; mouse), DEN (lung; mouse)	Sparnins et al. (1988); Wattenberg et al. (1989)
AMT	BP (forestomach; mouse)	Sparnins et al. (1988)
AM	DEN (lung; mouse)	Wattenberg et al. (1989)
SAC	DMH (colon; mouse), MNU (mammary gland; rat)	Sumiyoshi and Wargovich (1990); Schaffer et al. (1996)
SMC	DEN (liver foci; rat)	Takada et al. (1997)
L-cysteine	DEN (liver foci; rat)	Takada et al. (1997)
Ajoene	DMBA+PMA (skin; mouse)	Belman et al. (1989)
Glucosinolates		
Sinigrin	DEN (liver; rat)	Tanaka et al. (1990)
Glucobrassicin	BP (forestomach, lung; mouse), DMBA (mammary gland; rat)	Wattenberg et al. (1980)
Glucosinalbin	BP (forestomach, lung; mouse)	Wattenberg et al. (1986)
Glucotropaeolin	DMBA (mammary gland; rat)	Wattenberg et al. (1986)
Isothiocyanates		
PEITC	DMBA (mammary gland; rat), DMBA (forestomach, lung; mouse), NNK (lung; rat), NMBA (oesophagus; rat), BOP (lung, pancreas; hamster)	Morse et al. (1989); Stoner et al. (1991); Nishikawa et al. (1996a); Wattenberg (1997)
BTC	DMBA (mammary gland; rat), DEN (liver foci; rat), MAM acetate (intestine, rat)	Wattenberg (1977); Sugie et al. (1993a, 1994)

BITC	DMBA (mammary gland; rat), DMBA (forestomach, lung; mouse), DEN (liver; rat), DEN (forestomach, lung; mouse), BP (forestomach, lung; mouse), MAM acetate (intestine, rat)	Wattenberg (1987)
MMTS	AOM (colon, rat), DEN+PB (liver; rat)	Kawamori et al. (1995); Sugie et al. (1997)
Sulphoraphene	DMBA (mammary gland; rat)	Zhang and Talalay (1994)
Miscellaneous compounds		
Tauline	AOM (colon, rat), DEN+PB (liver; rat)	Reddy et al. (1993); Okamoto et al. (1996)
NAC	AOM (colon, rat)	Reddy et al. (1993)

GSTs are a widely distributed family of enzymes that catalyse the conjugation reaction of electrophilic hydrophobic compounds with glutathione. Many carcinogens and their metabolites are known to be detoxified by these enzymes. Hence, GST activity is considered to contribute extensively to anticarcinogenesis. DAS, DADS, AMT and SAC are established inducers of GST activity in the liver, digestive tract and lung. Hatono *et al.* (1996) indicated that hepatic GST-α and GST-μ, but not GST-π, are increased significantly following oral administration of SAC. This compound suppresses induction of aberrant crypt foci, being regarded as a putative preneoplastic population, by exposure to DMH during the initiation phase but not promotion phase (Sumiyoshi and Wargovich, 1990). The same workers reported that the stimulation of hepatic GST by organosulphur compounds present in garlic and onion may require prolonged administration for the effect to be evident. There is an organospecificity for the GST response to the sulphur compounds. Organosulphur compounds containing allyl groups are more effective inducers of GST activity in the liver and colon, whereas their saturated analogues (propyl group) give rise to little or no induction. It is therefore possible that allyl sulphur compounds, such as DAS or DADS, partially inhibit carcinogenesis through both stimulation of detoxifying enzymes and inhibition of bioactivation enzymes.

Meanwhile, the antioxidant and radical scavenging effects of garlic extracts and its constituents have been established (Imai *et al.*, 1994). Recently, a positive correlation was found between DADS-induced apoptosis and its ability to increase intracellular free calcium levels, and the widespread effectiveness of DADS was evident by its ability to inhibit the growth of human colon, skin and lung tumour cells (Sundaram and Milner, 1996b). Furthermore, Belman (1983) reported that onion and garlic oils can inhibit tumour promotion. He subsequently observed that ajoene, a sulphur compound present in garlic and onions, inhibited skin tumour promotion in the phorbol myristate acetate (PMA) model (Belman *et al.*, 1989). These effects may be related to the activity of sulphur compounds on cell growth.

Glucosinolates and isothiocyanates

Organic isothiocyanates and their biosynthetic precursors, glucosinolates, are recognised as a promising group of effective chemopreventive agents against cancer. Glucosinolates are present in cruciferous vegetables, and more than 100 types have been isolated (Talalay and Zhang, 1996). In plants, isothiocyantes are invariably accompanied by much larger quantities of their glucosinolates (β-thioglucoside, N-hydroxysulphate). Sinigrin, a typical glucosinolate precursor of allyl isothiocyanates present in cabbage, Brussels sprouts and cauliflower as well as mustard and horseradish was already isolated in the past century (Sones *et al.*, 1984). Sinigrin was reported to decrease 7-methylguanosine formation in the liver DNA of rats given dimethylnitrosamine or the tobacco-specific nitrosamine (NNK) (Chung *et al.*, 1985; Morse *et al.*, 1988). Sinigrin exhibited a chemopreventive effect against DEN-induced hepatocarcinogenesis when administered to rats during the initiation phase (Tanaka *et al.*, 1990). Since plant products containing sinigrin are known to increase the activity of GST, the principal mechanism of the inhibitory effect of this glucosinolate is probably increased detoxification. Glucobrassicin (indolylmethyl glucosinolate), glucotropaeolin (benzyl glucosinolate) and glucosinalbin (4-hydroxybenzyl glucosinolate), are also glucosinolate compounds found in some cruciferous vegetables (Wattenberg, 1986). The effects of these glucosinolates on BP-induced neoplasms of the forestomach and lung in mice were investigated by Wattenberg *et al.* (1986). All of these glucosinolate compounds inhibited carcinogenesis in these organs, but the most striking suppressive effect was elicited with glucobrassin. Furthermore, glucobrassin and glucotropaeolin prevented the development of DMBA-induced mammary tumours in Sprague-Dawley rats (Wattenberg *et al.*, 1986). Although it is not clear whether these glucosinolates themselves or their hydrolysis products are the active chemical species responsible for the protective effects, glucosinolates like glucobrassin have been shown to be hydrolysed to indole-3-acetonitrile, indole-3-carbinol and 3,3'-di-indolyl-methane, all of which are inducers of aryl hydrocarbon hydroxylase (Wattenberg *et al.*, 1986). Thus, the chemopreventive activity of these glucosinolates would be dependent on such indole chemicals which induce microsomal mixed-function oxidase activity.

Organic isothiocyanates (R—N=C=S) arise in plants as a result of enzymic cleavage of glucosinolates by myrosinase (thioglucoside glucohydrolase), which is released when plants are injured. Myrosinase promotes the hydrolysis of glucosinolates and intramolecular rearrangement of intermediates to yield isothiocyanates, hydrogen sulphate and glucose as the major products (Hecht, 1995; Talalay and Zhang, 1996). The highly electrophilic central carbon atom of the –N=C=S group is known to react rapidly, and under mild conditions, with oxygen-, sulphur-, or nitrogen-centred nucleophiles, giving rise to carbamates, thiocarbamates, or thiourea derivatives, respectively (Talalay and Zhang, 1996).

Isothiocyanates are also known as mustard oil and are responsible for the pungent flavour and odour of condiments such as mustard and horseradish. In addition to characteristic flavours and odours, isothiocyanates have also a variety of pharmacological activities such as goitrogenic activity, antibacterial, antifungal and antiprotozoal activity, and the ability to attract or repel insects (Zhang and Talalay, 1994).

Phenethyl isothiocyanate (PEITC), a natural constituent of cruciferous vegetables, such as cabbage, cauliflower, Brussels sprouts and turnips, is a most extensively investigated isothiocyanate. Pretreatment of animals with PEITC inhibited the induction of mammary tumours induced by 7,12-dimethylbenz-[a]anthracene (DMBA) (Wattenberg, 1977). Dietary PEITC exposure also suppressed DMBA-induced lung and forestomach tumours in mice (Wattenberg, 1977). Moreover, PEITC suppressed NNK-induced lung tumours in rats (Morse et al., 1989) and oesophageal tumours induced by long-term treatment with NMBA in rats (Stoner et al., 1991). Recently, this isothiocyanate compound was also an effective chemopreventive agent against lung and pancreas tumorigenesis in N-nitrosobis (2-oxopropyl)amine-treated hamsters (Nishikawa et al., 1996b). Principal mechanisms underlying the chemopreventive effects of PEITC are related to its ability to attenuate the DNA alkylation levels induced by chemical carcinogens such as NMBA (Stoner et al., 1991; Morse et al., 1993), N-nitrosomethylamylamine (Huang et al., 1993) and NNK (Morse et al., 1988, 1989). It has been proposed that the decreased levels of DNA alkylation brought about by PEITC are mediated by its ability to modulate Phase I enzymes and induce Phase II enzymes (Guo et al., 1992; Smith et al., 1993). Recently, PEITC was found to activate c-jun N-terminal kinase 1, a mitogen-activated protein kinase, suggesting that PEITC is involved in the kinase-mediated regulation of Phase II enzyme gene expression (Yu et al., 1996). Synthetic analogue compounds such as 6-phenylhexyl isothiocyanate (PHITC), 3-phenylpropyl isothiocyanate (PPITC), 5-phenylpentyl isothiocyanate (PPeITC) and 4-phenylbutyl isothiocyanate (PBITC) inhibited NNK-induced-lung tumorigenesis in mice (Morse et al., 1991). These analogues, with the exception of PHITC, also reduced NMBA-induced oesophageal carcinogenesis in rats (Stoner and Morse, 1996), and PPITC was shown to have greater chemopreventive effects in lung carcinogenesis in mice and hamsters (Hecht, 1995; Nishikawa et al., 1996a). PHITC, in contrast, is known to exert an enhancing effect on oesophageal carcinogenesis (Stoner et al., 1995). These results suggest that the ability of isothiocyanates to inhibit or enhance chemical carcinogenesis may depend on the alkyl chain length of the isothiocyanate, the animal species and the specific carcinogens (Stoner et al., 1995).

Benzyl thiocyanate (BTC) and benzyl isothiocyanate (BITC) are constituents of cruciferous vegetables, being present as their glucosinolate precursors (Hecht, 1995; Talalay and Zhang, 1996). BITC has been shown to inhibit DMBA-induced mammary carcinogenesis in rats (Wattenberg, 1977) and to suppress the development of forestomach and lung tumours induced by DMBA, DEN and B[a]P in mice (Wattenberg, 1977, 1987). BTC also reduced DMBA-induced mammary carcinogenesis in rats (Wattenberg, 1977). In these studies, the aromatic thiocyanates were basically administered by oral intubation prior to carcinogen treatment. The inhibitory effects of dietary exposure to BTC and BITC on hepatocarcinogenesis were also illustrated by Sugie et al. (1993a) in a rat model using DEN. In this experiment, exposure to BITC (100-ppm) prevented the development of liver neoplasms and prenoplastic lesions such as GST-P-positive foci; the administration of BTC suppressed only the occurrence of the precursor lesions. Both cyanate compounds suppressed carcinogen-induced unscheduled DNA synthesis and replicative DNA synthesis (Sugie et al., 1993b). The same authors also investigated the chemopreventive effects of BITC or BTC on methylazoxymethanol (MAM) acetate-induced intestinal carcinogenesis and observed that BITC was an effective anticarcinogen in both the large intestine and small intestine, whereas BTC was effective only in the small bowel (Sugie et al., 1994). Hecht (1995) has proposed employing a combination of BITC and PEITC to prevent tobacco-related lung cancer, since PEITC can inhibit the metabolic activation and carcinogenicity of NNK in rat and mouse lung, and BITC has similar effects on BaP activation and tumorigenicity in mouse lung.

S-Methyl methanethiosulphonate (MMTS) is an organosulphur compound recently isolated from cauliflower, Brassica oleracea L. var botrytis, and its chemical structure was established by Nakamura et al. (1993). MMTS inhibited the UV-induced mutation in Escherichia coli B/r WP2 by activating the excision–repairing systems (Nakamura et al., 1993). Modifying effects of MMTS on AOM-induced rat intestinal carcinogenesis were investigated by Kawamori et al. (1995). In this study, MMTS suppressed the AOM-induced large bowel carcinogenesis following post-initiation exposure at a dose level of 100 ppm. Furthermore, MMTS suppressed the occurrence of aberrant crypt foci. Recently, the antitumorigenic activity of this compound in rats was also confirmed by Sugie et al. (1997) using the DEN-initiated and phenobarbital-promoted model.

Sulphoraphene [1-isothiocyanato-4-(methylsulphinyl)butane] was isolated from broccoli (Brassica olearacea italica) as a potent inducer of Phase II enzymes (Zhang et al., 1992), monitored using the quinone reductase activity in murine hepatoma cells grown in microtitre plate wells (Prochaska et al., 1992). This thiocyanate does not induce aryl hydrocarbon receptor-dependent cytochrome P450 activity. Sulphoraphane and its sulphide and sulphone analogues induce both quinone reductase and glutathione transferase activity. The anticarcinogenic activity of sulphoraphane and of the structurally related synthetic norbornyl isothiocyanates (exo-2-acetyl-exo-6-isothiocyanatonorbornane, endo-2-acetyl-exo-6-isothiocyanatonorbornane and exo-2-acetyl-exo-5-isothiocyanatonorbornane) on DMBA-induced mammary carcinogenesis in rats was studied by Zhang and Talalay (1994). They reported that exposure to these thiocyanate compounds by gavage (75 or 150 μmol per day for 5 days) around the time of administration of the carcinogen, significantly suppressed the incidence, multiplicity and size of mammary tumours. The effects were prominent with sulphorphane and exo-2-acetyl-exo-6-isothiocyanatonorbornane (Zhang and Talalay, 1994).

Thus, the major mechanism proposed for the chemopreventive activity of isothiocyanates is the modulation of carcinogen metabolism, both depression of carcinogen bioactivation by Phase I enzymes and enhanced detoxification by Phase II enzymes, as in the case of allyl sulphur compounds. Recently, however, an increasing amount of evidence has been accumulated indicating that isothiocyanates modify cell proliferation. Some isothiocyanates suppress carcinogen-induced cell hyperproliferation in vitro (Sugie et al., 1994;

Kawamori et al., 1995; Mori et al., 1995). Benzyl thiocyanates and phenyl ethyl thiocyanates were shown to delay the cell cycle progression of cultured cells (Hasegawa et al., 1993). Furthermore, protective effects of thiocyanate compounds against lipid peroxidation have been reported (Mori et al., 1996a). There may also be other mechanisms contributing to the chemopreventive activities of isothiocyanates.

Other organosulphur compounds

Some organosulphur compounds are formed endogenously in the body. Tauline (2-aminoethanesulphonate) and N-acetylcysteine (NAC) are such examples. They have been shown to ameliorate the toxicity induced by a variety of chemicals in various organs. NAC inhibits cyclophosphamide-induced toxicity (Levy and Vredevoe, 1983). Oral administration of tauline afforded partial protection against lipid peroxidation, suggesting that this naturally occurring organosulphur compound aids by inhibiting lipid peroxidation and the consequent deterioration of membrane phospholipids (Pierson et al., 1985). Modifying effects of tauline and NAC on AOM-induced colon carcinogenesis in rats were investigated by Reddy et al. (1993). They found that oral administration of tauline or NAC suppressed AOM-induced large bowel carcinogenesis, although the effects were somewhat marginal, and both NAC and tauline increased hepatic GST activity (Reddy et al., 1993). Recently, Umemura et al. (1996) demonstrated in rats that NAC inhibited renal oxidative damage induced by ferric nitrilotriacetate as exemplified by 4-hydroxy-2-noneal and 8-hydroxydeoxyguanosine levels. The modifying effect of tauline on DEN and phenobarbital-induced hepatocarcinogenesis was studied by Okamoto et al. (1996). They reported that tauline prevented the induction of GST-P-positive foci as well as liver neoplasms. Furthermore, they also noted that tauline treatment reduces the level of ornithine decarboxylase activity in non-neoplastic liver tissues (Okamoto et al., 1996). Finally, tauline was also capable of inhibiting prostaglandin E_2 synthesis (Kimura et al., 1985). Tauline is an organosulphur compound which is not only formed endogenously in the human body but is also present in a variety of animals and plants. Such organosulphur compound may be promising agents in the prevention of neoplasia in digestive organs, especially cancers of the large bowel and liver.

It is known that cabbage and other cruciferous vegetables contain dithiolthiones (Jirousek and Starka, 1958). Dithiolthiones present in vegetables have been suggested to have anticarcinogenic activity by increasing GSH and quinone reductase activity that catalyse the inactivation of toxic chemicals including carcinogens (Ansher et al., 1986). Anticarcinogenic effects of this class of compounds have been demonstrated with some synthetic chemicals such as oltipraz, being used as an antischistosomal drug (Wattenberg and Bueding, 1986). However, the extent to which inhibition of carcinogenesis by cruciferous vegetables can be ascribed to their dithiolthione constituents is not clear (Ansher et al., 1986).

Conclusions

Cancer chemoprevention basically refers to the prevention of cancer prior to the malignant stage of carcinogenesis. Since the mechanisms for the occurrence of cancer are considered to originate from multiple factors, prevention of cancer should relate to the different stages of carcinogenesis, i.e. the formation of carcinogens, their activation or detoxification, oncogene activation and progression. Major naturally occurring organosulphur compounds are allium sulphur compounds derived from garlic or onion, and isothiocyanates and their precursors glucosinolates derived from cruciferous vegetables.

References

Amagase H and Milner JA (1993) Impact of various sources of garlic and their constituents on 7,12-dimethylbenz(a)anthracene binding to mammary cell DNA. *Carcinogenesis*, **14**, 1627–1631.

Ansher SS, Dolan P and Bueding E (1986) Biochemical effects of dithiolthiones. *Food and Cosmetics Toxicology*, **24**, 405–415.

Belman, S (1983) Onion and garlic oils inhibit tumor promotion. *Carcinogenesis*, **4**, 1063–1065.

Belman S, Solomon J, Segal A, Block E and Barany G (1989) Inhibition of soybean lipoxygenase and mouse skin tumor promotion by onion and garlic components. *Journal of Biochemical Toxicology*, **4**, 151–160.

Brady JF, Li D, Ishizuka H and Yang CS (1988) Effects of diallyl sulfide on rat liver microsomal nitrosamine metabolism and other monooxygenase activities. *Cancer Research*, **48**, 5937–5940.

Brady JF, Ishizaki H, Fukuto JM, Lin MC, Fadel A, Gapac JM and Yang CS (1991a) Inhibition of cytochrome P-450 2E1 by diallyl sulfide and its metabolites. *Chemical Research in Toxicology*, **4**, 642–647.

Brady JF, Wang M-H, Hong J-Y, Xiao F, Li Y, Yoo J-S H, Ning SM, Fukuto JM, Gapac JM and Yang CS (1991b) Modulation of rat hepatic microsomal monooxygenase activities and cytotoxicity by diallyl sulfide. *Toxicology and Applied Pharmacology*, **108**, 3423–354.

Chung F-L, Wang M and Hecht SS (1985) Effects of dietary indoles and isothiocyanates on *N*-nitrosodimethylamine and 4-(methylnitrosamino)-1-(3-pyridyl)-1-butanone alpha-hydroxylation and DNA methylation in rat liver. *Carcinogenesis*, **6**, 539–543.

Committee on diet, nutrition and cancer (1982). In *Diet, Nutrition and Cancer*, National Academy Press, Washington, DC, pp. 358–370.

Guo Z, Smith TJ, Wang E, Sadrieh N, Ma Q, Thomas PE and Yang CS (1992) Effects of phenylhexyl isothiocyanate, a carcinogenesis inhibitor, on xenobiotic-metabolizing enzymes and nitrosamine metabolism in rats. *Carcinogenesis*, **13**, 2205–2210.

Habermignard D, Suschetet M, Bergers R, Astorg P and Siess MH (1996) Inhibition of aflatoxin B_1- and *N*-nitrosodiethylamine-induced liver preneoplastic foci in rats fed naturally occurring allyl sulfides. *Nutrition and Cancer*, **25**, 61–70.

Hasegawa T, Nishino H and Iwashima A (1993). Isothiocyanates inhibit cell cycle progression of Hela cells at G_2/M phase. *Anti-Cancer Drugs*, **4**, 273–279.

Hatano S, Jimenez A and Wargovich MJ (1996). Chemopreventive effect of S-allylcysteine and its relationship to the detoxification enzyme glutathione S-transferase. *Carcinogenesis*, **17**, 1041–1044.

Hecht S (1995) Chemoprevention by isothiocyanates. *Journal of Cellular Biochemistry*, **22**, 195–209.

Imai J, Ide N, Nagae S, Moriguchi T, Matsuura H and Itakura Y (1994) Antioxidant and radical scavenging effects of aged garlic extract and its constituents. *Planta Medica*, **60**, 417–420.

Ip C and Lisk DJ (1995) Efficacy of cancer prevention by high-selenium garlic is primarily dependent on the action of selenium. *Carcinogenesis*, **16**, 2649–2652.

Jang JJ, Cho KJ, Myong NH, Kim SH and Lee SJ (1989). Effects of allyl sulfide, germanium and NaCl on the development of glutathione S-transferase P-positive rat hepatic foci initiated by diethylnitrosamine. *Anticancer Research*, **9**, 273–276.

Jirousek L and Starka J (1958) Uber das vorkommen von trithionen (1,2-dithiocyclopent-4-en-3-thione) in Brassicapflanzen. *Naturwissenschaften*, **45**, 386–387.

Kawamori T, Tanaka T, Ohnishi M, Hirose Y, Nakamura Y, Satoh K, Hara A and Mori H (1995) Chemoprevention of azoxymethane-induced colon carcinogenesis by dietary feeding of S-methyl methane thiosulfonate in male F344 rats. *Cancer Research*, **55**, 4053–4058.

Kimura H, Okamoto K and Sakai Y (1985) Modulatory effects of prostaglandin D_2, E_2 and $F_{2\alpha}$ on the postsynaptic actions of inhibitory and excitatory amino acids in cerebellar Purkinje cell dendrites *in vitro*. *Brain Research*, **330**, 235–244.

Levy L and Vredevoe DL (1983) The effects of N-acetylcysteine on cyclophosphamide immunoregulation and antitumor activity. *Seminars in Oncology*, **10**, 7–16.

Mei X, Wang ML, Xu HX, Pan XY, Gao CY, Han N and Fu MY (1982) Garlic and gastric cancer I. The influence of gastric on the level of nitrate and nitrite in gastric juice. *Acta Nutritica Sinica*, **4**, 53–56.

Mori H, Tanaka T, Sugie S and Yoshimi N (1995) Chemopreventive effects of plant derived phenolics, organosulfur and other compounds on carcinogenesis in digestive organs. *Environmental Mutagen Research Communications*, **17**, 127–133.

Mori H, Sugie S, Tanaka T, Makita H and Yoshimi N (1996a) Suppressive effects of natural antioxidants on carcinogenesis in digestive organs. *Environmental Mutagen Research Communications*, **18**, 73–77.

Mori H, Yoshimi N, Tanaka T and Hirose Y (1996b) Experimental colorectal carcinogenesis; role of cell proliferation. In *Recent Advances in Gastroenterological Carcinogenesis I*, Tahara E, Sugimachi, Oohara T (eds), Monduzzi Editore, Bologna, pp. 249–254.

Morioka N, Sze LL, Morton DL and Irie RF (1993) A protein fraction from aged garlic extract enhances cytotoxicity and proliferation of human lymphocytes mediated by interleukin-2 and concanavalin A. *Cancer Immunology Immunotherapy*, **37**, 316–322.

Morse MA, Wang C-X, Amin SG, Hecht SS and Chung F-L (1988) Effects of dietary sinigrin or indole-3-carbinol on O^6-methylguanine-DNA transmethylase activity and 4-(methylnitrosamino)-1-(3-pyridyl)-1-butanone-induced DNA methylation and tumorigenicity in F344 rats. *Carcinogenesis*, **9**, 1891–1895.

Morse MA, Wang C-X, Stoner GD, Mandel S, Conran PB, Amin SG, Hecht SS and Chung F-L (1989) Inhibition of 4-(methylnitrosamino)-1-(3-pyridyl)-1-butanone-induced DNA adduct formation and tumorigenicity in the lung of F-344 rats by dietary phenethyl isothiocyanate. *Cancer Research*, **49**, 549–553.

Morse MA, Eklind KI, Hecht SS, Jordan KG, Chi C-I, Desai DH, Amin SG and Chung F-L (1991) Structure-activity relationships for inhibition of 4-(methylnitrosamino)-

1 (3-pyridyl)-1-butanone lung tumorigenesis by arylalkyl isothiocyanates in A/J mice. *Cancer Research*, **51**, 1846–1850.

Morse MA, Zu H, Galatini AJ, Schmidt CJ and Stoner GD (1993) Dose-related inhibition by dietary phenethyl isothiocyanate of esophageal tumorigenesis and DNA methylation induced by N-nitrosomethylbenzylamine in rats. *Cancer Letters*, **72**, 103–110.

Nakamura Y, Matsuo T, Shimoi K, Nakamura Y and Tomita I (1993) S-Methyl methane thiosulfonate, a new antimutagenic compound isolated from *Brassica oleracea* L. var. *botrytis*. *Biological and Pharmaceutical Bulletin*, **16**, 207–209.

Nishikawa A, Furukawa F, Ikezaki S, Tanakamaru Z, Chung FL, Takahashi M and Hayashi Y (1996a) Chemopreventive effects of 3-phenylpropyl isothiocyanate on hamster lung tumorigenesis initiated with N-nitrosobis(2-oxopropyl)amine. *Japanese Journal of Cancer Research*, **87**, 122–126.

Nishikawa A, Furukawa F, Uneyama C, Ikezaki S, Tanakamaru Z, Chung F-L, Takahashi M and Hayashi Y (1996b) Chemopreventive effects of phenethyl isothiocyanate on lung pancreatic tumorigenesis in N-nitrosobis(2-oxopropyl)amine-treated hamsters. *Carcinogenesis*, **17**, 1381–1384.

Okamoto K, Sugie S, Ohnishi M, Makita H, Kawamori T, Watanabe T, Tanaka T and Mori H (1996) Chemopreventive effects of tauline on diethylnitrosamine and phenobarbital-induced hepatocarcinogenesis in male F344 rats. *Japanese Journal of Cancer Research*, **87**, 30–36.

Pierson HF, Fisher JM and Rabinovitz M (1985) Modulation by tauline of the toxicity of taumustine, a compound with antitumor activity. *Journal of the National Cancer Institute*, **75**, 905–909.

Prochaska HJ, Santamaria AB and Talalay P (1992) Rapid detection of inducers of enzymes that protect against carcinogens. *Proceedings of the National Academy of Sciences*, **89**, 2394–2398.

Reddy BS, Rao CV, Rivenson A and Kellof G (1993) Chemoprevention of colon carcinogenesis by organosulfur compounds. *Cancer Research*, **53**, 3493–3498.

Reicks NM and Crankshaw DL (1996) Modulation of rat hepatic cytochrome P-450 activity by garlic organosulfur compounds. *Nutrition and Cancer*, **25**, 241–248.

Schaffer EM, Liu J-Z, Green J, Dangler CA and Milner JA (1996) Garlic and associated allyl sulfur compounds inhibit N-methyl-N-nitrosourea induced rat mammary carcinogenesis. *Cancer Letters*, **102**, 199–204.

Smith TJ, Guo Z, Li C, Ning SM, Thomas PE and Yang CS (1993) Mechanism of inhibition of 4-(methylnitrosamino)-1(3-pyridyl)-1-butanone bioactivation in mouse by dietary phenethyl isothiocyanate. *Cancer Research*, **53**, 3276–3282.

Sones K, Heaney RK and Fenwick GR (1984) An estimate of the mean daily intake of glucosinolates from cruciferous vegetables in the UK. *Journal of the Science Food and Agriculture*, **35**, 712–720.

Sparnins VL, Mott AW, Barany G and Wattenberg LW (1986) Effects of allyl methyl trisulfide on glutathione S-transferase activity and BP-induced neoplasia in the mouse. *Nutrition and Cancer*, **8**, 211–215.

Sparnins VL, Barany G and Wattenberg LW (1988) Effects of organo-sulfur compounds from garlic and onions on benzo(a)pyrene-induced neoplasia and glutathione S-transferase activity. *Carcinogenesis*, **9**, 131–134.

Steinmetz KA, Kushi LH, Bostick RM, Folsom AR and Potter JD (1994) Vegetables, fruit, and colon cancer in the Iowa Women's Health Study. *American Journal of Epidemiology*, **139**, 1–15.

Stoner GD and Morse M (1996) Isothiocyanates as inhibitors of esophageal cancer. In *Dietary Phytochemicals in Cancer Prevention and Treatment*, American Institute for Cancer Prevention and Treatment, Plenum Press, New York, pp. 13–23.

Stoner GD, Morrissey D, Heur Y-H, Daniel EM, Galati AJ and Wagner SA (1991) Inhibitory effects of phenethyl isothiocyanate on N-nitrosobenzylmethylamine carcinogenesis in the rat eosphagus. Cancer Research, 51, 2063–2068.

Stoner GD, Siglin JC, Morse MA, Desai D, Amin S, Kresty LA, Toburen AL, Heffner EM and Francis DJ (1995) Enhancement of oesophageal carcinogenesis in male F344 rats by dietary phenylhexyl isothiocyanate. Carcinogenesis, 16, 2473–2476.

Sugie S, Okumura A, Tanaka T and Mori H (1993a) Inhibitory effects of benzyl isothiocyanate and benzyl thiocyanate on diethylnitrosamine-induced hepatocarcinogenesis in rats. Japanese Journal of Cancer Research, 84, 865–870.

Sugie S, Yoshimi N, Okumura A, Tanaka T and Mori H (1993b) Modifying effects of benzyl isothiocyanate and benzyl thiocyanate on DNA synthesis in primary cultures of rat hepatocytes. Carcinogenesis, 14, 281–283.

Sugie S, Okamoto K, Okumura A, Tanaka T and Mori H (1994) Inhibitory effects of benzyl thiocyanate and benzyl isothiocyanate on methylazoxymethanol acetate-induced intestinal carcinogenesis in rats. Carcinogenesis, 15, 1555–1560.

Sugie S, Okamoto K, Ohnishi M, Makita H, Kawamori T, Watanabe T, Tanaka T, Nakamura YK, Nakamura Y, Tomita I and Mori H (1997) Suppressive effects of S-methyl methanethiosulfonate on promotion stage of diethylnitrosamine-initiated and phenobarbital-promoted hepatocarcinogenesis model. Japanese Journal of Cancer Research, 88, 5–11.

Sundaram SG and Milner JA (1993) Impact of organosulfur compounds in garlic on canine mammary tumor cells. Cancer Letters, 74, 85–90.

Sundaram SG and Milner JA (1996a) Diallyl disulfide inhibits the proliferation of human tumor cells in culture. Biochimica et Biophysica Acta, 1315, 15–20.

Sundaram SG and Milner JA (1996b) Diallyl disulfide induces apoptosis of human colon tumor cells. Carcinogenesis, 17, 669–673.

Sumiyoshi H and Wargovich MJ (1990) Chemoprevention of 1,2-dimethylhydrazine induced colon cancer in mice by naturally occurring organosulfur compounds. Cancer Research, 50, 5084–5087.

Suzui N, Sugie S, Rahman KMW, Ohnishi M, Yoshimi N, Wakabayashi K and Mori (1997) Inhibitory effects of diallyl disulfide or aspirin on 2-amino-1-methyl-6-phenylimidazo[4,5-b]pyridine-induced mammary carcinogenesis in rats. Japanese Journal of Cancer Research, 88, 705–711.

Takada N, Kitano M, Chen T, Yano Y, Otani S and Fukushima S (1994a) Enhancing effects of organosulfur compounds from garlic and onions on hepatocarcinogenesis in rats: association with increased cell proliferation and elevated ornithine decarboxylase activity. Japanese Journal of Cancer Research, 85, 1067–1072.

Takada N, Matsuda T, Otoshi T, Yano Y, Otani S, Hasegawa T, Nakae D, Konishi Y and Fukushima S (1994b) Enhancement by organosulfur compounds from garlic and onions of diethylnitrosamine-induced glutathione S-transferase positive foci in the rat liver. Cancer Research, 54, 2895–2899.

Takada N, Yano Y, Wanibuchi H, Otani S and Fukushima S (1997) S-Methylcysteine and cysteine are inhibitors of induction of glutathione S-transferase placental form-positive foci during initiation and promotion phases of rat hepatocarcinogenesis. Japanese Journal of Cancer Research, 88, 435–442.

Takahashi S, Hakoi K, Yada H, Hirose M, Ito N and Fukushima S (1992) Enhancing effects of diallyl sulfide on hepatocarcinogenesis and inhibitory actions of the related diallyl disulfide on colon and renal carcinogenesis in rats. Carcinogenesis, 13, 1513–1518.

Talalay P and Zhang Y (1996) Chemoprevention against cancer by isothiocyanates and glucosinolates. Biochemical Society Transactions, 24, 806–810.

Tanaka T, Mori Y, Morishita Y, Hara A, Ohno T, Kojima T and Mori H (1990) Inhibitory effect of sinigrin and indole-3-carbinol on diethylnitrosamine-induced hepatocarcinogenesis in male ACI/N rats. *Carcinogenesis*, **11**, 1403–1406.

Umemura T, Hasegawa R, Sai-Kato K. Nishikawa A, Furukawa F, Toyokuni S, Uchida K, Inoue T and Kurokawa Y (1996) Prevention by 2-mercaptoethane sulfonate and N-acetylcysteine of renal oxidative damage in rats treated with ferric nitrilotriacetate. *Japanese Journal of Cancer Research*, **87**, 882–886.

Wargovich MJ (1987) Diallyl sulfide, a flavor component of garlic (*Allium sativum*), inhibits dimethylhydrazine-induced colon cancer. *Carcinogenesis*, **8**, 487–489.

Wargovich MJ (1992) Inhibition of gastrointestinal cancer by organosulfur compounds in garlic. In *Cancer Chemoprevention*, Wattenberg LW, Lipkin M, Boone CW, Kellof GJ (eds), CRC Press, Boca Raton, FL, pp. 195–203.

Wargovich MJ, Woods, C, Eng VWS, Stephens LC and Gray K (1988) Chemoprevention of N-nitrosomethylbenzylamine-induced esophageal cancer in rats by the naturally occurring thioether, diallyl sulfide. *Cancer Research*, **48**, 6872–6875.

Wattenberg LW (1977) Inhibition of carcinogenic effects of polycyclic hydrocarbons by benzyl isothiocyanate and related compounds. *Journal of the National Cancer Institute*, **58**, 295–298.

Wattenberg LW (1985) Chemoprevention of cancer. *Cancer Research*, **45**, 1–8.

Wattenberg LW (1987) Inhibitory effects of benzyl isothiocyanate administered shortly before diethylnitrosamine on pulmonary and forestomach neoplasia in A/J mice. *Carcinogenesis*, **12**, 1971–1973.

Wattenberg LW (1992a) Inhibition of carcinogenesis by minor dietary constituents. *Cancer Research*, **52**, 2085–2091.

Wattenberg LW (1992b) Chemoprevention of cancer by naturally occurring and synthetic compounds. In *Cancer Chemoprevention*, Wattenberg LW, Lipkin M, Boone CW, Kellof GJ (eds), CRC Press, Boca Raton, FL, pp. 19–39.

Wattenberg LW and Bueding E (1986) Inhibitory effects of 5-(2-pyrazinyl)-4-methyl-1,2-dithiol-3-thione (Oltipraz) on carcinogenesis induced by benzo(a)pyrene, diethylnitrosamine and uracil mustard. *Carcinogenesis*, **17**, 1379–1381.

Wattenberg LW, Hanley AB, Barany G, Sparnins VL, Lam LK and Fenwick GR (1986) Inhibition of carcinogenesis by some minor dietary constituents. In *Diet, Nutrition and Cancer*; Hayashi Y, Nagao M, Sugimura T, Takayama S, Tomatis L, Wattenberg LW, Wogan G (eds), Japan Sci. Soc. Press Tokyo/Vnu. Science Press, Utrecht, pp. 193–203.

Wattenberg LW, Sparnins VL and Barany G (1989) Inhibition of N-nitrosamine carcinogenesis by naturally occurring organosulfur compounds and monoterpenes. *Cancer Research*, **49**, 2689–2692.

Yu R, Jiano J-J, Duh J-L, Tan T-H and Kong AT (1996) Phenyl isothiocyanate, a natural chemopreventive agent, activates c-Jun N-terminal kinase 1. *Cancer Research*, **56**, 2954–2959.

Zhang Y and Talalay P (1994) Anticarcinogenic activities of organic isothiocyanates: chemistry and mechanisms. *Cancer Research*, **54**, 1976–1981.

Zhang Y, Talalay P, Cho C-G and Posner GH (1992) A major inducer of anticarcinogenic protective enzymes from broccoli: isolation and elucidation of structure. *Proceedings of the National Academy of Sciences, USA*, **89**, 2399–2403.

13 Cancer Chemoprevention by Tea Polyphenols

Nihal Ahmad, Santosh K Katiyar and Hasan Mukhtar

Department of Dermatology, University Hospitals of Cleveland, Case Western Reserve University, Cleveland, OH 44106, USA

Introduction

Many strategies are possible to reduce cancer-related deaths, four of which are noteworthy: (i) prevention; (ii) early diagnosis and intervention; (iii) successful treatment of localised cancer; and (iv) improved management of non-localised cancer. Among these, prevention appears the most practical approach to deal with the cancer problem. One approach for preventing the occurrence of cancer is through chemoprevention which, by definition, is a means of cancer control in which the occurrence of the disease can be entirely prevented, slowed or reversed by the administration of one or more naturally occurring and/or synthetic compounds (Ames, 1983; Ames and Gold, 1990; Wattenberg, 1990; Sporn, 1991; Morse and Stoner, 1993; Kohlmeier *et al.*, 1997). The expanded definition of cancer chemoprevention also includes the chemotherapy of precancerous lesions which are called preinvasive neoplasia, dysplasia or intraephelieal neoplasia, depending on the organ system (Boone *et al.*, 1990, 1992). Such chemopreventive compounds are known as anticarcinogens, and ideally they should have: (i) little or no toxic effects; (ii) high efficacy in multiple sites; (iii) capability of oral consumption; (iv) a known mechanism of action; (v) low cost; and (vi) human acceptance. Chemoprevention of cancer thus differs from cancer treatment in that the goal of this approach is to lower the rate of cancer incidence. This approach is promising because therapy and surgery have not been fully effective against the high incidence or low survival rate of most of the cancer types. Furthermore, this approach appears to have practical implications in reducing cancer risk because, unlike the carcinogenic environmental factors that are difficult to control, individuals can make decisions to modify their choice for the food and beverage they consume. In recent

Nutrition and Chemical Toxicity. Edited by Costas Ioannides. © John Wiley & Sons Ltd. ISBN 0 471 97453 6

years, the naturally occurring compounds, especially the antioxidants, present in the common diet and beverages consumed by the human population have gained considerable attention as chemopreventive agents for potential human benefit (Ames, 1983; Ames and Gold, 1990; Wattenberg, 1990; Sporn, 1991; Morse and Stoner, 1993; Kohlmeier et al., 1997). Abundant epidemiological, experimental and metabolic studies have provided convincing evidence that nutrition plays an important causative role in the initiation, promotion and progression stages of several types of human cancers (Ames, 1983; Wattenberg, 1990; Boone et al., 1992). It has become clear that, in addition to substances that pose a cancer risk, the human diet also contains agents which are capable of affording protection against some forms of cancer (Ames, 1983; Ames and Gold, 1990; Kohlmeier et al., 1997). This collective information strongly suggest that the occurrence of cancer can be prevented or slowed by dietary intake of substances that have the capacity to afford protection against the occurrence of cancer.

The picture-perfect image of serenity can be viewed as relaxing with an interesting book, sipping a cup of hot tea. For many thousand years, the harvesting and processing of the leaves of *Camellia senensis*, probably known as tea in the whole world, has become an integral part of human society and culture. Because of its characteristic flavour and pharmacological properties, next to water, tea is the most popular beverage consumed worldwide (Harbowy and Balentine, 1997). The per capita consumption of tea in the USA is approximately 340 g. Although the largest total consumption of tea is registered in India (540 000 metric tons, 620 g per capita), Ireland has the largest per capita consumption of tea (3220 g). Tea contains several polyphenolic components, which are antioxidant in nature, and many studies have shown that tea polyphenols possess the ability to prevent oxidant-induced cellular damage (Katiyar and Mukhtar, 1996; Harbowy and Balentine, 1997). In recent years, studies from many laboratories worldwide, conducted in various organ-specific animal bioassay systems have shown that tea and the polyphenolic constituents isolated from it, are capable of affording protection against a variety of cancer types. Although the majority of the studies was conducted with green tea, a limited number of studies have also shown the anti-cancer efficacy of black tea. This chapter presents a critical evaluation of this topic. To introduce the subject we provide some information on the consumption, composition, basic chemistry of tea and its polyphenols, and epidemiological studies associated with cancer risk and tea usage. The reader is referred to our previous review on this subject (Katiyar and Mukhtar, 1996).

Consumption composition and chemistry of tea

CONSUMPTION

The tea plant originated in Southeast Asia and is presently cultivated in over 30 countries around the globe. Currently, tea beverage is consumed worldwide, although at greatly varying levels. Consumption of tea is far from uniform as a large segment of the world's population virtually consumes no tea. Not only does the tea consumption vary from country to country, but also there is enormous variation in any given population. This ranges from none to as many as 20 or more cups per day. Although firm data are not available, it is generally accepted that next to water, tea is the most consumed beverage in the world; with a per capita worldwide consumption of approximately 120 ml per day (Katiyar and Mukhtar, 1996). Approximately 2.5 million metric tonnes of dried tea are manufactured annually in the whole world, of which 78% is black tea, 20% is green tea and less than 2% is oolong tea. Green tea is produced in relatively few countries, and is mainly consumed in China, Japan, India and a few countries in North Africa and the Middle East. About 78% of the world's total tea consumed is black tea, which is mainly consumed in western countries and some Asian countries. Oolong tea production and consumption is confined to Southeastern China and Taiwan (Katiyar and Mukhtar, 1996).

COMPOSITION

The composition of tea-leaf varies with climate, season, horticultural practices, variety of the plant and age of the leaf, i.e. the position of the leaf on the harvested shoot. Three main varieties of the commercial tea are available: Green (unfermented), Oolong (partially fermented) and Black (fully fermented) (Katiyar and Mukhtar, 1996). Their composition varies according to the manufacturing process which differs in the degree of 'enzymic oxidation' or fermentation. The principal polyphenolic components present in a typical green and black tea beverage are shown in Table 13.1, but variations may be considerable (Katiyar and Mukhtar, 1996). Oolong tea composition in general falls in between green and black teas.

Green tea

The manufacturing process of green tea involves rapid steaming or pan frying of freshly harvested leaves to inactivate enzymes, preventing fermentation and thereby producing a dry stable product. Green teas are generally produced in two different varieties: White tea and Yellow tea, the latter being less fermented because of the wilting process. There is also some difference between Chinese and Japanese green tea manufacture. Because of the increasing popularity of green tea, a wide variety of green tea products are entering the market.

Table 13.1 Major polyphenolic constituents present in green and black tea (%wt/wt)

Components	Green tea	Black tea
Catechins	30–42	3–10
Flavonols	5–10	6–8
Other flavanoids	2–4	–
Theogallin	2–3	–
Gallic acid	0.5	–
Quinic acid	2.0	–
Theanine	4–6	–
Methylxanthines	7–9	8–11
Theaflavins	–	3–6
Thearubigens	–	12–18

Epicatechins are the main constituent compounds in green tea, giving it the characteristic colour and flavour.

Black tea and Oolong tea

In the production process of black and oolong tea, the fresh leaves are allowed to wither until the moisture content of leaves is reduced to about 55% of the original leaf-weight that results in the concentration of polyphenols in the leaves and the deterioration of leaf-structural integrity. This step gives the typical aroma to the tea. The withered leaves are rolled and crushed, initiating fermentation of the polyphenols. This process is known as maceration and the fermenting mass is known as 'dhool'. The process used to macerate the leaf plays an important role in the final grading of tea. During these processes the catechins are converted to theaflavins and thearubigins. Theaflavins are astringent compounds contributing importantly to the colour and taste of the black tea. The thearubigen fraction is a mixture of substances, with a molecular weight distribution of 1000 to 40 000 Da and account for 15% of dry weight solids of black tea.

Oolong teas are prepared by firing the leaves shortly after rolling to terminate the oxidation and dry the leaves. Normal oolong tea is considered to be about half-fermented compared with black tea. Oolong tea extracts contain catechins at a level of 8–20% of the total dry matter. The fermentation process results in the oxidation of simple polyphenols to more complex condensed polyphenols to give black and oolong teas their characteristic colours and flavours (Harbowy and Balentine, 1997).

CHEMISTRY

The chemical composition of green tea is approximately similar to that of the fresh leaf with regard to the major components. Green tea contains polyphenolic compounds, which include flavanols, flavandiols, flavonoids and phenolic acids. These compounds account up to 60% of the dry weight of green tea leaves. Most of the polyphenols present in green tea are flavanols, commonly known as catechins. Some major catechins present in green tea are (-)-epicatechin (EC), (-)-epicatechin-3-gallate (ECG), (-)-epigallocatechin (EGC) and (-)-epigallocatechin-3-gallate (EGCG). The chemical structures of these compounds are given in Figure 13.1. In addition, caffeine, theobromine, theophylline and phenolic acids such as gallic acids are also present in green tea (Table 13.1).

During the fermentation process involved in the manufacture of black tea, the monomeric flavan-3-ols undergo polyphenol oxidase-dependent oxidative polymerisation leading to the formation of bisflavanols, theaflavins, thearubigins and some other oligomers. Theaflavins (1–2%, on a dry weight basis) contains benzotropolone rings with dihydroxy or trihydroxy substitution systems. About 10–20% of the dry weight of black tea is due to thearubigens, which are even more extensively oxidised and polymerised. The structures of theaflavins and thearubigins are shown in Figure 13.1.

Oolong tea contains monomeric catechins, theaflavins and thearubigins. In addition, epigallocatechin esters, theasinensins, dimeric catechins and dimeric proanthocyanidins are also the characteristic components of oolong tea.

Tea and cancer: epidemiological studies

In recent years, because of the availability of increasingly sophisticated biochemical approaches of molecular epidemiology, a better understanding of the process of cancer formation has been possible (Wright, 1991). Such understanding undoubtedly offers opportunities for defining the risk to individuals and for modulating this risk by means of agents that alter critical steps in the multistage process of cancer formation. The epidemiological studies published in 1991 by the International Agency for Research on Cancer (IARC) on tea-consumption and its effects on various types of cancer did not find conclusive results. The study concluded that there is inadequate evidence for the carcinogenicity of tea in humans and in experimental animals (IARC, 1991). It was also concluded that the available epidemiological data do not provide sufficient indication that tea consumption has a statistically significant causative effect on human cancers. However, the possible harmful effects of excessive tea consumption, tea consumption at very high temperature, or the consumption of salted tea were not ruled out, and this is an area in which as yet virtually no study has been conducted. Since the publication of this position paper by IARC, many laboratories as well as epidemiological studies defining an association between tea consumption and cancer risk and prevention have been published. Here, a general overview of the pertinent epidemiological studies on tea consumption and cancer prevention at different sites is provided. It is important to mention that a few studies have shown either no effect or

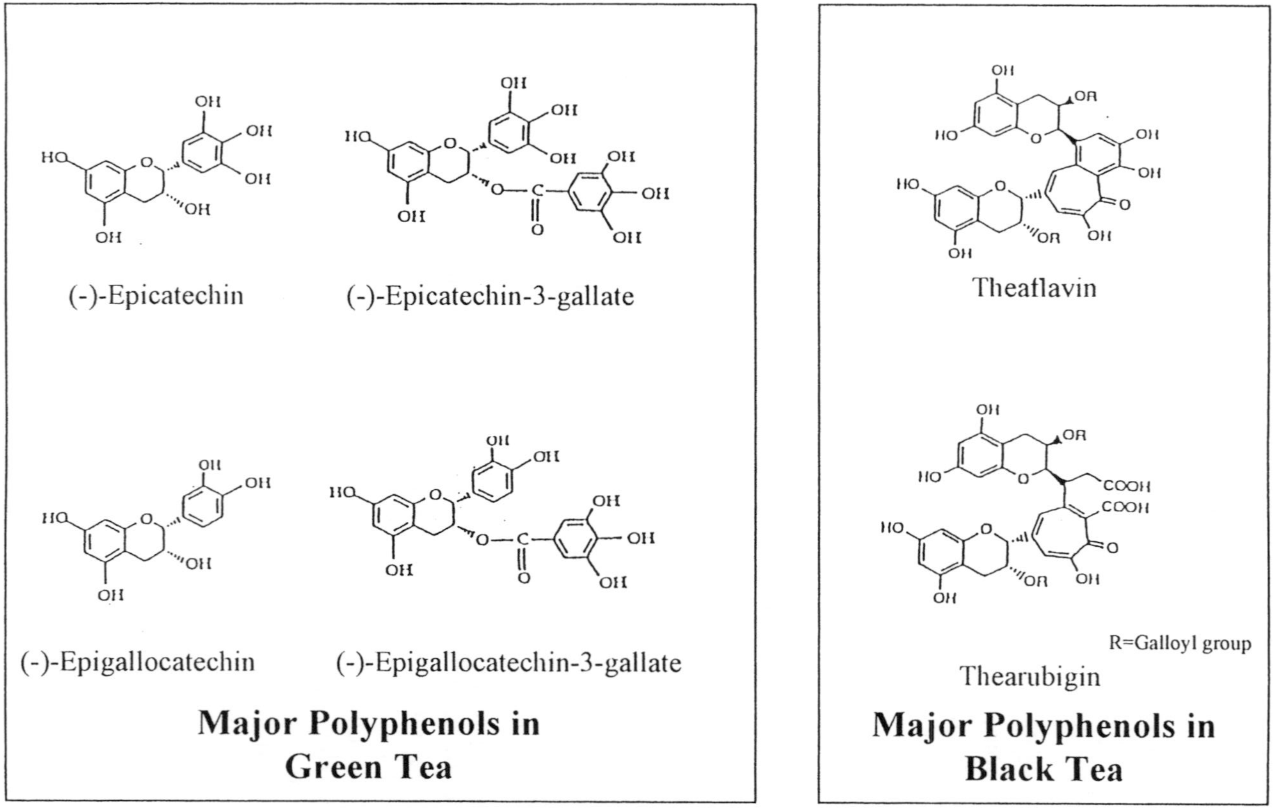

Figure 13.1 Major polyphenols present in green and black tea.

enhanced effect of tea consumption on cancer risk. A summary of the epidemiological studies based on organ site is provided below.

CANCER OF THE OESOPHAGUS AND NASOPHARYNX

The epidemiological studies conducted in China revealed that most of the areas with higher oesophageal cancer mortality rates are in the northern provinces where tea is either not produced or is infrequently consumed. In a case-control study, Gao et al. (1994) showed that the consumption of green tea reduces the risk of oesophageal cancer. This population based case-control study of oesophageal cancer in urban Shanghai, People's Republic of China, suggested a protective effect of green tea consumption. The authors concluded, 'Although these findings are consistent with studies in laboratory animals, indicating that green tea can inhibit esophageal carcinogenesis, further investigations are definitely needed'. Zheng et al. (1995) have conducted a cohort study in postmenopausal women in Iowa which revealed inverse associations between tea consumption and cancer risk for oropharyngeal and oesophageal cancers. The daily consumption of tea was found to be associated with an over 50% lower risk of these cancers.

In Linxian, which is a high-incidence area in northern China, the consumption of tea is rare and is believed not to be a contributing factor (Yang, 1980). Two case-control studies in southern Brazil (Victoria et al., 1987) and northern Italy (La Vecchia et al., 1992) also indicated that there was no relationship between oesophageal cancer risk and the frequency of tea consumption. Case-control studies conducted by several investigators (Kaufman et al., 1965; Bashirov et al., 1968; De Jong et al., 1974; Cook-Mozaffari et al., 1979) showed no association between drinking of tea at normal temperatures (35–47°C) and oesophageal cancer, but ingestion of tea at hot temperatures (55–67°C) was associated with an increased risk of oesophageal cancer. In another study conducted in Singapore, no association between tea drinking and oesophageal cancer was found (De Jong et al., 1974). Yang and Wang (1993) have suggested that the high temperature of tea or hot tea itself, rather than the components present in tea, may be an important factor in human oesophageal cancer. In three case-control studies (Lin et al., 1973; Henderson et al., 1976; Shanmugaratnam et al., 1978), no correlation between tea consumption and nasopharyngeal cancer was observed.

A limited number of studies suggested a positive association between tea consumption and the occurrence of oesophageal cancer. Morton (1986) and Kapadia et al. (1983) suggested that the excessive consumption of tea in the geographical zone between Iran to northern China may be a causative factor for the high incidence of oesophageal cancer. A geographical correlation study in the Caspian littoral of Iran (Lubin et al., 1985) indicated that individuals in the high-incidence area consumed more tea than in low-incidence areas. The case-control studies conducted in Kazakhastan (Kaufman et al., 1965; Bashirov *et al.*, 1968) revealed that only the consumption of very hot tea was associated with higher risk of oesophageal cancer. Another case-control study by Cook-Mozaffari *et al.* (1979) indicated that only the ingestion of very hot tea had a statistically significant association with oesophageal cancer.

CANCER OF THE STOMACH

In an epidemiological study (Oguni *et al.*, 1992) conducted in Shizuoka Prefecture, Japan, indicated that the cancer death rate in this tea-producing area, especially from stomach cancer, was lower than the national average. A case-control study in Kyushu, Japan showed that individuals consuming green tea frequently or in larger quantities have a lower risk of gastric cancer (Kono *et al.*, 1988). A cohort study conducted in Iowa (Zheng *et al.*, 1995) showed an inverse relationship between tea consumption and stomach cancer. A population-based case-control study to evaluate risk factors of gastric cancer conducted in areas with contrasting incidence rates in Sweden confirmed that tea had a statistically significant preventive effect when it was consumed during adolescence (Hansson *et al.*, 1993).

To establish a correlation of tea consumption with stomach cancer, a number of case-control studies were conducted in Buffalo (Graham *et al.*, 1967), Kansas City (Higginson, 1966), Nagoya, Japan (Tazima and Tominaga, 1985), Piraeus, Greece (Trichopoulos *et al.*, 1985), Milan, Italy (La Vecchia *et al.*, 1992), Spain (Agudo *et al.*, 1992) and Turkey (Demirer *et al.*, 1990). These studies indicated that there was no statistically significant association between tea consumption and cancer of the stomach. A cohort study conducted in London (Kinlen *et al.*, 1988) showed a positive association between black tea consumption and stomach cancer. Another case control study in Taipei, Taiwan also suggested that green tea consumption is a risk factor for gastric cancer (Lee *et al.*, 1990).

In a study by Goldbohm *et al.* (1996) an association was sought between black tea consumption and the subsequent risk of stomach, colorectal, lung and breast cancers in The Netherlands Cohort Study on Diet and Cancer among 58 279 men and 62 573 women aged 55–69 years. The consumption of tea showed an inverse association with cancer. However, tea drinkers appeared to smoke less and to eat more vegetables and fruits than did non-drinkers. When smoking and dietary factors were taken into account, tea in itself did not appear to protect against stomach cancer.

CANCER OF THE BLADDER, KIDNEY AND URINARY TRACT

In a cohort study conducted in Iowa, it was found that daily tea consumption reduced the risk of kidney cancers in postmenopausal women (Zheng *et al.*, 1995). Several other case-control studies were conducted to identify any association between tea consumption and cancers of the bladder and urinary tract (Stocks, 1970; Morgan and Jain, 1974; Simon *et al.*, 1975; Armstrong *et al.*,

1976; Miller *et al.*, 1978; Howe *et al.*, 1980; Hartge *et al.*, 1983; Ohno *et al.*, 1985; Claude *et al.*, 1986; Heilbrun *et al.*, 1986; Jensen *et al.*, 1986; Iscovich *et al.*, 1987; Kinlen *et al.*, 1988; Risch *et al.*, 1988; Slattery *et al.*, 1988; La Vecchia *et al.*, 1989; Nomura *et al.*, 1991; D'Avanzo *et al.*, 1992; Kunze *et al.*, 1992), without observing any positive relationship. Similarly, in five other case-control studies, no association was found between green tea consumption and renal cell cancer (Armstrong *et al.*, 1976; Goodman *et al.*, 1986; Yu *et al.*, 1986; McCredie *et al.*, 1988; La Vecchia *et al.*, 1992). In a cohort study (Kinlen *et al.*, 1988), a positive correlation was observed between tea consumption and cancer of the kidney.

CANCER OF THE COLON, RECTUM AND UTERUS

A number of studies (Morgan and Jain, 1974; Simon *et al.*, 1975; Armstrong *et al.*, 1976; Miller *et al.*, 1978; Howe *et al.*, 1980; Hartge *et al.*, 1983; Ohno *et al.*, 1985; Claude *et al.*, 1986; Goodman *et al.*, 1986; Heilbrun *et al.*, 1986; Jensen *et al.*, 1986; Yu *et al.*, 1986; Iscovich *et al.*, 1987; Kinlen *et al.*, 1988; McCredie *et al.*, 1988; Risch *et al.*, 1988; Slattery *et al.*, 1988; La Vecchia *et al.*, 1989; Nomura *et al.*, 1991; D'Avanzo *et al.*, 1992; Kunze *et al.*, 1992; La Vecchia *et al.*, 1992) indicated that the consumption of black tea decreased the risk for rectal cancer, while several others (Higginson, 1966; Morgan and Jain, 1974; Dales *et al.*, 1979; Miller *et al.*, 1983; Phillips and Snowdon, 1985; Tazima and Tominaga, 1985) showed no correlation. Two more studies (Stocks, 1970; Oguni *et al.*, 1992) concluded that there was a possible negative association between tea consumption and cancer of uterus. These studies also indicated that more studies are required to draw a final conclusion. Three other studies (Stocks, 1970; Heilbrun *et al.*, 1986; La Vecchia *et al.*, 1992) indicated a positive association between tea consumption and colon and rectal cancer. Baron *et al.* (1997) used data from an adenoma prevention trial to investigate these associations. Patients with at least one recent large bowel adenoma were followed with colonoscopy one and four years after their qualifying examinations. Adenomas detected at the four-year colonoscopy were used as endpoints. The study showed that there was no apparent association between the intake of tea and the risk of recurrent colorectal adenomas.

In a large population-based case-control study (Ji *et al.*, 1997) conducted in Shanghai, China, newly diagnosed cancer cases (931 colon and 884 rectum) during 1990–1993, among residents 30–74 years of age were included. An inverse association with each cancer was observed with increasing amount of green tea consumption.

An association between black tea consumption and the subsequent risk of colorectal cancer was sought in The Netherlands Cohort Study on Diet and Cancer (Goldbohm *et al.*, 1996). No association was observed between tea consumption and risk of colorectal cancer. The risk among tea drinkers in each consumption category was similar to that among non-drinkers. The authors concluded that on one hand this study did not support the hypothesis that consumption of black tea protects against four of the major cancers in humans, and on the other hand the cancer-enhancing effect was also not evident.

CANCER OF THE LIVER, LUNG, BREAST, AND PANCREAS

In Shizuoka Prefecture of Japan, a negative association between green tea consumption and liver cancer incidence was observed (Oguni et al., 1992), while no relationship was observed in three other studies (Stocks, 1970; Heilbrun, 1986; La Vecchia et al., 1992). A number of studies have shown positive as well as negative associations between tea consumption and lung cancer (Stocks, 1970; Morgan and Jain, 1974; Tewes et al., 1990; Oguni et al., 1992). Several other case-control studies indicated no association between tea consumption and breast cancer (Lubin et al., 1985; Mabuchi et al., 1985; Rosenberg et al., 1985; La Vecchia et al., 1986; Schairer et al., 1987). No association between pancreatic cancer and tea consumption was observed in a number of individual studies (Morgan and Jain, 1974; MacMahon et al., 1981; Mabuchi et al., 1985; Heilbrun, 1986; Mack et al., 1986; Schairer et al., 1987; Hiatt et al., 1988; Bueno de Mesquita et al., 1992; La Vecchia et al., 1992), whereas one case-control study (Kinlen and McPherson, 1984) showed a positive correlation. In a recent large population-based case-control study (Ji et al., 1997) conducted in Shanghai, China, 451 newly diagnosed pancreas cancer cases among residents 30–74 years of age were included. This study showed an inverse association with cancer with increasing amount of green tea consumption.

Goldbohm et al. (1996), conducted an epidemiological study to define an association between black tea consumption and the subsequent risk of stomach, colorectal, lung and breast cancers in The Netherlands Cohort Study on Diet and Cancer. They found that the risk among tea drinkers in each consumption category was similar to that among non-drinkers. They further concluded that this investigation did not support the hypothesis that black tea consumption protects against four of the major cancers in humans. However, in this study a cancer-enhancing effect was also not evident. In another prospective study Harnack et al. (1997) tested the hypothesis that teak intake increases the risk of cancer of the exocrine pancreas. The results from a cohort of 33 976 white American women with nine years of follow-up showed that tea consumption is not related to the incidences of cancer.

On the basis of available epidemiological studies and careful observations made in laboratory animals, it is reasonable to conclude that tea consumption is likely to have preventive effects against cancer risk at some body sites and suggest that more case-controlled studies be undertaken (Katiyar and Mukhtar, 1996).

Anticarcinogenic effects of tea: experimental studies

PREVENTION AGAINST SKIN TUMORIGENESIS

Prevention against skin tumour initiation

Utilizing several tumour bioassay protocols, studies from laboratories all over the world (Shanmugaratnam *et al.*, 1978; Katiyar *et al.*, 1992a; Mukhtar *et al.*, 1992; Katiyar and Mukhtar, 1996) have shown that the topical application as well as the oral feeding of a polyphenolic fraction isolated from green tea, hereafter referred to as GTP, to SENCAR, CD-1 and BALB/C mice results in significant prevention against the occurrence of skin tumorigenesis. In a complete carcinogenesis protocol, the topical application of GTP on the backs of BALB/C mice for 7 days prior to that of 3-methylcholanthrene, was found to result in significant prevention against the development of skin tumours (Wang *et al.*, 1989b). Studies were also conducted to assess whether GTP possesses anti-tumour-initiating effects. In these studies a two-stage skin carcinogenesis protocol in SENCAR mice was employed. Topical application of GTP for 7 days prior to the single application of 7,12-dimethylbenz(a)anthracene (DMBA) as the initiating agent followed by twice-weekly applications of the tumour promoter 12-*O*-tetradecanoyl-phorbol-13-acetate (TPA) resulted in significant prevention in the occurrence of tumorigenesis (Wange *et al.*, 1989b). In this study, in GTP-treated animals considerable delay in the latency period for the appearance of the first tumour and subsequent tumour growth was also observed. Oral feeding of GTP (0.05%, w/v) in drinking water for 50 days prior to the DMBA-TPA treatment or its continuous feeding during the entire period of the tumour protocol was also found to result in significant prevention both in terms of the tumour incidence and tumour multiplicity. EGCG is the major constituent present in GTP (Katiyar *et al.*, 1992b), and in a cup of green tea its concentration ranges up to 200 mg; thus, the intake of EGCG in individuals who habitually consume green tea is substantial. For this reason, it was of interest to examine the utility of this tea component as a cancer chemopreventive agent. The topical application of EGCG prior to DMBA/TPA protocol resulted in significant prevention against skin tumour initiation in SENCAR mouse skin. In these experiments, skin application of EGCG to the SENCAR mouse prior to that of carcinogen treatment was found to result in 30% inhibition in carcinogen metabolite binding to epidermal DNA, suggesting that EGCG may be affording its inhibition by inhibiting the metabolism of the precarcinogen.

Prevention against skin tumour promotion

The phorbol type tumour promoter TPA is most widely employed in the two-stage skin tumorigenesis protocol (Agarwal and Mukhtar, 1991; DiGiovanni, 1992; Katiyar and Mukhtar, 1996). Studies from the laboratory of the authors of this chapter investigated the effect of GTP on TPA-induced skin tumour promotion in DMBA-initiated SENCAR mouse. Topical application of varying doses of GTP prior to that of TPA resulted in significant prevention against skin tumour promotion in a dose-dependent manner (Katiyar et al., 1992). The pretreatment of the animals with GTP showed substantially lower tumour body burden such as decrease in total number of tumours per group, number of tumours per animal, tumour volume per mouse and average tumour size, as compared with the animals that did not receive GTP. Another study has shown that the topical application of GTP to CD-1 mice also inhibited TPA-induced tumour promotion in DMBA-initiated skin (Huang et al., 1992). Topical application of GTP or its major component EGCG, has been shown to inhibit tumour promotion mediated by TPA as well as by other skin tumour promoters such as teleocidin and okadaic acid (Yoshizawa et al., 1987; Huang et al., 1992). Another study (Fujiki et al., 1990) showed that the topical application of EGCG to mouse skin also inhibited teleocidin-promoted tumorigenesis in mouse skin.

It was shown that EGCG inhibited a tumour promoting activity of okadaic acid in a two-stage carcinogenesis experiment on mouse skin. EGCG treatment, prior to okadaic acid, completely inhibited the tumour formation in mice up to 20 weeks of the treatment (Yoshizawa, 1996), the inhibitory effects being dose-dependent. This study further showed that a topical application of 5 mg EGCG immediately reduced the specific binding of [^{3}H]okadaic acid to a particulate fraction of mouse skin to as low as 30% of control. According to the Scatchard analysis, the reduction of specific [^{3}H]okadaic acid binding was mainly due to the reduction of the binding sites, not due to the change of the affinity. The reduction of the specific binding was closely related to the inhibitory effect of EGCG on tumour promotion of okadaic acid.

Prevention against stage I and stage II skin tumour promotion

Skin tumour promotion is often divided in two operational stages known as stage I and stage II. Experiments were performed to determine which of these two stages of tumour promotion is inhibited by GTP. The topical application of GTP concurrently with each application of either TPA (stage I) or mezerein (stage II) resulted in significant prevention against DMBA-initiated tumour formation in SENCAR mouse, in terms of tumour multiplicity by 42 and 50%, and in terms of tumour growth by 54 and 43% respectively in stage I and stage II (Katiyar et al., 1993). Furthermore, this study showed that the sustained inhibition of tumour promotion by GTP required an uninterrupted application of GTP in conjunction with each promotional treatment of either of the tumour promoters. Under this treatment regimen, compared with non-GTP-treated positive controls, the GTP treatment afforded a significant inhibition (74%) in the growth/development of the tumour. It can, therefore, be concluded that GTP is capable of inhibiting stage I as well as stage II skin tumour promotion, and that the inhibition of tumour promotion depends on the duration of GTP treatment.

Prevention against malignant conversion of benign skin papillomas to carcinomas

The progression of benign tumours to malignant cancer is the most critical step in carcinogenesis since malignant lesions are capable of metastatic spread that eventually results in fatal consequences (Athar et al., 1991). Studies were conducted to assess the possible role of GTP in prevention against the conversion of chemically induced benign skin papillomas to squamous cell carcinomas in SENCAR mice. An enhanced rate of malignant conversion was achieved in the stabilised papilloma yield by twice-weekly topical applications of either the free-radical-generating compound, benzoyl-peroxide or the genotoxic agent, 4-nitroquinoline-N-oxide, whereas spontaneous malignant conversion was associated with topical application of acetone. In these protocols, the pre-application of GTP 30 minutes prior to skin application of acetone, benzoyl peroxide or 4-nitroquinoline-N-oxide resulted in significant prevention when assessed for the conversion of papillomas to carcinomas. This study suggested a significant preventive effect of green tea against tumour progression induced by free-radical-generating compounds and genotoxic agents (Katiyar et al., 1993).

In a study from our laboratory (Katiyar et al., 1997), we evaluated the protective effect of GTP against the induction and subsequent progression of papillomas to squamous cell carcinomas (SCCs) in experimental protocols where papillomas were developed with a low or high probability of their malignant conversion. Topical application of GTP (6 mg/animal) 30 minutes prior to that of TPA either once a week for five weeks (high-risk TPA protocol) or once a week for 20 weeks (low-risk TPA protocol) or mezerein (MEZ) twice a week for 20 weeks (high-risk MEZ protocol) in DMBA-initiated mouse skin resulted in significant protection against skin tumour promotion in terms of tumour incidence (32–60%), multiplicity (49–63%) and tumour volume/mouse (73–90%) at the termination of the experiment at 20 weeks. In three separate malignant progression experiments when papilloma yield in DMBA-initiated and TPA- or MEZ-promoted low- and high-risk protocols was stabilised at 20 weeks, animals were divided into two subgroups. These animals were either topically treated twice weekly with acetone (0.2 ml/animal, spontaneous malignant conversion group) or with GTP (6 mg/animal in 0.2 ml acetone) for an additional period of 31 weeks. During these treatment regimens, all suspected carcinomas were recorded and each was verified histopathologically either at the time when tumour-bearing mouse died/moribund or at the termination of the experiment at 51 weeks. GTP resulted in significant protection against the malignant conversion of papillomas to SCC in all the protocols employed. At the termination of the experiment at 51 weeks, these protective effects were evident in terms of mice with carcinomas (35–41%), carcinomas per mouse (47–55%) and percent malignant conversion of papillomas to carcinomas (47–58%). The kinetics of malignant conversion suggested that a subset of papillomas formed in the early phase of tumour promotion in all the protocols had a higher probability of malignant conversion into SCCs because all the positive control groups (acetone-treated) produced nearly the same number of carcinomas (33–38 in a group of 20 animals) at the end of the progression period. In the GTP-treated group of animals the number of carcinomas formed was less (14–20 in a group of 20 animals), which shows the ability of GTP to protect against the malignant conversion of papillomas of higher probability of malignant conversion to SCCs. The results of this study suggested that, irrespective of the risk involved, GTP might be highly useful in affording protection against skin cancer risk.

Prevention against UVB radiation-induced photocarcinogenesis

Ultraviolet B (UVB) radiation (280–320 nm) present in the solar spectrum is the major risk factor for skin cancer in humans (Elmets, 1991). Studies in our laboratory assessed the effect of topical application as well as oral feeding (through drinking water) of GTP to SKH-1 hairless mice on UVB radiation-induced photocarcinogenesis (Wang et al., 1991). The chronic oral feeding of GTP (0.1%, w/v) in drinking water to mice during the entire period of UVB exposure was found to result in significantly lower tumour body burden as compared with non-GTP-fed animals. The topical application of GTP before UVB radiation exposure also afforded some prevention against photocarcinogenesis. However, the observed protection was lower as compared with the oral feeding of GTP in drinking water. This observation was validated in terms of percentage of mice with tumours and number of tumours per mouse. Another study (Wang et al., 1992c) showed that the infusion of green tea extracts (1.25%, w/v) as a sole source of drinking water to mice afforded substantial prevention against UVB radiation-induced intensity of red colour and area of skin lesions, as well as UVB radiation-induced tumour initiation and promotion. In a subsequent study, Wang et al. (1994) showed that black tea consumption by SKH-1 hairless mice markedly reduced tumour formation when the animals were initiated with DMBA followed by multiple UVB exposures. The oral administration of black tea, green tea and decaffeinated black or green tea (0.63% or 1.25%, w/v) as the sole source of drinking water two weeks prior to and during 31 weeks of UVB treatment was found to reduce tumour risk in terms of number of tumours per animal, and also the tumour size. These studies suggest that consumption of tea as a sole source of drinking water may reduce the risk of some forms of human cancers induced by solar UV-radiation. Liu et al. (1995) analysed p53 and H-ras mutations in UV- and UV/green tea-induced skin tumours in SKH-1 mice, and found that mutations in exon 6 of the p53 gene are unique for tumours from UV/green tea group. They suggested that green tea might, somehow, select certain p53 mutations during the chemoprevention process. However, there is a need for additional studies to validate the suggestion that tea consumption offers selective advantage during clonal expansion by the tumour promoting agents. The effect of topically or orally administered pure EGCG on photocarcinogenesis and immunosuppression induced by UVB-radiation in BALB/cAnNHsd mice was assessed (Gensler *et al.*, 1996). This study showed that the induction of skin tumours by UV radiation was significantly reduced by topical, but not by oral, administration of EGCG through a mechanism distinct from inhibition of photoimmunosupression.

In a study from our laboratory (Chatterjee *et al.*, 1996) a novel ^{32}P postlabelling method was employed to detect UVB-induced DNA lesions in the epidermis of mice and its prevention by GTP. This study showed that epidermal DNA from UVB-exposed mice at 24 hours contains up to five DNA lesions; the quantitation of these lesions showed that their formation increased in a UVB dose-dependent manner. Treatment of DNA samples with the bacteriophage DNA repair enzyme T4 endonuclease V confirmed that four of these lesions are pyrimidine dimers. While some of these lesions were repaired 18 hours after UVB irradiation, 30% of them persisted even 48 hours post-irradiation. Topical application of GTP to the skin of the mice prior to UVB exposure was found to prevent the formation of pyrimidine dimers.

Huang *et al.* (1997) showed an inhibitory effect of orally administered green and black tea on UVB-induced complete carcinogenesis, but the decaffeinated teas were either inactive at moderate dose levels or enhanced the tumorigenic effect of UVB at high dose level. The oral administration of caffeine was found to have an inhibitory effect on UVB-induced complete carcinogenesis. This study concluded that caffeine is a biologically important constituent of tea.

Effect on the growth of established skin tumours

In multistage skin tumorigenesis studies in SENCAR mice, we observed that in mice, GTP treatment results in a reduction of tumour size in terms of total tumour volume per group and total tumour volume per animal when compared with the non-GTP-treated animals (Katiyar *et al.*, 1992c, 1993). In another study (Wang *et al.*, 1992d), it was shown that the consumption of water extracts of green tea (WEGT) or GTP in addition to resulting in decreased tumour formation and multiplicity, also markedly reduced tumour size. In this study it was also shown that feeding WEGT, or GTP or EGCG given intraperitoneally, inhibited tumour growth and caused partial regression of established skin papillomas in female CD-1 mice. These observations suggest that green tea may also possess chemotherapeutic effects. Lu *et al.* (1997) evaluated the effect of oral administration of black tea on the growth of chemically induced or UV radiation-induced established skin papillomas, keratoacanthomas and squamous cell carcinoma in CD-1 mice. They also evaluated the effect of oral administration of black tea on apoptosis, mitotic index and incorporation of bromodeoxyuridine into DNA of these tumours. The results suggested that black tea inhibited the growth of papillomas in mice. The treatment also inhibited the proliferation and enhanced apoptosis in both non-malignant as well as malignant skin tumours.

PREVENTION AGAINST FORESTOMACH AND LUNG TUMORIGENESIS

In a study from our laboratory, WEGT (2.5%, w/v) was given to female A/J mice as the sole source of drinking water and diethylnitrosamine (DEN) 20 mg/kg body weight of animal) and benzo(α)pyrene (BαP; 2 mg/animal) were employed as test carcinogens (Katiyar et al., 1993a). It was observed that compared with only DEN-treated mice, those fed with WEGT and DEN showed significantly lower tumour yield both in the lungs and forestomach. In terms of appearance of total number of tumours per mouse, a significant prevention in the occurrence of tumorigenesis in forestomach (80–85%) and lung (41–61%), at all the stages of carcinogenesis (initiation, promotion and complete carcinogenesis protocols), was observed. In the case of BαP-induced tumorigenicity, WEGT also resulted in 60–75% and 25–35% prevention in the total number of tumours per mouse in forestomach and lung respectively at all the stages of carcinogenesis.

The same protocols (Katiyar et al., 1993b), were used to assess the protective effects of GTP against DEN- and BαP-induced tumorigenesis in the forestomach and lungs of female A/J mice. The data showed that oral feeding of GTP (0.2%, w/v) significantly afforded prevention against DEN-induced total number of tumours per mouse in the forestomach (68–82%) and lung tumorigenesis (37–45%) during initiation, promotion and complete carcinogenesis protocols. GTP also showed comparable chemopreventive effects when BαP was used as a carcinogen. In a further study (Katiyar et al., 1993c), we also demonstrated that the administration of GTP (5 mg/animal) by gavage 30 minutes before challenge with the carcinogen afforded significant prevention against both DEN- and BαP-induced forestomach and lung tumorigenesis in A/J mice.

Further studies (Wang et al., 1992a,b) showed that treatment of A/J mice with WEGT (0.63%, 1.2% or 1.25%, w/v) protects against DEN- and BαP-induced forestomach and lung tumorigenesis. In one study (Xu et al., 1992), it was shown that 2% green tea infusion or 560 ppm EGCG feeding in drinking water for 13 weeks afforded prevention against 4-(methylnitrosamino)-1-(3-pyridyl)-1-butanone (NNK)-induced lung tumorigenesis in A/J mice. In a subsequent study, Shi et al. (1994) showed that when decaffeinated green or black tea extracts were given to female A/J mice as the sole source of drinking water before an intraperitoneal injection of NNK (100 mg/kg body weight), a significant reduction in lung tumour multiplicity was observed. Shim et al. (1995) reported the chemopreventive effects of daily green tea consumption among cigarette smokers. In this study, the sister-chromatid exchange frequency in peripheral lymphocytes was used as a marker for mutagenic response and green tea was shown to block the cigarette-induced increase in sister chromatid exchange frequency.

PREVENTION AGAINST OESOPHAGEAL TUMORIGENESIS

The chemopreventive effects of five different varieties of Chinese tea, including green tea, against N-nitroso-methylbenzylamine (NMBzA)-induced oesophageal tumorigenicity in Wistar rats was assessed (Chen, 1992). The oral administration of 2% tea as the sole source of drinking water to rats during the entire experimental period resulted in the inhibition of oesophageal tumorigenesis induced by NMBzA. All the five types of green and black tea tested were found to be effective and resulted in a reduction of tumour incidence by 26–53%, and tumour multiplicity by 58–75%. The oral feeding of green tea resulted in inhibition of oesophageal tumour formation induced by precursors of NMBzA (Gao et al., 1990) or by nitrososarcosine in mice (Oguni et al., 1992).

PREVENTION AGAINST DUODENUM AND SMALL INTESTINE TUMORIGENESIS

Some studies (Fujita et al., 1989; Fujiki et al., 1992) assessed the chemopreventive effects of EGCG against N-ethyl-N'-nitro-N-nitrosoguanidine (ENNG)-induced duodenum tumorigenicity in C57BL/6 mice. In this study, compared with non-EGCG-fed animals, the oral feeding of EGCG (after treatment with the carcinogen) in drinking water resulted in significant prevention against ENNG-caused tumour promotion in duodenum as observed by a decrease in tumour incidence and number of tumours per mouse. In one study (Hirose et al., 1993), the authors used a multi-organ carcinogenesis model to assess the preventive effect of GTP. In this study, F344 rats were pretreated with a combination of five carcinogens for four weeks, and a diet supplemented with 1% GTP was given during or after the carcinogen exposure period. The GTP treatment resulted in an inhibition of adenoma and adenocarcinoma formation in the small intestine.

PREVENTION AGAINST COLON TUMORIGENESIS

Using a rat colon tumorigenicity model, it was shown (Yamane et al., 1991) that one week after subcutaneous administration of azoxymethane to Fischer rats, oral feeding of GTP (0.01 or 0.1%. w/v) in the drinking water for an additional 10 weeks resulted in the inhibition of azoxymethane-induced colon tumorigenesis. However, in another study (Hirose et al., 1993) with a multi-organ tumorigenesis model using F344 rats, the administration of GTP (1%) in the diet did not inhibit tumorigenesis in the colon. In a further study (Narisawa and Fukaura, 1993) a very low dose of GTP against colon carcinogenesis in F344 rats was tested. In this study a total of 129 female F344 rats were given an intrarectal instillation of 2 mg of N-methyl-N-nitrosourea three times weekly for two consecutive weeks, and drinking water was replaced with WEGT (0.05, 0.01 or 0.002%) throughout the experiment. Autopsies performed at the 35th week revealed significant lowering in the incidence of colon carcinomas in rats given WEGT as compared with control animals.

A pyrolysis product in cooked foods, 2-amino-1-methyl-6-phenylimida-zo [4,5-b]pyridine (PhIP), has been shown to be a rat colon carcinogen and has been implicated in the aetiology of human colon cancer. In order to identify chemoprotection strategies that could be carried out in humans, a pilot study (Huber et al., 1997) was conducted in which PhIP-DNA adduct levels were quantified in the colon of male F344 rats that had been subjected to 16 different putative chemoprotection regimens, followed by a gavage of PhIP (560 mg/ kg) and sacrifice 24 hours laters. Out of 16 chemopreventive agents used, the strongest inhibition (67%) of PhIP-DNA adduct formation in the colon was observed upon pretreatment with black tea.

The effect of black tea and milk in tea was evaluated on colon cancer induced by azoxymethane, in an F344 rat model (Weisburger et al., 1997). Foci of aberrant crypts in the colon were decreased in tea- or tea-and-milk-fed animals. The study showed that tea consumption decreases the production of foci of aberrant crypts in the colon and that milk potentiates these inhibitory effects.

PREVENTION AGAINST LIVER TUMORIGENESIS

The administration of 5% green tea leaf in the diet from 10 days prior to the treatment with the carcinogenic compound aflatoxin B_1 until three days after the treatment resulted in a significant inhibition of aflatoxin B_1-induced γ-glutamyl transpeptidase-positive foci in rat liver (Chen et al., 1987). In another study, it was also shown that addition of 2.5% green tea leaf in the diet given to rats produced significant inhibition of DEN-induced hepatocarcinogenesis (Li, 1991). Mao showed the inhibitory effect of an epicatechin complex on DEN-induced liver precancerous lesions, variant cell foci and nodule formation in rats (Mao, 1993). Treatment with epicatechin complex resulted in a marked decrease in the number of N-ras overexpressed lesions. In a further study, it was shown that the administration of decaffeinated black tea extract by oral gavage to male Swiss mice resulted in a decrease of tobacco-induced liver tumours (Nagabhushan et al., 1991).

In a study by Yang et al. (1997), the pathogenesis of pulmonary tumours induced by a tobacco carcinogen, 4-(methylnitrosamino)-1-(3-pyridyl)-1-butanone (NNK), and its inhibition by black tea have been characterised in female A/J mice. In this short-term model, the administration of black tea polyphenols (0.3%) through the drinking water significantly inhibited NNK-induced early bronchiolar cell proliferation, as measured immunohistochemically by the incorporation of bromodeoxyuridine (BrdUrd). Administration of black tea also inhibited the progression of adenoma to adenocarcinoma as determined by both malignant tumour incidence and multiplicity. The cell proliferation rate in adenomas was also suppressed by black tea treatment. This study demonstrated the antiproliferative activities of black tea and its polyphenols, and the authors suggested that such activities, at the early and late stages of lung tumorigenesis, might be important for the cancer-chemopreventive activities of black tea.

In another study (Qin et al., 1997) in the Fischer rat model, the effect of green tea (given through the diet) has been examined on the initiation of aflatoxin B_1 (AFB_1)-induced hepatocarcinogenesis as assessed by hepatic AFB_1-DNA binding in vivo, AFB_1 metabolism in vitro, and by the appearance of AFB_1-induced glutathione S-transferase placental form (GST-P)-positive hepatocytes detected by immunohistochemical method. Green tea feeding did not affect the microsome-mediated AFB_1 binding to exogenous DNA, but enhanced microsome-mediated formation of non-toxic hydroxylated metabolites of AFB_1. Hepatic nuclear AFB_1-DNA binding in vivo was significantly inhibited by green tea. AFB_1-induced GST-P-positive single hepatocytes were also inhibited significantly by green tea treatment. The authors concluded that green tea inhibits initiation of AFB_1-induced hepatocarcinogenesis in the rat by modulation of AFB_1 metabolism, thereby inhibiting AFB_1-DNA binding and AFB_1-induced GST-P-positive hepatocytes.

PREVENTION AGAINST MAMMARY CARCINOGENESIS

In a study by Hirose et al. (1994) the effect of 1% green tea catechins on mammary gland carcinogenesis in female Sprague-Dawley rats pretreated with DMBA was evaluated. This study showed that although the final incidence and multiplicity of mammary tumours were not significantly affected by the administration of green tea catechins, the number of survivors in the green tea fed group at the end of the experiment (36 weeks) were significantly higher than in the basal diet group. The average size of the palpable mammary tumours was significantly smaller in the green tea catechins-fed group. This study indicated that green tea catechins also inhibit rat mammary gland carcinogenesis after DMBA initiation. Sakamoto et al. (1995) have shown that GTP and BTP (black tea polyphenols) suppressed the growth of canine mammary tumour cells CMT-13 in culture when added at the level of 25 ppm or more for at least 24 hours. This study also showed that BTP is more effective inhibitor of mammary tumour cells than GTP. Komori et al. (1993) reported that EGCG and WEGT treatment inhibited the growth of lung and mammary cancer cell lines with almost identical potencies. The authors postulated that EGCG and the components present in WEGT would block the interaction of tumour promoters, hormones and growth factors with their receptors.

In another study (Weisburger et al., 1997), the effect of tea, or tea and milk, instead of drinking water, in rat models of mammary gland cancer was evaluated. Solutions of 1.25% (w/v) black tea, or 1.85% (v/v) milk in tea were prepared three times per week. Sprague-Dawley rats were given tea beginning at 42 days of age; one group was gavaged 5 μg DMBA at 49 days of age; another group received 8.4 mg 2-amino-3-methylimidazo[4,5-f]quinoline (IQ) twice per week beginning at age 49, then 14 mg twice a week for four more weeks. The groups given DMBA were killed 33 weeks later, and those on IQ 39 weeks later. Tea decreased the mammary gland tumour multiplicity and volume, and milk potentiated these inhibitory effects.

PREVENTION AGAINST PANCREATIC AND PROSTATE CARCINOGENESIS

In a study by Harada *et al.* (1991), Syrian golden hamsters were used as the carcinogenesis model. The hamsters were treated with *N*-nitroso-bis(2-oxypropyl)amine and fed with a protein-deficient diet consisting of DL-ethionine and L-methionine for tumour promotion. In this study, the dietary supplementation with GTP (500 mg/kg per day) during the promotion stage was found to reduce pancreatic tumorigenesis as compared with non-GTP-supplemented animals (Harada *et al.*, 1991).

Another study from our laboratory (Mohan *et al.*, 1995) has shown that pretreatment of the human prostate carcinoma cell line LNCaP with GTP for 1 hour resulted in a dose-dependent inhibition of testosterone-induced ornithine decarboxylase (ODC) activity and mRNA expression. ODC is the rate-limiting enzyme in polyamine biosynthesis and plays an important role in cellular proliferation and differentiation, which are important processes in the development of cancer. This study, though non-conclusive, suggests that the consumption of GTP may be an approach for prostate cancer chemo-prevention.

CELL-SPECIFIC BIOLOGICAL EFFECTS OF TEA

Many tumour promoters are known to inhibit gap junctional intercellular communication that is regarded as an important mechanism of promotion. Sigler and Ruch (1993) assessed WEGT and the individual constituents of green tea for their effects on gap junctional intercellular communication in *p,p*-dichloro-diphenyltrichloro ethane-, TPA- and dieldrin-treated WB-F344 rat liver epithelial cells. All the three tumour promoters showed inhibition of gap junctional intercellular communication in a dose-responsive manner at non-cytolethal concentrations. WEGT enhanced gap junctional intercellular communication (20–80%) in promoter-treated cells. EGCG and ECG also enhanced gap junctional intercellular communication in *p,p*-dichlorodiphenyltrichloroethane-treated cells. These data suggest that WEGT may inhibit tumour promotion by enhancing gap junctional intercellular communication. Studies by Mitsui *et al.* (1995) showed that tea polyphenols, specifically EGCG, killed 3Y1 cells transformed by E1A gene of human adenovirus type 12 (E1A-3Y1 cells) at 100 times lower concentration than the parental 3Y1 cells. EGCG was also found to exert a strong E1A-3Y1 cell-specific toxicity, while EC and ECG did not. EGCG (0.05–0.1%, w/w), when given in drinking water to C3H/HeNCrj mice for 65 weeks, reduced the incidence of hepatoma-bearing mice from 83.3% (non-EGCG) to 56.0–52.2% (EGCG), and also reduced the average number of hepatoma per mouse. Nishida *et al.* (1994) showed that EGCG inhibited the growth and secretion of α-foetoprotein by human hepatoma-derived PLC/PRF/5 cells without decreasing their viability. In another study (Lea *et al.*, 1993), the polyphenols extracted from green or black tea were found to be strong inhibitors of DNA synthesis in HTC rat hepatoma cells and DS19 mouse erythroleukaemia cells. The intraperitoneal administration of EGCG was found significantly to inhibit the metastasis of lung caused by intravenous injection of lung carcinoma cells (Taniguchi *et al.*, 1992). WEGT has also been shown to prevent the induction of male B6C3F1 mouse-derived hepatocyte cytolethality by glucose oxidase, xanthine oxidase and paraquat in a dose-dependent manner. WEGT also prevented gap junctional-mediated intercellular communication by phenobarbital, lindane and paraquat (Klaunig, 1992).

The influence of EGCG and EGC on doxorubicin-resistant murine sarcoma (S180-dox) and human colon carcinoma (SW620-dox) cell lines was studied (Stammler and Volm, 1997). Both polyphenols showed a sensitizing effect on the cell lines by treatment with doxorubicin. These results suggested that protein kinase C might be inhibited by EGCG and EGC, thereby reducing the expression of some drug resistance-related proteins.

Another study (Valcic *et al.*, 1996) showed the inhibitory effect of six green tea catechins on the growth of four selected human tumour cell lines (MCF-7 breast carcinoma, HT-29 colon carcinoma, A-427 lung carcinoma and UACC-375 melanoma). EGCG was the most potent of the seven green tea components against three out of the four cell lines (i.e. MCF-7 breast cancer, HT-29 colon cancer and UACC-375 melanoma).

Grinberg *et al.* (1997) addressed the question of whether tea polyphenols in green and black tea, at concentrations close to plasma levels, would impart antioxidant effects on red blood cells (RBC) subjected to oxidative stress. This study showed a substantial effect of tea polyphenols against oxidant-mediated biochemical and morphological alterations in RBCs. In another study Zhang *et al.* (1997) showed that the four polyphenols, *viz.* EC, EGC, ECG and EGCG, purified from jasmine green tea exhibited strong protection for RBC membrane to haemolysis induced by 2,2′-azo-bis(2-amidinopropane)dihydrochloride, an azo free radical initiator.

Anti-inflammatory effects of tea

PREVENTION AGAINST TPA-ELICITED INFLAMMATORY RESPONSES

In view of the fact that oedema and hyperplasia are often used as early markers of skin tumour promotion, we assessed the effect of pre-application of GTP on these parameters (Katiyar et al., 1992c). In this study we found that topical application of GTP to SENCAR mouse skin results in significant prevention against TPA-elicited effects on the enzyme activities of cyclooxygenase and lipoxygenase, which play a role in inflammatory responses. The prior application of GTP to the mouse dorsal skin was found to result in significant inhibition of TPA-induced epidermal oedema and hyperplasia. In further studies, we showed that single or multiple application of GTP to SENCAR mouse ear skin, prior to or after the application of TPA, affords significant prevention against TPA-induced oedema (Katiyar et al., 1993). This study also showed that pre-application of GTP affords significant prevention against TPA-induced hyperplasia in the ear skin. The occurrence of prevention by GTP was 75% and 90% in terms of epidermal thickness and vertical cell layers, respectively. GTP was also found to afford prevention against TPA-elicited infiltration of poly-morphonuclear leukocytes in the dermis.

PREVENTION AGAINST UVB RADIATION-ELICITED INFLAMMATORY RESPONSES

In our laboratories, experiments were performed to assess whether GTP possesses chemopreventive effects against UVB radiation-elicited inflammatory changes in murine skin (Agarwal et al., 1993). We showed that oral feeding of GTP (0.2%, w/v) through drinking water to SKH-1 hairless mice for 30 days followed by irradiation with UVB (900 mJ/cm^2) resulted in significant protection against UVB radiation-elicited cutaneous oedema and depletion of the antioxidant-defence system in epidermis. GTP also afforded prevention against UVB radiation-caused induction of epidermal ODC and cyclooxygenase activities in a time-dependent manner.

PREVENTION AGAINST UVB RADIATION-INDUCED IMMUNOSUPPRESSION

Chronic UV exposure to the skin is known to cause diverse biological effects, including induction of inflammation, alteration in cutaneous immune cells and impairment of contact hypersensitivity responses (Kripke, 1984; Elmets, 1991). There is strong evidence that UVB radiation can cause skin cancer in humans and laboratory animals (Noonan et al., 1981; DeFabo and Noonan, 1983). In experimental studies in mice, studies from our laboratory (Katiyar et al., 1995a) have shown that topical application of GTP (1–6 mg/animal), 30 minutes or more prior or after exposure to a single dose of UVB (2 kJ/m^2), resulted in significant prevention against local (25–90%) and systemic suppression (23–95%) of contact hypersensitivity and inflammation (70–80%) in C3H/HeN mice. The preventive effects of GTP were found to have an inverse correlation with the doses of UVB (2–32 kJ/m^2). Among the four main epicatechin derivatives present in GTP, EGCG was found to be the most effective in affording prevention against UVB-elicited suppression of contact hypersensitivity.

INHIBITION OF TUMOUR PROMOTER-ELICITED INDUCTION OF CYTOKINES

Cytokines are known to play an important role in a variety of physiological and pathological processes including inflammation, wound healing, immunity and haematopoiesis. Interleukin-1α (IL-1α) plays an important role in both immune and inflammatory reactions, and has been shown to be induced in response to various skin tumour promoters (Katiyar et al., 1995b). We conducted studies to assess whether pretreatment of animals with GTP can afford preventive effects against tumour promoter-elicited induction of IL-1α expression in the murine skin model system. Northern blot analysis of IL-1α gene expression in mouse skin revealed that the topical application of GTP or BTP prior to treatment with TPA results in signficant inhibition of TPA-induced expression of epidermal IL-1α mRNA. These inhibitory effects were found to be dependent on the dose of GTP or BTP used. GTP also inhibited IL-1α mRNA and protein expression induced by skin tumour promoters like mezerein, benzoyl peroxide and anthralin. In this study EGCG and ECG showed maximum inhibitory effects at equimolar dose as compared with other epicatechin derivatives. Recent studies from our laboratory (Challa et al., 1998) showed that GTP treatment ameliorates UVB-induced oxidative burst as measured by H$_2$O$_2$ and myeloperoxidase production. GTP treatment to mice also partially blocked UVB-induced infiltration of leukocytes and appeared to inhibit IL-10 production in skin, as shown by immunohistochemistry. In this study, GTP application to mice prior to UVB-irradiation was found to result in complete reversal of UVB-induced inhibition of contact hypersensitivity, but showed only partial reversal of induction of tolerance to 2,4-dinitrofluorobenzene. These data suggested that green tea and the polyphenols present therein might be useful against inflammatory dermatoses and immunosuppression caused by solar radiation in humans. The validation of these studies to human population exposed to low level of UV radiation chronically through solar radiation is an area for further study.

Mechanism(s) of the biological effects of tea

PREVENTION AGAINST MUTAGENICITY AND GENOTOXICITY

Tea has been shown to suppress the mutagenicity of products formed in a model nitrosation reaction system (Mukhtar et al., 1992). GTP and WEGT were found significantly to inhibit the mutagenicity induced by BαP, aflatoxin B$_1$, 2-aminofluorene and methanol extract of coal tar pitch in bacterial or mammalian cell test systems (Wang *et al.*, 1989a). In one study, Jain *et al.* (1989) showed that tea extracts inhibited *N*-methyl-*N*-nitro-*N*-nitrosoguanidine (MNNG)-induced mutagenicity *in vitro* as well as in the intragastric tract of rats. It was also observed that the galloyl group-containing compounds in green tea, such as EGCG, ECG and EGC were antimutagenic in nature in the *Escherichia coli* B/r WP$_2$ assay system (Kada *et al.*, 1985; Shimoi *et al.*, 1986). Oral feeding of green tea or black tea extracts to rats was shown to inhibit chromosomal aberrations in rat bone marrow cells if the extracts were given 24 hours prior to aflatoxin B$_1$ treatment (Ito *et al.*, 1989). Cheng *et al.* (1991) showed that, compared with other chemopreventive agents such as ellagic acid, ascorbic acid, α-tocopherol and β-carotene, GTP afforded stronger inhibitory effects against mutagenicity of cigarette smoke condensate as assessed using the Ames test.

Heterocyclic amines (HCAs), formed during the cooking of meats and fish, are thought to be the genotoxic carcinogens associated with important types of human cancer such as cancer of the breast, colon or pancreas in meat-eating populations (Weisburger *et al.*, 1994). These researchers studied the effect of black tea, green tea, theaflavin gallate (polyphenol in black tea) and EGCG (polyphenol in green tea) on the formation of typical HCAs, 2-amino-3,8-dimethylimidazo(4,5-f)quinoxaline and 2-amino-1-methyl-6-phenylimidazo (4,5-b)pyridine, using the model *in vitro* systems of Jagerstad. This study revealed that although the teas as such were either less effective or not effective, the polyphenols were inhibitory in the production of HCAs, 2-amino-3,8-dimethylimidazo(4,5-f)quinoxaline or 2-amino-1-methyl-6-phenylimidazo(4,5-b)pyridine. In this study, it was suggested that the tea polyphenols represent another approach to lower the formation of HCAs and its associated cancer risk.

INHIBITION OF BIOCHEMICAL MARKERS OF TUMOUR INITIATION: CYTOCHROME P450-DEPENDENT METABOLISM

The major enzyme system that is responsible for the metabolism of procarcinogens to their DNA binding metabolites is cytochrome P450 (P450) (Conney, 1982; Mukhtar *et al.*, 1991). This binding to DNA is considered essential for tumour initiation. Wang *et al.* (1988) studied the interaction of GTP and its constituent polyphenols EC, EGC, ECG, and EGCG with cytochrome P450 and associated monooxygenase activities. The addition of EC, EGC, ECG, EGCG and GTP to microsomes prepared from rat liver resulted in a concentration-dependent inhibition of cytochrome P450-dependent arylhydrocarbon hydroxylase, 7-ethoxycoumarin-O-de-ethylase and 7-ethoxyresorufin-O-de-ethylase activities. In this study it was also shown that epidermal arylhydrocarbon hydroxylase activity and epidermal enzyme-mediated binding of BαP and

DMBA to DNA were inhibited by these polyphenols. Sohn et al. (1994) found significant increase in hepatic CYP1A1, A2 and 2B1 activities in rats consuming green tea or black tea. Tea consumption, however, did not affect the CYP2E1 and 3A4 activities. Tea consumption also resulted in an increase in enzyme activity of the Phase II enzyme UDP-glucuronyltransferase but not in glutathione S-transferase. In another study, Shi et al. (1994) showed that EGCG inhibited the catalytic activities of several cytochrome P450 enzymes and was more potent against CYP1A and 2B1 than 2E1. Bu-Abbas et al. (1994) used aqueous extracts of tea (2.5%) as the sole source of drinking water to rats for four weeks and determined hepatic cytochrome P450 activity by using chemical probes with selectivity for particular isoforms. Feeding of green tea resulted in an increase in the O-demethylation of methoxyresorufin and O-depentylation of pentoxyresorufin. Immunoblot analysis revealed increases in the apoprotein levels of CYP1A2 and CYP4A1 following treatment with green tea.

Recently, Chen et al. (1996) reported a comparative study on the induction of CYP1A2 with different teas in male Fischer 344 rats. In this study, induction of the CYP1A2-dependent O-methoxyresorufin demethylase (MROD) activity in liver microsomes was observed. The induction was also shown by intragastric administration of caffeine (100 mg/kg). The CYP1A2 protein, as determined by immunoblot analysis, and the concentrations of tea polyphenols and caffeine in plasma were also measured. This study demonstrates that caffeine, not tea polyphenols, is the component in tea responsible for the induction of this enzyme.

INHIBITION OF BIOCHEMICAL MARKERS OF TUMOUR PROMOTION

A number of studies reported that the consumption of green tea inhibits tumour promotion as assessed by inhibition of the biochemical markers of tumour promotion (Katiyar and Mukhtar, 1996). Topical application of TPA on mouse skin resulted in induction of ODC activity followed by an increase in the levels of polyamines, epidermal hyperplasia, inflammation and increase in the number of dark basal keratinocytes (Agarwal and Mukhtar, 1991; DiGiovanni, 1992; Katiyar et al., 1992c). Which of these or other parameters are obligatory or sufficient for the process of tumour promotion, is not yet clear. ODC plays an essential role in cell proliferation and differentiation and its induction is considered to be closely associated, though not sufficient, with the tumour-promoting activity of a variety of tumour promoters (Agarwal and Mukhtar, 1991; DiGiovanni, 1992). TPA-mediated inflammation in skin is believed to be governed by cyclooxygenase- and lipoxygenase-catalysed metabolites of archidonic acid, specifically prostaglandins and hydroxyeicosatetraenoic acids respectively (Katiyar and Mukhtar, 1996 and references therein). The importance of induction of epidermal ODC, cyclooxygenase and lipoxygenase activities in skin tumour promotion is evident from the fact that several inhibitors of these enzymes inhibit the tumour promotion in murine skin (Katiyar and Mukhtar, 1996 and references therein).

Skin application of GTP in mouse was shown to inhibit TPA-mediated induction of epidermal ODC activity in a dose-dependent manner (Agarwal et al., 1992). The inhibitory effect of GTP was also dependent on the time of its application relative to the TPA treatment. Topical application of GTP to SENCAR mouse skin was also found to inhibit the induction of epidermal ODC activity caused by several structurally different mouse skin tumour promoters. Also, the prior application of GTP to mouse skin was found to result in significant inhibition of TPA-induced epidermal oedema and hyperplasia (Katiyar et al., 1992c, 1993a). As quantitated by the formation of prostaglandins and hydroxyeicosatetraenoic acid metabolites from respectively cyclooxygenase- and lipoxygenase-catalysed metabolism of arachidonic acid, skin application of GTP to SENCAR mice was also found to result in significant inhibition of TPA-elicited effects on these two enzymes (Katiyar et al., 1992). Inhibition of all of these pathways alone or in combination may contribute to the overall antitumour-promoting effects of green tea (Katiyar and Mukhtar, 1996).

EFFECTS ON DETOXICATION ENZYMES

Studies from our laboratory (Wang et al., 1992) have shown that the topical application or oral administration of GTP to SENCAR mice inhibited carcinogen–DNA adduct formation in epidermis after topical application of [^{3}H]BP or [^{3}H]DMBA. In another study from this laboratory (Khan et al., 1992), it was also shown that the chronic oral administration of 0.2% (w/v) GTP in drinking water to mice for four weeks resulted in significant enhancement in glutathione peroxidase (86–129%), catalase (59–92%), NADPH-quinone oxidoreductase (53–71%) and glutathione S-transferase (GST) (28–30%) activities in small bowel, lung and liver. Modulation by green tea of the enzymatic pathways which first, play a role in the detoxication of carcinogenic metabolites generated by cytochrome P450 and other enzymes and second, are key determinants for cancer initiation, may be expected to have cancer-chemopreventive functions (Katiyar and Mukhtar, 1996 and references therein). The Phase II enzyme GST not only catalyses the conjugation of hydroquinones and epoxides of PAH with reduced glutathione for their excretion, but also shows low activity towards organic hydroperoxides for their detoxication from cells/tissue (Laskin et al., 1992). These pathways alone or in combination may contribute to the overall chemopreventive effects of green tea against cancer.

TRAPPING OF ACTIVATED METABOLITES OF CARCINOGENS

Another important mechanism by which green tea prevents against cancer is by trapping the active metabolites of carcinogens (Katiyar and Mukhtar, 1996). Flavanols are a group of chemicals that possess strong nucleophilic centres at two positions. This property provides an opportunity for the flavanols to react with electrophilic carcinogenic species to form flavanol–carcinogen adducts which may result in the prevention of tumorigenesis. In general, the initial step in carcinogenesis is the metabolic activation of chemical carcinogens by the cytochrome P450-dependent biotransformation reactions. For example, the ubiquitous environment pollutant BαP is known to cause cancer in experimental animals only after its metabolic activation to highly reactive molecules (Agarwal and Mukhtar, 1993; Katiyar and Mukhtar, 1996). The ultimate carcinogenic metabolite of BαP is BαP diolepoxide-2 (BPDE-2), the formation of which is catalysed by successive enzymatic steps catalysed by cytochrome P450 and epoxide hydrolase (Conney, 1982; Mukhtar et al., 1991). Our studies have shown that tea polyphenols interact with BPDE-2 and that topical application of GTP prior to BPDE-2 treatment resulted in inhibition of skin tumour initiation (Khan et al., 1988).

ANTIOXIDANT AND FREE RADICAL-SCAVENGING ACTIVITY

The generation of reactive oxygen species (ROS) in biological systems, either by normal metabolic pathways or as a consequence of exposure to chemical carcinogens, has been extensively studied (Wattenberg, 1990). It is now universally agreed that the ROS generation contributes to the multistage process of carcinogenesis (Wattenberg, 1990; Agarwal and Mukhtar, 1993). It has been suggested that peroxides and superoxide anion ($O_2 \cdot^-$) produce cytotoxicity/genotoxicity in cellular systems (Perchellet and Perchellet, 1989). The source of hydrogen peroxide (H_2O_2) in cells/tissues is mainly through superoxide dismutase-mediated dismutation of $O_2 \cdot^-$, which is generated in the cells/tissues by endogenous enzyme systems as well as by the non-enzymatic pathways (Perchellet and Perchellet, 1989). Additionally, the highly reactive hydroxide radical ($\cdot$OH), generated from H_2O_2 is known to damage DNA and produce pathological alterations. The two-electron reduction of the metabolic products of PAH such as quinones, catalysed by NADPH quinone reductase (QR), has been considered to be a detoxication pathway, since the resulting hydroquinones may be conjugated with glutathione and excreted through mercapturic acid pathway (Katiyar and Mukhtar, 1996). Our studies have shown that the administration of chemopreventive agents results in an increase in the levels of antioxidant enzymes in various organs of the test animals (Khan et al., 1992). In view of this fact, we assessed the effect of oral feeding of GTP (0.2%, w/v) to SKH-1 hairless mice via drinking water for 30 days, on the activities of antioxidant enzymes, viz. glutathione peroxidase and catalase, and Phase II detoxifying enzymes, GST and QR (Khan et al., 1992). We found that GTP consumption resulted in a significant increase in glutathione peroxidase, catalase and QR activities in small bowel, liver and lungs, and GST activity in small bowel and liver. In another study, compared with DEN- or BαP-fed animals, feeding of WEGT (2.5%) or GTP (0.2%) in drinking water with

DEN or BαP to female A/J mice resulted in significant increase in GST activity in the liver and small bowel, and QR activity in the small bowel, lung and stomach (Katiyar et al., 1993). Such studies suggest that these may be contributing factors for the cancer chemopreventive effects of green tea.

It is becoming clear that the anticarcinogenic properties of tea are due to the antioxidant effect of epicatechins present therein (Katiyar and Mukhtar, 1996). In one study, Katiyar et al. (1994) found that EGCG, EGC and ECG from green tea significantly inhibited the Fe^{3+}/ADP-supported spontaneous lipid peroxidation in mouse epidermal microsomes. Interestingly, each of these epicatechins was also effective in inhibiting photo-enhanced lipid peroxidation generated by incubating epidermal microsomes in the presence of silicon phthalocyanine and 650 nm irradiation. EGCG, which is also the major constituent in GTP, showed maximum inhibitory effects compared with other epicatechins. This study provides the evidence for the antioxidant property of epicatechins. In another study, Terao et al. (1994) also showed the antioxidant property of EC and ECG by measuring the inhibition of lipid peroxidation in large unilamellar liposomes composed of egg yolk phosphatidylcholine. This study provided evidence that EC and ECG serve as powerful antioxidants against lipid peroxidation when phospholipid bilayers are exposed to aqueous oxygen radicals (Terao et al., 1994). The concept of antioxidant activities is also supported by the findings that EGCG inhibited the formation of 8-hydroxy-deoxyguanosine in HeLa cells (Bhimani and Frenkel, 1991). The oral administration of green tea inhibited the formation of 8-hydroxydeoxyguanosine in mice (Xu et al., 1992), and topically treated GTP inhibited TPA-induced hydrogen peroxide formation (Katiyar and Mukhtar, 1996).

The mechanism of the antioxidant properties of these epicatechins can be explained as follows:

- Tea polyphenols such as EGCG, ECG and EGC are strong scavengers against superoxide anion radicals and hydroxyl radicals which are two major reactive oxygen species considered to be responsible for the damage to DNA and other cellular molecules and can also initiate lipid peroxidation.
- Tea flavanols can react with and trap the peroxy radicals, thereby terminating lipid peroxidation chain reactions. The reactive oxygen species play an important role in carcinogenesis through damaging DNA, altering gene expression or affecting cell growth and differentiation (Cerruti, 1989; Namiki, 1990).

RECENT ADVANCES IN THE MECHANISM(S) OF THE BIOLOGICAL EFFECTS OF TEA

Green tea activates mitogen-activated protein kinases

In a recent study it was shown that the activation of mitogen-activated protein kinases (MAPK) by GTP may be a potential signalling pathway in the regulation of antioxidant-responsive element-mediated Phase II enzyme gene expression (Yu *et al.*, 1997). In this study it was shown that GTP induces chloramphenicol acetyltransferase (CAT) activity in human hepatoma HepG2 cells transfected with a plasmid construct which contains an antioxidant-responsive element (ARE) and a minimal glutathione S-transferase Ya promoter linked to the CAT reporter gene. This indicates that GTP stimulates the transcription of Phase II detoxifying enzymes through the ARE. The authors studied the involvement of MAPKs extracellular signal-regulated kinase 2 (ERK2) and c-Jun N-terminal kinase 1 (JNK1). Potent activation of ERK2 was seen following treatment of HepG2 cells with GTP. Similar to ERK2, JNK1 was also activated by treatment with GTP. GTP treatment also increased mRNA levels of the immediate-early genes c-*jun* and c-*fos*, as determined by reverse transcriptase-coupled polymerase chain reaction.

EGCG inhibits urokinase activity

In a publicised study, it was shown that the anticancer activity of EGCG in green tea might be due to the inhibition of the enzyme urokinase, one of the most frequently expressed enzymes in human cancers (Jankun *et al.*, 1997). The authors, using molecular modelling, demonstrated that EGCG binds to urokinase, blocking His57 and Ser195 of the urokinase catalytic triad and extending towards Arg35 from a positively charged loop of urokinase. They verified this computer-based calculation by assessing the inhibition of urokinase activity using an amidolytic assay in which the release of a chromogen, on specific cleavage by urokinase, was quantified spectrophotometrically.

Green tea induces apoptosis and cell cycle arrest

Apoptosis, in recent years, has become a challenging issue in biomedical research, and the life span of both normal and cancer cells within a living system is regarded to be significantly affected by apoptotic rate. In addition, cell death by apoptosis differs discretely from necrotic cell death and is regarded as an ideal means of cell elimination (Fesus *et al.*, 1995 and references therein). Thus, the chemopreventive agents, which can modulate apoptosis, may be able to affect the steady-state cell population that can be useful in the management and therapy of cancer. In recent years, many cancer chemopreventive agents have been shown to induce apoptosis and conversely several tumour promoters have also been shown to inhibit apoptosis (Wright *et al.*, 1994; Mills *et al.*, 1995; Boolbol *et al.*, 1996). Therefore, it is reasonable to assume that the chemopreventive agents which have proven effects in animal tumour bioassay systems and/or human epidemiology on one hand, and cause induction of apoptosis of cancer cells on the other hand, may have wider implication for cancer control. Only a limited number of chemopreventive agents are known to induce apoptosis (Jiang *et al.*, 1996). In our recent study

(Ahmad *et al.*, 1997), we found that the green tea constituent EGCG induced apoptosis and cell cycle arrest in human epidermoid carcinoma cells A431. A promising observation of this study was that the EGCG-mediated apoptotic response was specific to cancer cells, as the induction of apoptosis was also observed in human carcinoma keratinocytes HaCaT, human prostate carcinoma cells DU145 and mouse lymphoma cells LY-R, but not in normal human epidermal keratinocytes. The exact molecular mechanism responsible for the striking differences in apoptotic response between cancer versus normal cells by EGCG is unknown. This study, if validated in human clinical trials, could lend support to the anticancer activity of tea polyphenols.

EGCG suppresses extracellular signals and cell proliferation through EGF receptor binding

Liang *et al.* (1997), using a thymidine incorporation assay, demonstrated that EGCG could significantly inhibit DNA synthesis in A431 cells. EGCG also inhibited the protein tyrosine kinase activities of EGF-R, PDGF-R and FGF-R, but not of pp60^{v-src}, PKC and PKA. EGCG also inhibited the phosporylation of EGF-R by EGF and blocked the binding of EGF to its receptor. These findings suggest that EGCG might inhibit the process of tumour formation via blocking cellular signal transduction pathways.

EGCG blocks the induction of nitric oxide synthase by down-regulating the transcription factor nuclear factor-κB

Lin and Lin (1997) examined the effects of EGCG on nitric oxide production from murine peritoneal macrophages and sought the possible mechanisms. Their data suggested that EGCG blocked the early event of nitric oxide synthase induction via the inhibition of binding of the transcription factor NFκB to the iNOS promoter, thereby inhibiting the induction of iNOS transcription.

EGCG and theaflavins inhibit tumour promoter-induced activator protein 1 activation and cell transformation

Dong *et al.* (1997) used the JB6 mouse epidermal cell line, a system that has extensively been used as an *in vitro* model for tumour promotion studies, to examine the antitumour promotion effects of EGCG and theaflavins at the molecular level. EGCG and theaflavins inhibited EGF- TPA-induced cell transformation in a dose-dependent manner. EGCG and theaflavins also inhibited AP-1-dependent transcriptional activity and DNA-binding activity. This study further showed that the inhibition of AP-1 activation occurs through the inhibition of a c-Jun NH$_2$-terminal kinase-dependent pathway.

Conclusions and future directions

Although not adequately explained, it is estimated that almost one-third of cancers are caused by dietary substances. Thus, dietary habits are an important factor in the development of human cancer. The best example of this association is the fact that changes in dietary habits modulate the incidence of cancer in experimental animals, and epidemiological studies also suggest a similar association in the human population. The usefulness of dietary substances for prevention against the occurrence of cancer is increasingly recognised as one practical approach in this direction (Katiyar and Mukhtar, 1996). Changing life style, as reflected in dietary habits and culinary practices, has been recognised as a major factor for human cancer risk. There is suggestive evidence in humans that diets rich in fruits, or containing reduced levels of fats, particularly those derived from animal sources, are less likely to lead to cancer. Because tea is a popular beverage consumed worldwide, the relationship between tea consumption and human cancer incidence is an important concern, and epidemiological studies have indicated that tea consumption does not pose a causative effect on human cancers. Indeed, epidemiological observations as well as laboratory studies have indicated that tea consumption is likely to have beneficial effects in reducing certain cancer types in some populations. However, possible harmful effects of the consumption of excessive amounts of tea, tea at very high temperature or salted tea cannot be ruled out.

Although a considerable body of information provides compelling evidence for the preventive potential of tea against cancer, a clear understanding of the mechanisms by which tea polyphenols retard the induction, growth and subsequent progression of cancer is necessary for examining the effect of tea polyphenols on health and for devising better strategies against cancer. Black tea is the major form of tea consumed in western countries. The chemistry, biological activities and chemopreventive properties of black tea, especially the polyphenols present therein, however, are not well understood; thus, research in this area is needed.

In view of the available experimental data on the protection by tea polyphenols of mouse skin carcinogenesis and inflammation (Katiyar and Mukhtar, 1996), an intervention study on human skin carcinogenesis and inflammatory responses, including a dose–response effect, could be of great importance. Since only limited data are available on the bioavailability of tea polyphenols following the consumption of tea by the human population, studies on the absorption, distribution and metabolism of green and black tea polyphenols in animals and humans are of great importance. In this regard, a method has been developed for the analysis of plasma and urinary tea polyphenols in human subjects (Lee *et al.*, 1995). This methodology may prove valuable for studying the effects of tea consumption, bioavailability of polyphenols and an association of the two with human cancer.

Because the causative factors are different for different populations, tea consumption may affect carcinogenesis only in selected situations rather than have a general effect on all cancers. Thus, there is a need to define the population that could benefit from tea consumption. Such intervention studies in various populations may provide useful information on the protective effects of tea polyphenols on cancer of organ site or in specific populations. After careful evaluation of additional studies, recommendations may be made to consume tea polyphenols by humans. Such agent(s) do not necessarily have to be consumed by tea drinking. They can be supplemented in other food items, for example in cosmetic products, consumer items and in vitamin supplements and other products. This approach can be called 'designer items', for consumption by human population.

Because research findings in laboratory animals clearly point to a role of tea polyphenols in cancer chemoprevention, the well-defined naturally occurring polyphenols found in tea should be evaluated in clinical intervention in human trials. In this regard, the MD Anderson Cancer Center in collaboration with the Memorial Sloan-Kettering Cancer Center has obtained an investigational New Drug permit from USFDA to begin Phase I Clinical Trials where 30 cancer patients with advanced solid tumours will participate. The patients will take daily capsules of formulated powdered green tea for up to six months or possibly longer if the treatment appears beneficial. This clinical trial will examine, in a 'dose-escalation study', the safety and possible efficacy of consuming the equivalent of 10 cups or more of green tea a day. This is an important step that may prove to be a turning point in the area of cancer chemoprevention. Further research is needed to define the molecular mechanism(s) of green tea action that may result in devising better strategies against a variety of cancer types.

Acknowledgements

The author's work cited in this review was supported by American Institute for Cancer Research Grants 86A61, 90A47, 92B35 and 96B015, and by USPHS grant AR 39750.

References

Agarwal R and Mukhtar H (1991) Cutaneous chemical carcinogenesis. In *Pharmacology of the Skin*, Mukhtar H (ed), CRC Press, Boca Raton FL, pp. 371–387.

Agarwal R and Mukhtar H (1993) Oxidative stress in skin chemical carcinogenesis. In *Oxidative Stress in Dermatology*, Fuchs J and Packer L (eds), Marcel Dekker, Inc., New York, pp. 207–241.

Agarwal R, Katiyar SK, Zaidi SIA and Mukhtar H (1992) Inhibition of tumor promoter-caused induction of ornithine deacarboxylase activity in SENCAR mice by polyphenolic fraction isolated from green tea and its individual epicatechin derivatives. *Cancer Research*, **52**, 3582–3588.

Agarwal R, Katiyar SK, Khan SG and Mukhtar H (1993) Protection against ultraviolet B radiation-induced effects in the skin of SKH-1 hairless mice by a polyphenolic fraction isolated from green tea. *Photochemistry and Photobiology*, **58**, 695–700.

Agudo A, Gonzalez CA, Marcos G, Sanz M, Saigi E, Verge J, Boleda M and Ortego J (1992) Consumption of alcohol, coffee, and tobacco, and gastric cancer in Spain. *Cancer Causes and Control*, **3**, 137–143.

Ahmad N, Feyes DK, Nieminen A-L, Agarwal R and Mukhtar H (1997) Green tea constituent epigallocatechin-3-gallate and induction of apoptosis and cell cycle arrest in human carcinoma cells. *Journal of the National Cancer Institute*, **89**, 1881–1886.

Ames BN (1983) Dietary carcinogens and anticarcinogens. *Science*, **221**, 1256–1262.

Ames BN and Gold LS (1990) Too many rodent carcinogens: mitogenesis increases mutagenesis. *Science*, **5249**, 970–971.

Armstrong B, Garrod A and Doll RA (1976) Retrospective study of renal cancer with special reference to coffee and animal protein consumption. *British Journal of Cancer*, **33**, 127–136.

Athar M, Agarwal R, Wang ZY, Lloyd JR, Bickers DR and Mukhtar H (1991) All trans retinoic acid protects against free radical generating compounds-mediated conversion of chemically- and ultraviolet B radiation-induced skin papillomas to carcinomas. *Carcinogenesis*, **12**, 2325–2329.

Baron JA, Greenberg ER, Haile R, Mandel J, Sandler RS and Mott L (1997) Coffee and tea and the risk of recurrent colorectal adenomas. *Cancer Epidemiology Biomarkers and Prevention*, **6**, 7–10.

Bashirov MS, Nugmanov SN and Kolycheva NI (1968) On the epidemiology of cancer of the esophagus in the Aktiubinsk region of the Kazakhastan SSR. *Voprosy Onkologii*, **14**, 3–7.

Bhimani R and Frenkel K (1991) *Proceedings of the American Association for Cancer Research*, **32**, 126.

Boolbol SK, Dannenberg AJ, Chadburn A, Martucci C, Guo XJ, Ramonetti JT, Abreu-Goris M, Newmark H, Lipkin ML, DeCosse JJ and Bertgnolli MM (1996) Cyclooxygenase-2 overexpression and tumor formation are blocked by sulindac in murine model of familial polyposis. *Cancer Research*, **56**, 2556–2560.

Boone CW, Kelloff GJ and Malone WE (1990) Identification of candidate cancer chemopreventive agents and their evaluation in animal models and human clinical trials: a review. *Cancer Research*, **50**, 2–9.

Boone CW, Kelloff GJ and Steele VE (1992) Natural history of intraepithelial neoplasia in humans with implications for cancer chemoprevention strategy. *Cancer Research*, **52**, 1651–1659.

Bu-Abbas A, Clifford MN, Walker R and Ioannides C (1994) Selective induction of rat hepatic CYP1 and CYP4 proteins and of peroxisomal proliferation by green tea. *Carcinogenesis*, **15**, 2575–2579.

Bueno de Mesquita HB, Maisonneuve P, Moerman CJ, Runia S and Boyle P (1992) Lifetime consumption of alcoholic beverages, tea and coffee and exocrine carcinoma of the pancreas: a population-based case-control study in The Netherlands. *International Journal of Cancer*, **50**, 514–522.

Cerruti PA (1989) Mechanisms of action of oxidant carcinogens. *Cancer Detection and Prevention*, **14**, 281–284.

Challa A, Katiyar SK, Cooper KD and Mukhtar H (1998) Inhibition of UV-radiation-caused induction of oxidative stress and immunosuppression in C3H/HeN mice by polyphenols from green tea. *Journal of Investigative Dermatology*, **110**, 695.

Chatterjee ML, Agarwal R and Mukhtar H (1996) Ultraviolet B radiation-induced DNA lesions in mouse epidermis: an assessment using a novel 32P-postlabelling technique. *Biochemical Biophysical Research Communication*, **229**, 590–595.

Chen JS (1992) The effect of Chinese tea on the occurrence of esophageal tumors induced by N-nitrosomethylbenzylamine in rats. *Preventive Medicine*, **21**, 385–391.

Chen L, Bondoc FY, Lee MJ, Hussin AH, Thomas PE and Yang CS (1996) Caffeine induces cytochrome P4501A2: induction of CYP1A2 by tea in rats. *Drug Metabolism and Disposition*, **24**, 529–533.

Chen ZY, Yan RQ, Qin GZ and Chia KB (1987) Effect of six edible plants on the development of aflatoxin B$_1$-induced γ-glutamyltranspeptidase positive hepatocyte foci in rats. *Chung Hua liu Tsa Chih*, **9**, 109–111.

Cheng S, Lin P, Ding L, Hu X, Oguni I and Hara Y (1991) Inhibition of green tea extract on mutagenicity and carcinogenicity. *Proceedings of the International Symposium on Tea Science, Japan*, pp. 195–199.

Claude J, Kunze E, Frentzel-Beyme R, Paczkowski K, Schneider J and Schubert H (1986) Life-style and occupational risk factors in cancer of the lower urinary tract. *American Journal of Epidemiology*, **124**, 578–589.

Conney AH (1982) Induction of microsomal enzymes by foreign chemicals and carcinogenesis by polycyclic aromatic hydrocarbons. *Cancer Research*, **42**, 4875–4917.

Cook-Mozaffari PJ, Azordegan F, Day NE, Ressicand A, Sabai C and Aramesh B (1979) Oesophageal cancer studies in the Caspian Littoral of Iran: results of a case-control study. *British Journal of Cancer*, **39**, 293–309.

Dales LG, Friedman GD, Ury HK, Grossman S and Williams SR (1979) A case-control study of relationships of diet and other traits to colorectal cancer in American blacks. *American Journal of Epidemiology*, **109**, 132–144.

D'Avanzo B, La Vecchia C, Franceschi S, Negri E, Talamani R and Buttino I (1992) Coffee consumption and bladder cancer risk. *European Journal of Cancer*, **28A**, 1480–1484.

De Jong UW, Breslow N, Hong JGE, Sridharan M and Shanmugaratnam K (1974) Aetiological factors in oesophageal cancer in Singapore Chinese. *International Journal of Cancer*, **13**, 291–303.

DeFabo EC and Noonan FP (1983) Mechanism of immune suppression by ultraviolet radiation in vivo. I. Evidence for the existence of a unique photoreceptor in skin and its role in photoimmunology. *Journal of Experimental Medicine*, **157**, 84–98.

Demirer T, Icli F, Uzunalimoglu O and Kucuk O (1990) Diet and stomach cancer incidence. A case-control study in Turkey. *Cancer*, **65**, 2344–2348.

DiGiovanni J (1992) Multistage carcinogenesis in mouse skin. *Pharmacology and Therapeutics*, **54**, 63–128.

Dong Z, Ma W-y, Huang C and Yang CS (1997) Inhibition of tumor promoter-induced activator protein 1 activation and cell transformation by tea polyphenols, (-)-epigallocatechin gallate and theaflavins. *Cancer Research*, **57**, 4414–4419.

Elmets CA (1991) Cutaneous photocarcinogenesis. In *Pharmacology of the Skin*, Mukhtar H (ed), CRC Press, Boca Raton, FL, pp. 389–416.

Fesus L, Szondy Z and Uray I (1995) Probing the molecular program of apoptosis by cancer chemopreventive agents. *Journal of Cellular Biochemistry (Supplement)*, **22**, 151–161.

Fujiki H, Suganuma M, Suguri H, Takagi K, Yoshizawa S, Ootsuyama A, Tanooka H, Okuda T, Kobayashi M and Sugimura T (1990) New antitumor promoters: (-)-epigallocatechin gallate and sacrophytols A and B. *Basic Life Sciences*, **52**, 205–212.

Fujiki H, Yoshizawa S, Horiuchi T, Suganuma M, Yatsunami S, Nishiwaki S, Okabe S, Nishiwaki MR, Okuda T and Sugimura T (1992) Anticarcinogenic effect of (-)-epigallocatechin gallate. *Preventive Medicine*, **21**, 503–509.

Fujita Y, Tamane T, Tanaka M, Kuwata K. Okuzumi J, Takahashi T, Fujiki H and Okuda T (1989) Inhibitory effect of (-)-epigallocatechin gallate on carcinogenesis with N-ethyl-N'-nitro-N-nitrosoguanidine in mouse duodenum. *Japanese Journal of Cancer Research*, **80**, 503–505.

Gao GD, Zhou LF and Qi G (1990) Initial study of antitumorigenesis of green tea: animal test and flow cytometry. *Tumor*, **10**, 42–44.

Gao YT, McLaughlin JK, Blot WJ, Ji BT, Dai Q and Fraumeni JF Jr (1994) Reduced risk of esophageal cancer associated with green tea consumption. *Journal of the National Cancer Institute*, **86**, 855–858.

Gensler HL, Timmermann BN, Valcic S, Wachter GA, Door R, Dvorakova K and Alberts DS (1996) Prevention of photocarcinogenesis by topical administration of pure epigallocatechin gallate isolated from green tea. *Nutrition and Cancer*, **26**, 325–335.

Goldbohm RA, Hertog MG, Brants HA, van-Poppel G and van-den-Brandt-PA (1996) Consumption of black tea and cancer risk: a prospective cohort study. *Journal of the National Cancer Institute*, **88**, 93–100.

Goodman MT, Morgenstern H and Wynder EL (1986) A case-control study of factors affecting the development of renal cell cancer. *American Journal of Epidemiology*, **124**, 926–941.

Graham S, Lilienfeld AM and Tidings JE (1967) Dietary and purgation factors in the epidemiology of gastric cancer. *Cancer*, **20**, 2224–2234.

Grinberg LN, Newmark H, Kitrossky N, Rahamim E, Chevion M and Rachmilewitz EA (1997) Protective effects of tea polyphenols against oxidative damage to red blood cells. *Biochemical Pharmacology*, **54**, 973–978.

Hansson L-E, Nyren O, Bergstrom R, Wolk A, Lindgren A, Baron J and Adami H-O (1993) Diet and risk of gastric cancer. A population-based case-control study in Sweden. *International Journal of Cancer*, **55**, 181–189.

Harada N, Takabayashi F, Oguni I and Hara Y (1991) Anti-promotion effect of green tea extracts on pancreatic cancer in golden hamster induced by N-nitroso-bis(2-oxyopropyl)amine. *International Symposium on Tea Science, Japan*, pp. 200–204.

Harbowy ME and Balentine DA (1997) Tea chemistry. *Critical Reviews in Plant Science*, **16**, 415–480.

Harnack LJ, Anderson KE, Zheng W, Folsom AR, Sellers TA and Kushi LH (1997) Smoking, alcohol, coffee, and tea intake and incidence of cancer of the exocrine pancreas: the Iowa women's health study. *Cancer Epidemiology, Biomarkers and Prevention*, **6**, 1081–1086.

Hartge P, Hoover R, West DW and Lyon JL (1983) Coffee drinking and risk of bladder cancer. *Journal of the National Cancer Institute*, **70**, 1021–1026.

Heilbrun LK, Nomura A and Stemmermann GN (1986) Black tea consumption and cancer risk: a prospective study. *British Journal of Cancer*, **54**, 677–683.

Henderson BE, Louie E, Soo Hoo Jing J, Buell P and Gardner MB (1976) Risk factors associated with nasopharyngeal carcinoma. *New England Journal of Medicine*, **295**, 1101–1106.

Hiatt RA, Klatsky AL and Armstrong MA (1988) Pancreatic cancer, blood glucose and beverage consumption. *International Journal of Cancer*, **41**, 794–797.

Higginson J (1966) Etiological factors in gastrointestinal cancer in man. *Journal of the National Cancer Institute*, **37**, 527–545.

Hirose M, Hoshiya T, Akagi K, Takahashi S, Hara Y and Ito N (1993) Effects of green tea catechins in a rat multi-organ carcinogenesis model. *Carcinogenesis*, **14**, 1549–1553.

Hirose M, Hoshiya T, Akagi K, Futakuchi M and Ito N (1994) Inhibition of mammary gland carcinogenesis by green tea catechins and other naturally occurring antioxidants in female Sprague-Dawley rats pretreated with 7,12,dimethylbenz(a)anthracene. *Cancer Letters*, **83**, 149–156.

Howe GR, Burch JD, Miller AB, Cook GM, Esteve J, Morrison B, Gordon P, Chambers LW, Fodor G and Winsor GM (1980) Tobacco use, occupation, coffee, various nutrients, and bladder cancer. *Journal of the National Cancer Institute*, **64**, 701–713.

Huang M-T, Ho C-T, Wang ZY, Ferraro T, Finnegan-Olive T, Lou Y-R, Mitchell JM, Laskin JD, Newmark H, Yang CS and Conney AH (1992) Inhibitory effect of topical application of a green tea polyphenol fraction on tumor initiation and promotion in mouse skin. *Carcinogenesis*, **13**, 947–954.

Huang M-T, Xie J-G, Wang ZY, Ho C-T, Lou Y-R, Wang C-X, Hard GC and Conney AH (1997) Effects of tea, and caffeine on UVB light-induced complete carcinogenesis in SKH-1 mice: demonstration of caffeine as a biologically important constitutent of tea. *Cancer Research*, **57**, 2623–2629.

Huber WW, McDaniel LP, Kaderlik KR, Teitel CH, Lang NP and Kadlubar FF (1997) Chemoprotection against the formation of colon DNA adducts from the food-borne carcinogen 2-amino-1-methyl-6-phenylimidazo[4,5-b]pyridine (PhIP) in the rat. *Mutation Research*, **376**, 115–122.

IARC Monographs (1991) The evaluation of the carcinogenic risk to humans: coffee, tea, mate, methylxanthines and methylglyoxal. *International Agency for Research on Cancer Working Group Lyon*, **51**, pp. 1–513.

Iscovich J, Castelleto R, Esteve J, Munoz N, Colanzi R, Coronel A, Deamezola I, Tassi V and Arslan A (1987) Tobacco smoking, occupational exposure and bladder cancer in Argentina. *International Journal of Cancer*, **40**, 734–740.

Ito Y, Ohnishi S and Fujie K (1989) Chromosome aberrations induced by aflatoxin B1 in rat bone marrow cells in vivo and their suppression by green tea. *Mutation Research*, **222**, 253–261.

Jain AK, Shimoi K, Nakamura Y, Kada T, Hara Y and Tomita I (1989) Crude tea extracts decrease the mutagenic activity of N-methyl-N'-nitro-N-nitrosoguanidine in vitro and in intragastric tract of rats. *Mutation Research*, **210**, 1–8.

Jain M, Howe GR and St Louis P (1991) Coffee and alcohol as determinants of risk of pancreas cancer: a case-control study from Toronto. *International Journal of Cancer*, **47**, 384–389.

Jankun J, Selman SH, Swiercz R and Skrzypczak-Jankun E (1997) Why drinking green tea could prevent cancer. *Nature*, **387**, 561.

Jensen OM, Wahrendorf J, Knudsen JB and Sorensen BL (1986) The Copenhagen case-control study of bladder cancer. II. Effect of coffee and other beverages. *International Journal of Cancer*, **37**, 651–657.

Ji BT, Chow WH, Hsing AW, McLaughlin JK, Dai Q, Gao YT, Blot WJ and Fraumeni JF Jr (1997) Green tea consumption and the risk of pancreatic and colorectal cancers. *International Journal of Cancer*, **70**, 255–258.

Jiang MC, Yang-Yen HF, Yen JJY and Lin JK (1996) Curcumin induces apoptosis in immortalized NIH 3T3 and malignant cancer cell lines. *Nutrition and Cancer*, **26**, 111–120.

Kada T, Kaneko K, Matsuzaki S, Matsuzaki T and Hara Y (1985) Detection and chemical identification of natural bio-antimutagens, a case of the green tea factor. *Mutation Research*, **150**, 127–132.

Kapadia GJ, Rao S and Morton JF (1983) Herbal tea consumption and esophageal cancer. In *Carcinogens and Mutagens in the Environment*, Stich HF (ed), CRC Press, Boca Raton, FL, pp. 3–12.

Katiyar SK and Mukhtar H (1996) Tea in chemoprevention of cancer: epidemiologic and experimental studies (review). *International Journal of Oncology*, **8**, 221–238.

Katiyar SK, Agarwal R and Mukhtar H (1992a) Green tea in chemoprevention of cancer. *Comprehensive Therapy*, **18**, 3–8.

Katiyar SK, Agarwal R, Wang ZY, Bhatia AK and Mukhtar H (1992b) (-)-Epigal-locatechin-3-gallate in *Camellia sinensis* leaves from Himalayan region of Sikkim: inhibitory effects against biochemical events and tumor initiation in SENCAR mouse skin. *Nutrition and Cancer*, **18**, 73–83.

Katiyar SK, Agarwal R, Wood GS and Mukhtar H (1992c) Inhibition of 12-O-tetra-decanoylphorbol-13-acetate-caused tumor promotion in 7,12-dimethylbenz[a]-anthracene-initiated SENCAR mouse skin by a polyphenolic fraction isolated from green tea. *Cancer Research*, **52**, 6890–6897.

Katiyar SK, Agarwal R, Ekker S, Wood GS and Mukhtar H (1993a) Protection against 12-O-tetradecanoylphorbol-13-acetate-caused inflammation in SENCAR mouse ear skin by polyphenolic fraction isolated from green tea. *Carcinogenesis*, **14**, 361–365.

Katiyar SK, Agarwal R, Zaim MT and Mukhtar H (1993b) Protection against N-nitroso-diethylamine and benzo(a)pyrene-induced forestomach and lung tumorigenesis in A/J mice by green tea. *Carcinogenesis*, **14**, 849–855.

Katiyar SK, Agarwal R and Mukhtar H (1993c) Protective effects of green tea polyphe-nols adminstered by oral intubation against chemical carcinogen-induced fore-stomach and pulmonary neoplasia in A/J mice. *Cancer Letters*, **73**, 167–172.

Katiyar SK, Agarwal R and Mukhtar H (1994) Inhibition of spontaneous and photo-enhanced lipid peroxidation in mouse epidermal microsomes by epicatechin deriva-tives from green tea. *Cancer Letters*, **79**, 61–66.

Katiyar SK, Elmets CA, Agarwal R and Mukhtar H (1995a) Protection against ultraviolet B radiation-induced local and systemic suppression of contact hypersensitivity in mice by green tea polyphenols. *Photochemistry and Photobiology*, **62**, 855–861.

Katiyar SK, Agarwal R, Korman NJ, Rupp CO and Mukhtar H (1995b) Inhibition of tumor promoter-caused induction of interleukin-1 (IL-1)-alpha, tumor necrosis factor (TNF)-alpha, and ornithtine decarboxylase (ODC) gene expression in SENCAR mouse skin by tea polyphenols. *Proceedings of American Association for Cancer Research*, **36**, 594.

Katiyar SK, Mohan RR, Agarwal R, Mukhtar H (1997) Protection against induction of mouse skin papillomas with low and high risk of conversion to malignancy by green tea polyphenols. *Carcinogenesis*, **18**, 497–502.

Kaufman BD, Liberman IS and Tyshetskii VI (1965) Data concerning the incidence of oesophageal cancer in the Gurjev region of the Kazakh SSR (Russ). *Voprosy Onkologii*, **11**, 78–85.

Khan SG, Katiyar SK, Agarwal R and Mukhtar H (1992) Enhancement of antioxidant and phase II enzymes by oral feeding of green tea polyphenols in drinking water to SKH-1 hairless mice: possible role in cancer chemoprevention. *Cancer Research*, **52**, 4050–4052.

Khan WA, Wang ZY, Athar M, Bickers DR and Mukhtar H (1988) Inhibition of the skin tumorigenicity of (+)-7β,8α-dihydroxy-9α,10α-epoxy-7,8,9,10-tetrahydrobenzo(a) pyrene by tannic acid, green tea polyphenols and quercetin in SENCAR mice. *Cancer Letters*, **42**, 7–12.

Kinlen LJ and McPherson K (1984) Pancreas cancer and coffee and tea consumption: a case-control study. *British Journal of Cancer*, **49**, 93–96.

Kinlen LJ, Willows AN, Goldblatt P and Yudkin J (1988) Tea consumption and cancer. *British Journal of Cancer*, **58**, 397–401.

Klaunig JE (1992) Chemopreventive effects of green tea components on hepatic carci-nogenesis. *Preventive Medicine*, **21**, 510–519.

Kohlmeier L, Weterings KGC, Steck S and Kok FJ (1997) Tea and cancer prevention: an evaluation of the epidemiologic literature. *Nutrition and Cancer*, **27**, 1–13.

Komori A, Yatsunami J, Okabe S, Abe S, Hara K, Suganuma M, Kim SJ and Fujiki H (1993) Anticarcinogenic activity of green tea polyphenols. *Japanese Journal of Clinical Oncology*, **23**, 186–190.

Kono S, Ikeda M, Tokudome S and Kuratsune M (1988) A case-control study of gastric cancer and diet in northern Kyushu, Japan. *Japanese Journal of Cancer Research*, **79**, 1067–1074.

Kripke ML (1984) Immunological unresponsiveness induced by ultraviolet radiation. *Immunology Reviews*, **80**, 87–102.

Kunze E, Chang-Claude J and Frentzel-Beyme R (1992) Life style and occupational risk factors for bladder cancer in Germany: a case-control study. *Cancer*, **69**, 1776–1790.

Laskin JD, Heck D and Laskin DL (1992) Inhibitory effects of a green tea polyphenol fraction on 12-O-tetradecanoylphorbol-13-acetate-induced hydrogen peroxide formation in mouse epidermis. In *Phenolic Compounds in Foods and Health II: Antioxidant and Cancer Prevention*, Huang MT, Ho CT and Lee CY (eds), Washington DC, pp. 308–314.

La Vecchia C, Talamini R, Decarli A, Franceschi S, Parazzini F and Tognoni G (1986) Coffee consumption and the risk of breast cancer. *Surgery*, **100**, 477–481.

La Vecchie C, Negri E, Decarli A, D'Avanzo B, Liberati C and Franceschi S (1989) Dietary factors in the risk of bladder cancer. *Nutrition and Cancer*, **12**, 93–101.

La Vecchia C, Negri E, Franceschi S, D'Avanzo B and Boyle P (1992) Tea consumption and cancer risk. *Nutrition and Cancer*, **17**, 27–31.

Lea MA, Xiao Q, Sadhukhan AK, Cottle S, Wang ZY and Yang CS (1993) Inhibitory effects of tea extracts and -(-)-epigallocatechin gallate on DNA synthesis and proliferation of hepatoma and erythroleukemia cells. *Cancer Letters*, **68**, 231–236.

Lee HH, Wu HY, Chuang YC, Chang AS, Chao HH, Chen KY, Chen HK, Lai GM, Huang HH and Chen CJ (1990) Epidemiological characteristics and multiple risk factors of stomach cancer in Taiwan. *Anticancer Research*, **10**, 875–881.

Lee MJ, Wang ZY, Li H, Chen L, Sun Y, Gobbo S, Balentine DA and Yang CS (1995) Analysis of plasma and urinary tea polyphenols in human subjects. *Cancer Epidemiology Biomarkers and Prevention*, **4**, 393–399.

Liang Y-C, Lin-shiau S-Y, Chen C-F and Lin J-K (1997) Suppression of extracellular signals and cell proliferation through EGF receptor binding by (-)-epigallocatechin gallate in human A431 epidermoid carcinoma cells. *Journal of Cellular Biochemistry*, **67**, 55–65.

Li Y (1991) Comparative study on the inhibitory effect of green tea, coffee and levamisole on the hepatocarcinogenic action of diethylnitrosamine. *Chung Hua Chung liu Tsa Chih (Chinese Journal of Cancer)*, **13**, 193–195.

Lin TM, Chen KP, Lin CC, Hsu MM, Tu SM, Chaing TC, Jung PF and Hirayama T (1973) Retrospective study on nasopharyngeal carcinomas. *Journal of the National Cancer Institute*, **51**, 1403–1408.

Lin YL and Lin JK (1997) (-)-Epigallocatechin-3-gallate blocks the induction of nitric oxide synthase by down-regulating lipopolysaccharide-induced activity of transcription factor nuclear factor-kappaB. *Molecular Pharmacology*, **52**, 465–472.

Liu Q, Wang Y, Crist KA, Huang M-T, Conney AH and You M (1995) Analysis of p^{53} and H-*ras* mutations in UV- and UV/green tea-induced tumorigenesis in the skin of SKH-1 mice. *Proceedings of American Association for Cancer Research*, **36**, 591.

Lu Y-P, Lou Y-R, Xie J-G, Yen P, Huang M-T and Conney AH (1997) Inhibitory effect of black tea on the growth of established skin tumors in mice: effects on tumor size, apoptosis, mitosis and bromodeoxyuridine incorporation into DNA. *Carcinogenesis*, **18**, 2163–2169.

Lubin F, Ron E, Wax Y and Modan B (1985) Coffee and methylxanthines and breast cancer: a case-control study. *Journal of the National Cancer Institute*, **74**, 569–573.

Mabuchi K, Bross DS and Kessler YE (1985) Epidemiology of cancer of the vulva. A case-control study. *Cancer*, **55**, 1843–1848.

Mabuchi K, Bross DS and Kessler YE (1985) Risk factors for male breast cancer. *Journal of the National Cancer Institute*, **74**, 371–375.

Mack TM, Yu MC, Hanisch R and Henderson BE (1986) Pancreas cancer and smoking, beverage consumption, and past medical history. *Journal of the National Cancer Institute*, **76**, 49–60.

MacMahon B, Yen S, Trichopoulos D, Warren K and Nardi G (1981) Coffee and cancer of the pancreas. *New England Journal of Medicine*, **304**, 630–633.

Mao R (1993) The inhibitory effects of epicatechin complex on diethylnitrosamine induced initiation of hepatocarcinogenesis in rats. *Chung Hua Yu Fang I Hsueh Tsa Chih*, **27**, 201–204.

McCredie M, Ford JM and Stewart JH (1988) Risk factors for cancer of the renal parenchyma. *International Journal of Cancer*, **42**, 13–16.

Miller AB, Howe GR, Jain M, Craib KJ and Harrison L (1983) Food items and food groups as risk factors in a case-control study of diet and colo-rectal cancer. *International Journal of Cancer*, **32**, 155–161.

Miller CT, Neutel CI, Nair RC, Marrett LD, Last JM and Collins WE (1978) Relative importance of risk factors in bladder carcinogenesis. *Journal of Chronic Diseases*, **31**, 51–56.

Mills JJ, Chari RS, Boyer IJ, Gould MN and Jirtle RL (1995) Induction of apoptosis in liver tumors by the monoterpene perillyl alcohol. *Cancer Research*, **55**, 979–983.

Mitsui T, Yamada K, Yamashita K, Matuso N, Okuda A, Kimura G and Sugano M (1995) E1A-3Y1 cell-specific toxicity of tea polyphenols and their killing mechanism. *International Journal of Oncology*, **6**, 377–383.

Mohan RR, Khan SG, Agarwal R and Mukhtar H (1995) Testosterone induces ornithine decarboxylase (ODC) activity and mRNA expression in human prostate carcinoma cell line LNCaP: inhibition by green tea. *Proceedings of American Association for Cancer Research*, **36**, 274.

Morgan RW and Jain MG (1974) Bladder cancer: smoking, beverages and artificial sweeteners. *Canadian Medical Association Journal*, **111**, 1067–1070.

Morse MA and Stoner GD (1993) Cancer chemoprevention: principles and prospects. *Carcinogenesis*, **14**, 1737–1746.

Morton JF (1986) The potential carcinogenicity of herbal tea. *Environmental Carcinogenesis Reviews (Journal of Environmental Science and Health)*, **C4**, 203–223.

Mukhtar H, Agarwal R and Bickers DR (1991) Cutaneous metabolism of xenobiotics and steroid hormones. In *Pharmacology of the Skin*, Mukhtar H (ed), CRC Press, Boca Raton, FL, pp. 89–110.

Mukhtar H, Wang ZY, Katiyar SK and Agarwal R (1992) Tea components: antimutagenic and anticarcinogenic effects. *Preventive Medicine*, **21**, 351–360.

Mukhtar H, Katiyar SK and Agarwal R (1994) Green tea and skin-Anticarcinogenic effects. *The Journal of Investigative Dermatology*, **102**, 3–7.

Nagabhushan M, Sarode AV, Nair J, Amonkar AJ, D'Souza AV and Bhide SV (1991) Mutagenicity and carcinogenicity of tea, *Camellia sinensis*. *Indian Journal of Experimental Biology*, **29**, 401–406.

Namiki M (1990) Antioxidants/antimutagens in foods. *CRC Critical Review in Food Science and Nutrition*, **29**, 273–300.

Narasiwa T and Fukaura Y (1993) A very low dose of green tea polyphenols in driking water prevents N-methyl-N-nitrosourea-induced colon carcinogenesis in F344 rats. *Japanese Journal of Cancer Research*, **84**, 1007–1009.

Nishida H, Omori M, Fukutomi Y, Ninomiya M, Nishiwaki S, Suganuma M, Moriwaki H and Muto Y (1994) Inhibitory effects of (-)-epigallocatechin gallate on spontaneous hepatoma in C3H/HeNCrj mice and human-derived PLC/PRF/5 cells. *Japanese Journal of Cancer Research*, **85**, 221–225.

Nomura AM, Kolonel LN, Hankin JH and Yoshizawa CN (1991) Dietary factors in cancer of the lower urinary tract. *International Journal of Cancer*, **48**, 199–205.

Noonan FP, DeFabo EC and Kripke ML (1981) Suppression of contact hypersensitivity by UV radiation and its relationship to UV-induced suppression of tumor immunity. *Photochemistry and Photobiology*, **34**, 683–689.

Oguni I, Chen SJ, Lin PZ and Hara Y (1992) Protection against cancer risk by Japanese green tea. *Preventive Medicine*, **21**, 332.

Ohno Y, Aoki K, Obata K and Morrison AS (1985) Case-control study of urinary bladder cancer in metropolitan Nagoya. *Monograph of National Cancer Institute*, **69**, 229–234.

Perchellet J and Perchellet EM (1989) Antioxidants and multistage carcinogenesis in mouse skin. *Free Radicals in Biology and Medicine*, **7**, 377–408.

Phillips RL and Snowdon DA (1985) Dietary relationships with fatal colorectal cancer among Seventh-Day Adventists. *Journal of the National Cancer Institute*, **74**, 307–317.

Qin G, Gopalan-Kriczky P, Su J, Ning Y and Lotlikar PD (1997) Inhibition of aflatoxin B1-induced initiation of hepatocarcinogenesis in the rat by green tea. *Cancer Letters*, **112**, 149–154.

Risch HA, Burch JD, Miller AB, Hill GB, Steele R and Howe GR (1988) Dietary factors and the incidence of cancer of the urinary bladder. *American Journal of Epidemiology*, **127**, 1179–1191.

Rosenberg L, Miller DR, Helmrich SP, Kaufman DW, Schottenfeld D, Stolley PD and Shapiro S (1985) Breast cancer and the consumption of coffee. *American Journal of Epidemiology*, **122**, 391–399.

Sadzuka Y, Sugiyama T and Hirota S (1998) Modulation of cancer chemotherapy by green tea. *Clinical Cancer Research*, **4**, 153–156.

Sakamoto K, Reddy D, Hara Y and Milner JA (1995) Impact of green or black tea polyphenols on canine mammary tumor cells in culture. *Proceedings of American Association for Cancer Research*, **36**, 595.

Schairer C, Brinton LA and Hoover RN (1987) Methylxanthines and breast cancer. *International Journal of Cancer*, **40**, 469–473.

Shanmugaratnam K, Tye CY, Goh EH and Chia KB (1978) Etiological factors on naso-pharyngeal carcinoma: a hospital-based, retrospective, case-control, questionnaire study. In *Nasopharyngeal Carcinoma, Etiology and Control*, Ito Y (ed), IARC, Lyon, pp. 199–212.

Shi ST, Wang ZY, Theresa JS, Hong JY, Chen WF, Ho CT and Yang CS (1994) Effect of green tea and black tea on 4-(methylnitrosamino)-1-(3-pyridyl)-1-butanone bioactiva-tion, DNA methylation and lung tumorigenesis in A/J mice. *Cancer Research*, **54**, 4641–4647.

Shim JS, Kang MH, Kim YH, Roh JK, Toberts C and Lee IP (1995) Chemopreventive effects of green tea (*Camellia sinensis*) among cigarette smokers. *Cancer Epidemiology Biomarkers and Prevention*, **4**, 387–391.

Shimoi K, Nakamura Y, Tomita I, Hara Y and Kada T (1986) The pyrogallol related compounds reduce UV-induced mutations in *Escherichia coli* B/r WP2. *Mutation Research*, **173**, 239–244.

Sigler K and Ruch RJ (1993) Enhancement of gap junctional intercellular communication in tumor promoter-treated cells by components of green tea. *Cancer Letters*, **69**, 15–19.

Simon D, Yen S and Cole P (1975) Coffee drinking and cancer of the lower urinary tract. *Journal of the National Cancer Institute*, **54**, 587–591.

Slattery ML, West DW and Robison LM (1988) Fluid intake and bladder cancer in Utah. *International Journal of Cancer*, **42**, 17–22.

Sohn OS, Surace A, Fiala ES, Richie Jr JP, Colosimo S, Zang E and Weisburger JH (1994) Effects of green and black tea on hepatic xenobiotic metabolizing systems in the male F344 rat. *Xenobiotica*, **24**, 119–127.

Sporn MB (1991) Carcinogenesis and cancer: different perspectives on the same disease. *Cancer Research*, **51**, 6215–6218.

Stammler G and Volm M (1997) Green tea catechins (EGCG and EGC) have modulating effects on the activity of doxorubicin in drug-resistant cell lines. *Anti-Cancer Drugs*, **8**, 265–268.

Stocks P (1970) Cancer mortality in relation to national consumption of cigarettes, solid fuel, tea and coffee. *British Journal of Cancer*, **24**, 215–225.

Taniguchi S, Fujiki H, Kobayashi H, Go H, Miyado K, Sadano H and Shimokawa R (1992) Effect of (-)-epigallocatechin gallate, the main constituent of green tea, on lung metastasis with mouse B16 melanoma cell lines. *Cancer Letters*, **65**, 51–54.

Tazima K and Tominaga S (1985) Dietary habits and gastro-intestinal cancers: a comparative case-control study of stomach and large intestinal cancers in Nagoya, Japan. *Japanese Journal of Cancer Research*, **76**, 705–716.

Terao J, Piskula M and Yao Q (1994) Protective effect of epicatechin, epicatechin gallate, and quercetin on lipid peroxidation in phospholipid bilayers. *Archives of Biochemistry and Biophysics*, **308**, 278–284.

Tewes FJ, Koo LC, Meisgen TJ and Rylander R (1990) Lung cancer risk and mutagenicity of tea. *Environmental Research*, **52**, 23–33.

Trichopoulos D, Ouranos G, Day NE, Tzonou A, Manousos O, Papadimitriou C and Trichopoulos A (1985) Diet and cancer of the stomach: a case-control study in Greece. *International Journal of Cancer*, **36**, 291–297.

Valcic S, Timmermann BN, Alberts DS, Wachter GA, Krutzsch M, Wymer J and Guillen JM (1996) Inhibitory effect of six green tea catechins and caffeine on the growth of four selected human tumor cell lines. *Anticancer-Drugs*, **7**, 461–468.

Victoria CG, Munoz N, Day NE, Barcelos LB, Peccin DA and Braga NM (1987) Hot beverages and oesophageal cancer in southern Brazil: a case-control study. *International Journal of Cancer*, **39**, 710–716.

Wang ZY, Das M, Bickers DR and Mukhtar H (1988) Interaction of epicatechins derived from green tea with rat hepatic cytochrome P-450. *Drug Metabolism and Disposition*, **16**, 98–103.

Wang ZY, Cheng SJ, Zhou ZC, Athar M, Khan WA, Bickers DR and Mukhtar H (1989a) Antimutagenic activity of green tea polyphenols. *Mutation Research*, **223**, 273–285.

Wang ZY, Khan WA, Bickers DR and Mukhtar H (1989b) Protection against polycyclic aromatic hydrocarbon-induced skin tumor initiation in mice by green tea polyphenols. *Carcinogenesis*, **10**, 411–415.

Wang ZY, Agarwal R, Bickers DR and Mukhtar H (1991) Protection against ultraviolet B radiation-induced photocarcinogenesis in hairless mice by green tea polyphenols. *Carcinogenesis*, **12**, 1527–1530.

Wang ZY, Agarwal R, Khan WA and Mukhtar H (1992a) Protection against benzo(a)-pyrene and N-nitrosodiethylamine-induced lung and forestomach tumorigenesis in A/J mice by water extracts of green tea and licorice. *Carcinogenesis*, **13**, 1491–1494.

Wang ZY, Hong JY, Huang M-T, Reuhl KR, Conney AH and Yang CS (1992b) Inhibition of N-nitrosodiethylamine- and 4-(methylnitrosamino)-1-(3-pyridyl)-1-butanone-induced tumorigenesis in A/J mice by green tea and black tea. *Cancer Research*, **52**, 1943–1947.

Wang ZY, Huang M-T, Ferraro T, Wong C-Q, Lou Y-R, Reuhl K, Iatropoulos M, Yang CS and Conney AH (1992c) Inhibitory effect of green tea in the drinking water on tumorigenesis by ultraviolet light and 12-*O*-tetradecanoylphorbol-13-acetate in the skin of SKH-1 mice. *Cancer Research*, **52**, 1162–1170.

Wang ZY, Huang M-T, Ho C-T, Chang R, Ma W, Ferraro T, Reuhl KR, Yang CS and Conney AH (1992d) Inhibitory effect of green tea on the growth of established skin papillomas in mice. *Cancer Research*, **52**, 6657–6665.

Wang ZY, Huang M-T, Lou Y-R, Xie J-G, Reuhl KR, Newmark HL, Ho C-T, Yang CS and Conney AH (1994) Inhibitory effects of black tea, green tea, decaffeinated black tea, and decaffeinated green tea on ultraviolet B light-induced skin carcinogenesis in 7,12-dimethylbenz(a)anthracene-initiated SKH-1 mice. *Cancer Research*, **54**, 3428–3435.

Wattenberg LW (1990) Inhibition of carcinogenesis by naturally occurring and synthetic compounds. In *Antimutagenesis and Anticarcinogenesis, Mechanisms II*, Kuroda Y, Shankel DM and Waters MD (eds), Plenum Publishing Corp., New York, pp. 155–166.

Weisburger JH, Nagao M, Wakabayashi K and Oguri A (1994) Prevention of heterocyclic amine formation by tea and tea polyphenols. *Cancer Letters*, **83**, 143–147.

Weisburger JH, Rivenson A, Garr K and Aliaga-C (1997) Tea, or tea and milk, inhibit mammary gland and colon carcinogenesis in rats. *Cancer Letters*, **114**, 323–327.

Wright AS (1991) Emerging strategies for the determination of human carcinogens: detection, identification, exposure monitoring, and risk evaluation. In *Human Carcinogen Exposure, Biomonitoring and Risk Assessment*, Garner RC, Farmer B, Steel GT and Wright AS (eds), IRL Press, Oxford, UK, pp. 3–23.

Wright SC, Zhong J and Larrick JW (1994) Inhibition of apoptosis as a mechanism of tumor promotion. *FASEB Journal*, **8**, 654–660.

Xu Y, Ho C-T, Amin SG, Han C and Chung FL (1992) Inhibition of tobacco-specific nitrosamine-induced lung tumorigenesis in A/J mice by green tea and its major polyphenol as antioxidants. *Cancer Research*, **52**, 3875–3879.

Yamane T, Hagiwara N, Tateishi M, Akachi S, Kim M, Okuzumi J, Kitao Y, Inagake M, Kuwata K and Takahashi T (1991) Inhibition of azoxymethane-induced colon carcinogenesis in rat by green tea polyphenol fraction. *Japanese Journal of Cancer Research*, **82**, 1336–1339.

Yang CS (1980) Research on esophageal cancer in China: a review. *Cancer Research*, **40**, 2633–2644.

Yang CS and Wang ZY (1993) Tea and cancer. *Journal of the National Cancer Institute*, **85**, 1038–1049.

Yang G, Wang ZY, Kim S, Liao J, Seril DN, Chen X, Smith TJ and Yang CS (1997) Characterization of early pulmonary hyperproliferation and tumor progression and their inhibition by black tea in a 4-(methylnitrosamino)-1-(3-pyridyl)-1-butanone-induced lung tumorigenesis model with A/J mice. *Cancer Research*, **57**, 1889–1894.

Yoshizawa-S (1996) (-)-Epigallocatechin gallate, the main constituent of Japanese green tea, inhibits tumor promotion of okadaic acid. *Fukuoka Igaku Zasshi*, **87**, 215–221.

Yoshizawa S, Horiuchi T, Fujiki H, Yoshida T, Okuda T and Sugimura T (1987) Antitumor promoting activity of (-)-epigallocatechin gallate, the main constituent of 'tannin' in green tea. *Phytotherapy Research*, **1**, 44–47.

Yu MC, Mack TM, Hanisch R, Cicioni C and Henderson BE (1986) Cigarette smoking, obesity, diuretic use, and coffee consumption as risk factors for renal cell carcinoma. *Journal of the National Cancer Institute*, **77**, 351–356.

Yu R, Jiao JJ, Duh JL, Gudehithlu K, Tan TH and Kong AN (1997) Activation of mitogen-activated protein kinases by green tea polyphenols: potential signaling pathways in the regulation of antioxidant-responsive element-mediated phase II enzyme gene expression. *Carcinogenesis*, **18**, 451–456.

Zhang A, Zhu QY, Luk YS, Ho KY, Fung KP and Chen ZY (1997) Inhibitory effects of jasmine green tea epicatechin isomers on free radical-induced lysis of red blood cells. *Life Sciences*, **61**, 383–394.

Zheng W, Doyle TJ, Hong CP, Kushi LH, Sellers TA and Folsom AR (1995) Tea consumption and cancer incidence in a prospective cohort study of postmenopausal women. *Proceedings of the American Association for Cancer Research*, **36**, 278.

14 Animal Diets in Safety Evaluation Studies

Ghanta N Rao[1] and Joseph J Knapka[2]

[1]*National Institute of Environmental Health Sciences, National Institutes of Health, Research Triangle Park, North Carolina, 27709, USA*
[2]*National Center for Research Services, National Institutes of Health, Bethesda, Maryland, 20892, USA (retired)*

Introduction

Genetic and environmental factors can influence the physiological processes and pharmacological/toxicological responses of animal models to chemicals and other agents. Diet is one of the most important environmental factors in safety evaluation with experimental animals. The ingredients, major nutrient composition, vitamin and mineral concentrations, microbial and chemical contaminants and energy density of diets could effect the health, severity of ageing diseases, life span and toxic responses to chemicals and other agents under investigation. Therefore, the composition and quality of diets for safety studies should be defined, standardised and controlled (Sontag *et al.*, 1976; Institute of Laboratory Animal Resources, 1978; US National Research Council (NRC), 1978a).

Types of diets

Diets available for safety studies with laboratory animals may be classified as 'cereal-based' natural ingredient diets and 'purified' diets (American Institute of Nutrition (AIN), 1977). Natural ingredient diets can be further classified as 'open formula' in which the ingredient composition is published or known and 'closed formula' or 'proprietary' in which the ingredient composition is confidential (AIN, 1977). The advantages and limitations of each of these Diet

Nutrition and Chemical Toxicity. Edited by Costas Ioannides. © John Wiley & Sons Ltd. ISBN 0 471 97453 6

types are listed in Table 14.1 (Institute of Laboratory Animal Resources, 1978; Rao, 1988).

Cereal-based diets contain mostly non-purified products of cereal grains, plants, single cell (yeast) proteins and some animal products such as dried milk, fish meal, bone, blood and meat meal. Cereal-based diets may contain naturally occurring enzyme inducers such as indoles and flavones from the ingredients of plant origin (Campbell and Hayes, 1974) and environmental contaminants. However, they are economical to produce in large quantities and will have a longer shelf life at room temperature. The nutrient concentrations, especially the trace minerals and vitamins, may vary from batch to batch of cereal-based diets (Rao and Knapka, 1987) due to nutrient variability in different batches of each ingredient. It is preferable to use the 'open formula' diets to minimise the variability in response that can be introduced when the ingredients and their proportions are altered (AIN, 1977) due to availability and cost considerations. However, the essential nutrient concentrations of properly formulated cereal-based diets will be equivalent to or greater than the estimated minimum requirements as recommended by the US NRC (NRC, 1995). Cereal-based diets, by inducing drug-metabolising enzymes in various tissues may decrease the toxic and carcinogenic potential of chemicals inactivated by these enzymes in the liver (Shively et al., 1986) and may increase the toxicity and carcinogenicity of chemicals that are activated by these enzymes.

Purified diets may be more appropriate for safety studies because of less variability in nutrient composition as they contain refined ingredients such as purified casein, soy protein isolates, purified carbohydrates such as starches and sugars. However, they are more expensive than the cereal-based diets. Furthermore, the purified diets may deteriorate (become rancid due to accumulation of lipid peroxides) rapidly at room temperature and should be stored

Table 14.1 Advantages and limitations of different types of diets

Cereal-based diets	Purified diets
Advantages	
Most commonly used, economical and routinely available	Reproducible nutrient concentrations
Several months of shelf life at room temperature	Low levels of contaminants
Extensive historical data	Low levels of enzyme inducers
Limitations	
Variable essential nutrient concentrations	Limited historical data
Contaminants	May cause lesions in control animals
Enzyme inducers	5 to 10 times more expensive
	Require refrigeration for storage

at 4°C to extend the shelf life (Fullerton *et al.*, 1982). The purified diets, due to refined ingredients, may be low in contaminants and enzyme inducers (Rao, 1991), and the nutrient concentrations can be controlled without much variability between batches. Standardised purified diets appropriate for safety studies with all species are not established. The most commonly used purified diet for rodent studies up to 1994 was AIN-76, formulated by the American Institute of Nutrition (AIN), and this diet was reformulated as AIN-93 (AIN, 1977; Reeves *et al.*, 1993). Due to high digestibility of nutrients, purified diets have high caloric value and may cause higher body weights (AIN, 1977; Medinsky *et al.*, 1982; Fullerton *et al.*, 1991, 1992) and increase the carcinogenic potential of chemicals (Kritchevsky, 1977; Fullerton *et al.*, 1991, 1992). Purified diets also cause periportal lipidosis (Medinsky *et al.*, 1982) calcification of heart and kidneys (Woodard, 1971; Nguyen, 1982), haemorrhagic disease (Medinsky *et al.*, 1982; Roebuck *et al.*, 1979) and dystrophic calcification of heart and other organs (Everitt *et al.*, 1988). Purified diets may cause substantial changes in the physiological processes by altering the hydration of intestinal contents (Rao, 1988). Changes may also occur in gut flora (Rowland *et al.*, 1985) that may lead to altered endogenous vitamin synthesis, lower concentrations of unconjugated serum bile acids (Rao, 1988) and alterations in chemical disposition (Shively *et al.*, 1986).

Scientific considerations favour the use of purified diets. However, safety studies are intended for extrapolation to human effects and cereal-based, non-purified diets are more similar to human diets than purified diets. Cereal-based diets are the most commonly used diets for safety studies due to economic reasons and practical considerations. Extensive historical databases on physiology and background/spontaneous lesions are available on most commonly used stocks and strains of experimental animals fed cereal-based diets in safety studies. Historical data on physiology and spontaneous lesions of commonly used experimental animals fed purified diets are limited. However, when the chemical under investigation is a nutrient or a common contaminant such as fluorine or selenium, found in cereal-based diets, and its concentration in the natural ingredient diet cannot be controlled, it may be appropriate to use a purified diet.

Dietary ingredients

Commonly used ingredients in cereal-based, non-purified diets include but are not limited to wheat, corn (maize), rice, oats, barley and their products; soybean meal (bean cake), fish meal or fish powder (menhaden), dried skim milk, dried whey, dried egg, single cell (yeast) protein, meat meal, blood meal, bone meal, alfalfa meal, brans of various cereal grains, oat hulls, beet pulp, cellulose, animal fats, soy oil, corn oil, fish oil, ground nut oil, cane or beet molasses, dried brewer's yeast, rock salt, limestone (stone powder), and some binders for making pellets. However, various cereal, animal and plant products used in human foods may be used in diets for experimental animals, albeit at different proportions than selected for human consumption. Approximate concentrations of nutrients and non-nutrients of various ingredients available for animal feeds were published by the US NRC (NRC, 1982). However, the composition of major ingredients used in formulation of 'cereal-based' diets may vary depending upon the country of origin, season, strain of seed grains, unusual weather conditions, curing/drying and other processes involved in preparing ingredients for storage and transportation in world commerce.

Major ingredients often used in purified diets include but are not limited to various grades of casein, soy protein isolates, lactalbumin, ovalbumin, cornstarch, modified starches from different sources, purified or semipure oils or animal fats, purified celluloses, surcrose, dextrose and purified mineral ingredients such as sodium chloride and dicalcium phosphate. However, various purified food ingredients appropriate for human consumption, including individual amino acids, fatty acids, sugars, etc., may also be used in formulation of purified diets for experimental animals.

Nutrients

Various dietary nutrients may interact with chemicals under investigation and influence their toxic responses in animals (Conner and Newberne, 1984; Omaye, 1986). Nutrients with potential to influence significantly the toxic responses of chemicals include proteins, fats, minerals and vitamins. Nutrient requirements for most species of experimental animals may differ by strain or stock and stage of life cycle such as growth, reproduction, maintenance of adult and aged animals (NRC, 1995). The nutrient requirements for maintenance of laboratory animals in safety assessment studies beyond the growth and reproductive stages have not been well established. Furthermore, the recommended nutrient requirements for growth, reproduction and lactation (NRC, 1995) were selected for maximum growth and reproductive capacity, which may not be appropriate in some or most safety assessment studies as they may not be compatible with long life span.

PROTEINS

Protein provides the essential amino acids arginine, histidine, isoleucine, leucine, lysine, methionine, cystine, phenylalanine, threonine, tryptophan, valine and others for growth and maintenance (NRC, 1995). Concentration and quality of protein in the diet are known to influence the levels of hepatic drug-metabolising enzymes (Hietanen, 1980; Bidlack et al., 1986), which can metabolise chemicals to less toxic or more toxic intermediates (Williams and Millburn, 1975). Various investigators evaluated the effects of high- and low-protein diets on drug-metabolising enzymes (Hayes and Campbell, 1974; Bidlack et al., 1986) and toxic effects of drugs (McLean and McLean, 1966;

Shakman, 1974; Butler and Dauterman, 1988). However, protein concentrations within the range to support growth and reproduction (15–22%) may not consistently influence the toxic responses of chemicals. High-protein (25%) diets may decrease the toxic effects of some pesticides and aflatoxin B_1 (Rogers and Newberne, 1971). Low protein concentrations (3–8%) may depress the activity of hepatic drug-metabolising enzymes (McLean and McLean, 1966) and increase the toxicity of cholinesterase inhibitors, chlorinated hydrocarbons (Shakman, 1974) bromobenzene and procaine (Butler and Dauterman, 1988) as compared with diets containing 22–26% protein. The effect of dietary protein concentration on the toxicity of selected chemicals is shown in Table 14.2. Individual amino acid concentrations of dietary proteins may influence the toxic potential of some chemicals. The amino acid glycine is essential for detoxication and elimination of the food additive, benzyl acetate (Abdo *et al.*, 1998), and related compounds. High protein intake due to high (>15%) concentration of protein in the diet may markedly increase the severity of kidney lesions in rats (Newberne, 1978; Klahr *et al.*, 1983) and hamsters (Feldman *et al.*, 1982). Most diets used in safety assessment studies were formulated for fast growth and maximum reproduction, and may contain excess of some nutrients such as protein. Diets containing an ideal protein such as whole-egg protein, at about 12%, are considered adequate for growth and maintenance (NRC, 1978a). A diet with approximately 15% crude protein derived from cereal grains and animal proteins (soybean, wheat, corn, fish

Table 14.2 Influence of dietary protein concentration on toxicity of chemicals in male rats

Chemical	Protein content as casein	
	3.5–8%	22–26%
LD_{50} mg/kg body weight[a]		
Endosulfan	24	102
Toxaphene	80	293
Carbaryl	89	575
Diazinon	215	466
Malathion	759	1401
Diuron	437	2390
Captan	480	12 600
Hexobarbital sleeping time at 10 mg/kg i.p. (min)[b]	142	38
Bromobenzene mortality at 1570 mg/kg i.p. (%)[b]	0	50
Procaine mortality at 230 mg/kg i.p. (%)[b]	86	17

[a]Modified from Shakman (1974). LD_{50}, single oral dose required for mortality of 50% rats in 28 days.
[b]i.p., intraperitoneal injection. Modified from Butler and Dauterman (1988).

meal), supplemented with essential amino acids if necessary, will be adequate for growth without causing high protein-related lesions in rodents (Rao *et al.*, 1993; Rao, 1996, 1997).

FATS

Dietary fats provide the essential fatty acids, linoleic and linolenic acids, as well as other polyunsaturated fatty acids for growth and maintenance and aid in the absorption of fat-soluble vitamins. A fat content of $5 \pm 2\%$ from soybean oil is considered to be appropriate with regard to linoleic:linolenic (essential fatty acids) and polyunsaturated:saturated fatty acid ratios that are optimal for growth and maintenance of rodents (Reeves *et al.*, 1993). Dietary fat concentrations in the 5–10% range have not caused consistent changes in toxicity and tumour development by chemicals in rodents (Haseman *et al.*, 1985). Feeding diets containing 20–25% fat was associated with increased incidence of mammary tumours in rats (Conner and Newberne, 1984). Fat has 2.25 times the caloric value of carbohydrate or protein, and various studies have indicated that fat, due to such high caloric value, increased the adult body weight and body weight-associated tumours, such as anterior pituitary and mammary tumours (Rao *et al.*, 1987, 1990; Rao and Haseman, 1993). Methionine, choline, folic acid and vitamin B_{12} are the essential lipotropic methyl-donating nutrients and these may influence the toxicity of some chemicals (Conner and Newberne, 1984). High fat content (>10%) will increase caloric intake, obesity and some tumour incidences with no consistent advantage in evaluating the safety of chemicals. Low fat content (<2%) may decrease palatability and may not provide adequate concentrations of essential fatty acids necessary for the growth and well-being of rodents. Absorption, bioavailability and toxic responses of fat-soluble chemicals administered by incorporation into the diet may be effected by the fat content of diets.

CARBOHYDRATES

Digestible carbohydrates are the most efficient and major sources of energy in animal diets available for safety studies. Complex carbohydrates (starch) account for most of the carbohydrate in the cereal-based diets. The purified diets may contain complex carbohydrate and simple carbohydrates (sucrose and glucose) in various proportions. When proteins and fats are major sources of energy instead of carbohydrates, some blood chemistry values such as urea nitrogen and ketones, the by-products of protein and fat energy metabolism, could be substantially higher. However, definite requirements for carbohydrates in diets have not been established (NRC, 1995). Most commonly used carbohydrates in purified diets include glucose, fructose, sucrose, starch, dextrins and maltose. Feeding fructose and sucrose may cause increases in the weight and lipid and glycogen contents of the liver of rats (NRC, 1995). Poor growth and cataract formation were observed in rats fed lactose or galactose (Day and Pigman, 1957). Animals fed high amounts of simple carbohydrates, such as sucrose and glucose, had a reduced ability to metabolise drugs. These changes include prolonged barbiturate sleeping time in mice (Strother *et al.*, 1971) and increased toxicity of benzylpenicillin in rats (Boyd *et al.*, 1970).

FIBRE

There are no specific requirements or recommendations for the fibre content of rodent diets. However, dietary fibre may be potentially beneficial (NRC, 1995). Some fibres, such as cellulose, may provide mostly bulk to the intestinal contents, whereas other fibres derived from brans and alfalfa may actively bind to chemicals and nutrients. Dietary fibre may increase faecal bulk, decrease gastrointestinal transit time and increase the weight of caecum and colon (Fleming and Lee, 1983). Dietary fibre may alter the gut flora and gut flora-associated metabolism and toxicity of chemicals (Kritchevsky, 1977; Maciorowski *et al.*, 1997). Fibre may also reduce the absorption of chemicals by decreasing the gastrointestinal transit time and, depending on the type of fibre, may bind some nutrients and chemicals. Most cereal-based diets contain approximately 5% fibre from natural ingredient sources. Some diets with ~ 10% fibre delayed the development of mammary tumours (Rao, 1995; Rao *et al.*, 1996, 1997).

MINERALS

Various minerals are necessary for survival and growth and may be classified as macrominerals and trace minerals. The macrominerals calcium, phosphorus, chloride, magnesium, potassium and sodium are present in living tissues in substantial amounts (NRC, 1985). Iron, copper, manganese, zinc, molybdenum, iodine and selenium are considered to be essential trace minerals. A number of minerals such as chromium, fluorine, arsenic, boron, nickel, vanadium, silicon, lead, cadmium, lithium and others are classified as ultratrace minerals and are considered to be potentially beneficial minerals at very low concentrations in diets of experimental animals (Reeves *et al.*, 1993; NRC, 1995).

Macrominerals

Recommended concentrations of macrominerals in diets for experimental animals commonly used in safety studies are listed in Table 14.3. The physiological basis for the recommended concentrations of minerals was discussed in various publications (AIN, 1977; Reeves *et al.*, 1993; NRC, 1977, 1978a, 1985, 1995). Ingredients of cereal-based diets contain varying concentrations of essential minerals; however, the bioavailability of these minerals is not known. To ensure that there are adequate concentrations of macrominerals

Table 14.3 Recommended concentrations of essential minerals in diets for growth and maintenance

Mineral	Unit[a]	Rat[b]	Mouse[b]	Rabbit[c]	Dog[d]	Monkey[e]
Calcium	g	5.0	5.0	4.0	0.32	5.0
Phosphorus	g	3.0	3.0	2.2	0.24	4.0
Potassium	g	3.6	2.0	6.0	0.24	8.0
Sodium	g	0.5	0.5	2.0	0.03	3.0
Chloride	g	0.5	0.5	3.0	0.046	3.5
Magnesium	g	0.5	0.5	0.3	0.022	1.5
Iron	mg	35	35	ND	1.74	180
Zinc	mg	12	10	ND	1.94	10
Manganese	mg	10	10	8.5	0.28	40
Copper	mg	5	6	3.0	0.16	ND
Iodine	μg	150	150	200	32	ND
Molybdenum	μg	150	150	ND	ND	ND
Selenium	μg	150	150	ND	6	ND

[a] Amount per kg diet (for dog the units are amount per kg body weight for growth).
[b] Adapted from NRC (1995).
[c] Adapted from NRC (1977).
[d] Adapted from NRC (1985); note that the recommended concentrations are per kg body weight.
[e] Adapted from NRC (1978); recommended concentrations were based on concentrations in commercial diets that were considered adequate.
ND, quantitative requirements not determined.

in diets, minimum recommended levels are generally added to the diets. However, some ingredients, such as fish meal, may contain high concentrations of the macrominerals calcium and phosphorus, so that added concentrations may have to be adjusted to prevent large excesses. In addition, the calcium to phosphorus ratio appears to be important to prevent calcification of tissues such as kidney (nephrocalcinosis). A calcium:phosphorus molar ratio of >1 and <2 may prevent abnormal calcification of tissues.

Trace minerals

Estimated requirements or recommended concentrations of trace minerals in experimental animal diets are listed in Table 14.3. Physiological and toxicological considerations for the selected concentrations were discussed in various publications (AIN, 1977; Reeves *et al.*, 1993; NRC, 1977, 1978a, 1985, 1995). Consistent changes in the toxicity of chemicals have not been demonstrated within the range of trace mineral concentrations adequate for growth, reproduction and maintenance. However, either too low or too high concentrations of some minerals such as selenium may influence the toxicity of chemicals because the concentration difference between deficiency and toxicity of selenium in diets is narrow. High or low concentrations of copper and selenium may interact with other trace minerals such as iron, manganese, molybdenum and zinc and may influence the toxic effects of arsenic, cadmium, fluorine, lead and others (Conner and Newberne, 1984). Due to its relationship with vitamin E to enhance antioxidant effect, selenium may influence the toxicity of chemicals. Diets containing very low or high (<0.1 or >4 ppm) concentrations of selenium appear to increase the hepatotoxic effects of aflatoxin B_1 (Newberne and Conner, 1974). Beneficial effects of optimum concentration of selenium ($\sim$ 1 ppm) appear to be due to maximisation of liver glutathione peroxidase (Sunde et al., 1992), an enzyme that detoxifies the peroxides formed by agents such as ozone and carbon tetrachloride (Bus and Gibson, 1979) and prevents cell membrane damage. Many minerals, especially essential trace minerals that are required at low concentrations in the diet, are the components of active enzymes and metabolic cofactors necessary for metabolic processes. The essential trace minerals may influence the metabolism and toxicity of chemicals, if the diets are deficient or contain lower than optimal concentrations.

Ultratrace minerals

Many ultratrace minerals are present at very low concentrations in tissues and body fluids. Recommended concentrations of these elements in diets are listed in Table 14.4. Chromium and vanadium may enhance glucose metabolism, but the mechanism is not known. Even though biochemical functions for most of these ultratrace minerals are not well established, feeding diets with less than the recommended levels may negatively influence growth, reproduction and various physiological parameters in animals (Mertz and Roginski, 1969; Reeves et al., 1993). Beneficial effects of these ultratrace minerals may be due to an indirect effect on and by the microbial population of the gut (Yoshida et al., 1993; NRC, 1995). Most of the ultratrace minerals are present at more than adequate concentrations in the non-purified natural ingredient cereal-based diets. However, only certain ingredients may contribute specific elements.

Table 14.4 Recommended concentrations and analysed concentrations of ultratrace minerals in rodent diets

Mineral (mg/kg)	Recommended[a]	NIH-07[b]	NTP-2000[b]
Sulphur	300	2660	1760
Silicon	5.0	1140	2200
Chromium	1.0	1.6	1.0
Fluoride	1.0	13.1	3.3
Nickel	0.5	2.5	2.5
Boron	0.5	7.4	5.5
Lithium	0.1	1.0	4.1
Vanadium	0.1	1.4	0.8

[a]From Reeves et al. (1993); NRC (1995).
[b]From the National Toxicology Program (NTP) database.

Molasses, for example, may be the major source of chromium in animal diets; thus, if molasses is not one of the ingredients, chromium may have to be added to the cereal-based diets (Rao, 1996). Concentrations of selected ultratrace minerals contributed by the ingredients of some cereal-based diets are given in Table 14.4.

VITAMINS

Fat-soluble vitamins A, D, E and K are essential for many critical functions of the body. Vitamin E is one of the best natural antioxidants (Scott, 1978). The water-soluble B complex vitamins biotin, cyonocabalamin (B_{12}), folic acid, niacin, pantothenic acid, pyridoxine and riboflavin are coenzymes or cofactors in various metabolic processes in energy metabolism and tissue synthesis. The gut flora of rodents synthesise many of the B complex vitamins, and coprophagy contributes to the vitamin requirements of rodents (Daft et al., 1963). Substantial alteration of gut flora by drugs and chemicals in safety studies may cause subclinical B vitamin deficiency. Vitamin C is not required by experimental animals, except guinea pigs and primates. Recommended concentrations of vitamins in diets for animal models used in safety studies are listed in Table 14.5. Consistent effects on toxicity and tumour development have not

Table 14.5 Recommended concentrations of essential vitamins in diets

Vitamin	Unit/kg[a]	Rat[b]	Mouse[b]	Rabbit[c]	Dog[d]	Monkey[e]
A (retinol)	IU	2300	2400	580	202	12 500
D_3 (cholecalciferol)	IU	1000	1000	ND	22	2000
E (*RRR*-α-Tocopherol)	IU	27	32	40	1.2	50
K (phylloquinone)	μg	1000	1000	NR	ND	ND
C (ascorbic acid)	mg	0	0	0	0	100
Choline	mg	750	2000	1200	50	ND
Niacin	mg	15	15	180	0.45	50
Pantothenate	mg	10	16	NR	0.40	15
Pyridoxine	mg	6	8	39	0.06	2.5
Thiamin	mg	4	5	NR	0.054	ND
Riboflavin	mg	3	7	NR	0.10	5
Folic acid	μg	1000	500	NR	0.008	200
Biotin	μg	200	200	NR	ND	100
B_{12}	μg	50	10	NR	1.0	ND

[a]Amount per kg diet (for dog the units are amount per kg body weight for growth).
[b]Adapted from NRC (1995); concentrations in AIN-93 diets (Reeves et al., 1993) were higher than the NRC recommendations.
[c]Adapted from NRC (1977).
[d]Adapted from NRC (1985); note that the recommended concentrations are per kg body weight.
[e]Adapted from NRC (1978); recommended concentrations were based on concentrations in commercial diets that were considered adequate.
ND, quantitative requirement not established; NR, dietary supplementation may not be necessary as intestinal microbial synthesis may be adequate.

been observed within the range of vitamin concentrations adequate for growth, reproduction and maintenance. However, marked or prolonged deficiency of vitamins A, C and E or several-fold higher than the recommended concentrations of these vitamins may influence the toxic and carcinogenic responses of some chemicals and agents (Welsh *et al.*, 1981). Some diets may contain several-fold higher than the recommended concentrations of vitamins A and C (see Tables 14.3, 14.15 and 14.16). Vitamin A deficiency may enhance the lesions caused by chemicals affecting the epithelial cells of the respiratory tract (Nettesheim and Williams, 1976), and may increase the colon tumours caused by chemicals such as dimethylhydrazine (Rogers *et al.*, 1973). High intakes of vitamin A may protect against squamous metaplasia and lung tumours caused by benzo[a]pyrene (Saffiotti *et al.*, 1967), but many not protect against colon cancer (Rogers *et al.*, 1973). High intake of vitamin A may decrease the absorption of vitamin E (Blakeley *et al.*, 1990), while high dietary intake of vitamins A and E has been shown to accelerate the deficiency of vitamin K (Beri, 1979), and may lead to an increase in the toxicity of chemicals affecting blood clotting. Vitamin C appears to lower the potency of nitrite to induce methaemoglobinaemia in animals, such as guinea pigs, which require dietary vitamin C (Stoewsend *et al.*, 1973). Vitamin C may decrease drug-metabolising enzyme activities in liver (Zannoni *et al.*, 1972). As an antioxidant, vitamin E may act similar to vitamin C in reducing the formation of nitrosamines (Megens *et al.*, 1979). A higher fat content ('>5%) and higher phytates such as soybean meal in the diet may require highe concentrations of vitamin E in the diet (Johnston and Fritsche, 1989; NRC, 995). Vitamin E concentrations in diets may influence the toxic responses of chemicals affecting the skeletal muscle and the myocardium (Van Fleet *et al.*, 1981). In addition, Vitamin E appears to have a significant influence on the toxicity of metals, except selenium (Van Fleet, 1976).

OTHER NUTRIENTS

Choline is an essential nutrient because it is a component of lecithin, sphingomyelin and acetylcholine. Since choline is a methyl-donating lipotrope, choline requirement is a function of methionine, folic acid, vitamin B_{12} and lipid concentrations of diets. Choline deficiency may increase the carcinogenic potential of chemicals such as aflatoxins and nitrosamines (Rogers, 1983; Newberne and Conner, 1986). Sphingolipids are structurally diverse membrane lipids that may be essential for cell growth, differentiation, apoptosis and other cell functions and are present in various ingredients of the cereal-based diets (Merrill *et al.*, 1997). Feeding of sphingomyelin reduced the incidence of colon cancer caused by 1,2-dimethylhydrazine (Dillehay *et al.*, 1994), indicating that dietary sphingolipid content may influence the toxicity of chemicals.

Dietary nucleotides may influence cell proliferation and differentiation (Jackson *et al.*, 1997). Mice and rats fed purified diets appear to be more sensitive to dimethylbenzanthracene-induced mammary cancer (Ip, 1987), to liver and bladder tumours induced by 2-acetylaminofluorene (Fullerton *et al.*, 1991), and to azaserine-induced pancreatic cancer (Longnecker *et al.*, 1981), as compared with rodents fed natural ingredient diets. The natural ingredients, especially the fish meal, animal by-products (blood meal, meat meal), milk products and brewer's yeast are the major sources of nucleotides in cereal-based diets. The above information indicates that the availability of nucleotides in diet may influence the carcinogenic potential of chemicals though, in general, the natural ingredient diets appears to provide adequate concentrations of the above classes of nutrients.

Dietary contaminants

Chemical and biological contaminants in the diet may influence the biological responses of experimental animals (Newberne, 1975; Greenman *et al.*, 1980; Rao, 1991) to chemicals and other agents, and may complicate the interpretation of toxicity and carcinogenicity studies.

Sources of contaminants

Dietary ingredients, especially the non-purified natural ingredients, may contribute various chemical and biological contaminants. Some contaminants in the natural ingredient cereal-based diets are due to accumulation of chemicals from the soil, the use of pesticides and to the environmental conditions during the cereal's growing and harvest seasons. Some are intentional additives such as preservatives (antioxidants), while others are accidental contaminants included during processing, storage and transportation or by-products of processing. Possible sources of contaminants in experimental animal diets are described in Table 14.6. Concentrations of contaminants will vary with the type and proportion of ingredients, especially non-purified ingredients. Diets high in fish meal content such as NIH-07 (Knapka *et al.*, 1974) may have higher concentrations of nitrates, nitrosamines, metals and antioxidants (Rao and Knapka, 1987; Rao, 1991) than diets with a lower proportion of fish meal (Rao, 1996). Diets high in ingredients such as alfalfa, corn and wheat may contain high concentrations of nitrates, selenium and mycotoxins (Rao, 1991). Since the ingredients of purified diets such as casein, soy protein, albumin, sucrose, starch, etc., are refined or semipurified (AIN, 1977), the concentrations of chemical contaminants in purified diets are generally lower than in cereal-based diets (Rao, 1991).

Concentrations of contaminants

Most frequently measured contaminants of cereal-based diets include the metals lead, arsenic, cadmium and mercury; nitrates, volatile nitrosamines

Table 14.6 Sources of contaminants in cereal-based diets[a]

Ingredient	Contaminants
Fish meal	Nitrosamines, Pb, As, Hg, Cd, Se, organophosphorus and organochlorine insecticides including DDT and its metabolites, fluoride, nitrate, nitrite
Blood, meat and bone meal	Nitrosamine, nitrate, nitrite, Pb
Corn and wheat	Mycotoxins including aflatoxins, vomitoxins, fumonisins; insecticides especially malathion, As, Se, fluoride
Soybean products[b]	Oestrogenic activity
Alfalfa meal	Nitrate, nitrite, Pb
Vegetable oils	Mycotoxins, peroxides, preservatives
Animals fats	Insecticides, preservatives
Beet pulp and molasses	Se, As, insecticides
Lime stone, salt and dicalcium phosphate	Pb, As, Se, Cd, fluoride

[a] Adapted from Rao (1991).
[b] Not due to contaminants but due to natural phytates.

such as nitrosodimethylamine (NDMA) and nitrosopyrrolidine; pesticides such as DDT or its degradation products, and other chlorinated insecticides, malathion and ethylene dibromide. Other contaminants of cereal-based diets include the essential nutrients fluorine and selenium, which can be toxic at relatively low concentrations. Fish meal and mineral ingredients are the major sources of fluorine in cereal-based diets (Rao and Knapka, 1987; Rao, 1991). One or more preservatives or antioxidants such as BHA, BHT and ethoxyquin, may also be present depending on the ingredients and their origin. Concentrations of contaminants in various cereal-based open formula diets, proprietary diets and purified diets were published in various reports (Greenman *et al.*, 1980; Rao and Knapka, 1987; Rao, 1991, 1996). Concentrations of selected contaminants in cereal-based diets and purified diets are listed in Table 14.7. Concentrations of contaminants in diets fed to the animal models in safety studies should be as low as possible to prevent modification of toxic and carcinogenic responses of the chemicals or agents under investigation. Limits of contaminant concentrations or action levels of selected contaminants in diets for safety studies recommended by various organisations are listed in Table 14.8.

Biological effects of contaminants in diet

The effects of common chemical contaminants include molecular level changes to carcinogenicity, teratological changes and mortality. The effects of some common contaminants with minimum dietary concentrations to

Table 14.7 Concentrations of selected contaminants in cereal-based and purified diets

Contaminant (mg/kg)[a]	Open formula			Closed formula		Purified
	NIH-07[b]	NIH-31[c]	NTP-2000[d]	Purina 5002[e]	Kocanda[f]	AIN-76A[g]
Arsenic	0.47 (0.23)	0.44 (0.17)	0.27 (0.09)	0.31	0.15	0.15 (0.11)
Cadmium	0.09 (0.05)	0.13 (0.09)	0.05 (0.02)	0.14	0.13	0.06 (0.02)
Lead	0.46 (0.41)	0.31 (0.15)	0.17 (0.09)	0.32	0.26	0.26 (0.21)
Selenium[h]	0.34 (0.11)	0.47 (0.33)	0.21 (0.12)	0.24	0.19	0.21 (0.07)
Total volatile						
Nitrosamines (µg/kg)	11.1 (23.1)	7.0 (2.7)	6.6 (2.8)	NA	3.8	1.5 (NA)
Malathion	0.16 (0.28)	0.25 (0.25)	0.10 (0.11)	< 0.1 – 1.18[i]	< 0.02	< 0.05
BHA	2.4 (2.9)	1.76 (3.28)	1.07 (1.02)	NA	<1.0	NA
BHT	1.8 (1.6)	1.76 (3.01)	0.97 (0.90)	NA	<1.0	NA

[a] Mean (SD).
[b] From 197 lots over a 17-year period.
[c] From 35 lots over a 6-year period.
[d] From 30 lots over a 3-year period.
[e] From 300 lots over a 6-year period, SD not available (Rao, 1991).
[f] From one lot made by Mill Kocanda in Czech Republic.
[g] From 22 lots over a 3-year period (Rao, 1991).
[h] Also an essential nutrient.
[i] Range, mean not available.
NA, not available; BHA, butylated hydroxyanisole; BHT, butylated hydroxytoluene.

Table 14.8 Limits or action levels of common dietary contaminants recommended by various organisations[a]

Contaminant	Concentration	NTP	NCTR	ILAR	EPA	Purina[b]
As	mg/kg	0.60	1.00	0.25	1.0	1.0
Cd	mg/kg	0.25	0.25	0.05	0.26	0.5
Hg	mg/kg	0.05	0.10	0.05	0.10	0.2
Pb	mg/kg	1.0	1.5	1.0	1.5	1.5
Se	mg/kg	0.50	0.65	0.5	0.6	0.5
Aflatoxins	µg/kg	5[c]	5	1	5	5
Nitrosamines	µg/kg	25[d]	20	NS	10	NS
Lindane	mg/kg	0.02	0.10	0.01	0.02	0.05
Heptachlor	mg/kg	0.02	0.02	0.01	0.02	0.03
Methoxychlor	mg/kg	0.05	NS	NS	NS	0.5
DDT	mg/kg	0.02	0.10	0.05	0.10	0.15
Dieldrin	mg/kg	0.02	0.01	0.01	0.02	0.03
Malathion	mg/kg	0.5	5.0	0.5	2.5	0.5
BHA	mg/kg	10	50	NS	NS	NS

[a]Only the contaminants detected in cereal-based natural ingredient diets were included.
[b]Courtesy of Purina Mills, Inc., St. Louis, Missouri, USA.
[c]Aflatoxin B_1 limit is 2 µg/kg.
[d]Methylnitrosamine limit is 15 µg/kg.
NTP, National Toxicology Program; NCTR, National Center for Toxicological Research; ILAR, Institute of Laboratory Animal Resources, US NRC; EPA, Environmental Protection Agency, USA; NS, not specified; BHA, Butylated hydroxyanisole.

cause biological effects are listed in Table 14.9 (Anderson *et al.*, 1979; Greenman *et al.*, 1980; Rao, 1991). Even at the recommended maximum limits listed in Table 14.8, some of the chemical contaminants may cause biological changes or influence the toxic effects of chemicals and agents under investigation. Common effects of dietary contaminants include changes in the induction of drug-metabolising enzymes, leading to changes in the metabolism of test chemicals by various tissues, morphological changes in liver and kidney cells, alterations in haematopoiesis, impairment of liver and kidney functions and changes in behaviour. Other consequences of dietary chemical contaminants include changes in tumour induction and spontaneous tumour rates, impairment of growth, reproduction, survival; and teratological and development changes in the offspring.

Control of dietary chemical contaminants

Based on the ingredients of the selected diet, maximum limits of contaminant concentrations expected not to complicate the interpretation of safety studies should be established. Contaminant levels below the limits can be achieved with most batches/lots of diet, if the batches of ingredients such as fish meal are prescreened for heavy metals and nitrosamines, and corn, wheat and alfalfa meal for mycotoxins, selenium and nitrates before being selected for the diet formulation (Rao and Knapka, 1987; Rao, 1991).

Table 14.9 Biological effects of common dietary contaminants[a]

Contaminant	Concentration[b] (ppm)	Biological effects[c]
As	5	Growth, reproduction, and mortality. Decreased tumour incidence, and may be carcinogenic
Cd	0.2	Renal vasculature, hypertension reproduction, mortality and tumours
Hg	2.0	Renal vasculature, hypertension, behaviour, learning, growth and mortality
Pb	5	Haematopoiesis, antibody formation, growth and mortality
Se	2	Hepatic lesions, reproduction, growth and mortality. Decreased tumour incidence
Nitrosamines (NDMA)	0.01	Hepatic lesions and tumours. Increased spontaneous tumours
Aflatoxin B_1	0.001	Liver hyperplasia and tumours
Heptachlor, DDT methoxychlor, dieldrin, lindane	1	Microsomal enzymes, liver weight, brain lesions, liver tumours, lung tumours, growth, reproduction and mortality
Malathion	100	Liver weight and cholinesterase
BHA	5	Enzyme induction, decreased incidence of tumours and may be carcinogenic
Fumonisin B_1	9^d	Kidney lesions, liver lesions and may be carcinogenic

[a] Adapted from Rao (1991).
[b] Minimum concentration with some biological effect.
[c] From Greenman *et al.* (1980) and the references cited therein.
[d] Voss *et al.* (1995).

Formulations and nutrient composition of diets

The ingredient concentrations (formulations) of various cereal-based, natural ingredient open formula diets available for safety studies with rats, mice, rabbits and non-human primates are listed in Tables 14.10–14.12. Closed formula or proprietary natural ingredient diet formulations are confidential; therefore, their details are not available for publication. Selected nutrient concentrations of the open formula rabbit and non-human primate diets as determined by analysis are listed in Table 14.13. Complete nutrient profiles as determined by analysis of several lots of two open formula rat and mouse diets used for safety studies are listed in Table 14.14. Selected nutrient concentrations of some open formula and closed formula natural ingredient diets available for safety studies with different species of laboratory animals, compiled from various sources are listed in Tables 14.15 and 14.16. Ingredient and nutrient compositions of open formula purified diets such as AIN-76, AIN-93G (for growth and reproduction) and AIN-93M (for maintenance) are listed in various publications (AIN, 1977; Reeves *et al.*, 1993; NRC, 1995).

Table 14.10 Ingredient composition of cereal-based, open formula rat and mouse diets for safety studies

Ingredient	Amount by weight (%)		
	NIH-07[a]	NIH-31[a,b]	NTP-2000
Ground wheat	23.0	35.5	22.26
Ground corn	24.5	21.0	22.18
Wheat middlings	10.0	10.0	15.0
Soybean meal (49% protein)	12.0	5.0	5.0
Fish meal (60% protein)	10.0	4.0	9.0
Dried skim milk	5.0	0.0	0.0
Corn gluten meal (60% protein)	3.0	2.0	0.0
Dried brewer's yeast	2.0	1.0	1.0
Dry molasses	1.5	0.0	0.0
Alfalfa meal (17% protein)	4.0	2.0	7.5
Oat hulls	0.0	0.0	8.5
Purified cellulose	0.0	0.0	5.5
Corn oil (without preservatives)	0.0	0.0	3.0
Soy oil (without preservatives)	2.5	1.5	3.0
Sodium chloride	0.5	0.5	0.3
Calcium phosphate, dibasic (USP)	1.25	1.5	0.4
Calcium carbonate (USP)	0.5	0.5	0.9
Choline chloride (70% choline)	0.09[c]	0.11[c]	0.26
Methionine	0.0	0.0	0.2
Vitamin premix	0.13	0.25	0.5[d]
Mineral premix	0.12	0.25	0.5[e]

[a] Vitamin and mineral premix composition was given by NRC (1995).
[b] NIH-31 is an autoclavable diet. NIH-07 and NTP-2000 diets are not autoclavable.
[c] Included in the vitamin premix.
[d] Vitamin premix per kg diet contained: vitamin A (stabilised palmitate or acetate), 4000 IU; vitamin D (activated animal sterol) 1000 IU; vitamin K (menadione sodium bisulphite complex), 1 mg; α-tocopheryl acetate (vitamin E), 100 mg; folic acid, 1.1 mg; niacin, 2.3 mg; D-pantothenic acid (D-calcium pantothenate, 10 mg); riboflavin, 3.3 mg; thiamine (thiamine mononitrate), 4 mg; B_{12}, 52 µg; pyridoxine (pyridoxine hydrochloride), 6.3 mg; D-biotin, 0.2; with wheat middlings as carrier (From Rao, 1997).
[e] Mineral premix per kg diet contained: magnesium (oxide), 514 mg; iron (sulphate), 35 mg; zinc (oxide), 12 mg; manganese (oxide), 10 mg; copper (sulphate), 2mg; iodine (calcium iodate), 0.2 mg; chromium (acetate), 0.2 mg; with calcium carbonate as carrier (From Rao, 1997).

Physical forms of diets and feeding of diets

Diets for safety studies are available in different physical forms. The most common form is the pelleted diet. Pelleted diet is appropriate for safety studies where the chemical under investigation is administered by oral (gavage), dermal, inhalation or parenteral routes. If the chemical under investigation, such as nutrients, food additives and environmental chemicals, is to be incorporated into the diet (dosed feed), and fed to the experimental animals, meal or powder forms of the diet may be convenient or necessary. Pelletisation of diets facilitates feeding, decreases dust from feed and may decrease wastage. Meal form of diet may lead to excess wastage and dust if not provided in special feeders to

Table 14.11 Ingredient composition of open formula rabbit and monkey diets

Ingredient	Amount by weight (%)	
	Rabbit[a] (NIH-09)	Non-human primate[b]
Wheat	0.0	28.0
Ground oat mill by-product	0.0	22.5
Ground whole kernel yellow corn	0.0	17.0
Soybean meal (49% protein)	13.0	8.0
Fish meal (70% protein)	0.0	6.0
Sucrose	0.0	2.9
Alfalfa meal (17% protein)	28.0	3.0
Ground oat hulls	22.5	0.0
Ground barley	14.75	0.0
Wheat bran	7.0	0.0
Wheat middlings	6.0	0.0
Dried whey	2.0	3.0
Dried molasses	1.5	0.0
Brewer's dried yeast	1.0	2.0
Soybean oil	0.5	3.6
Calcium carbonate	1.5	1.2
Dicalcium phosphate	1.25	0.50
Sodium chloride	0.50	0.30
Vitamin premix[c]	0.25	1.0
Mineral premix[c]	0.25	1.0

[a]National Institutes of Health (NIH), USA, NIH-09 diet specification NIH-11-136f (1986).
[b]National Institutes of Health (NIH), USA, Specification NIH-11-152d (1993).
[c]Composition of premixes is listed in Table 14.12.

decrease wastage. Commonly available feeders for rodent diet in meal form may allow the rodents to nest in the feeders and urinate and defecate on the feed. Urination and defecation on the feed may complicate collection of accurate feed/compound consumption data and may affect the stability of the chemical under investigation. Feeders designed to decrease the wastage and prevent nesting and therefore, decreasing the contamination of dosed feed with urine and faeces, were described by various investigators (Fullerton *et al.*, 1981; Miller, 1990; Lambert *et al.*, 1991).

Treatment of diets by heat and ionising energy

Since most ingredients of cereal-based diets are natural or non-purified, some could also be sources of biological contaminants bacteria, molds, parasites and insects. Bacteria such as *Salmonella* sp. and coliforms may be pathogenic not only to the experimental animals but also to the animal care personnel. Pelletisation of diets will involve forcing the mixture of ground ingredient formulation through diets with water or steam injection. The pelleting process will subject the feed ingredients to temperatures of ~ 80°C for a minute or longer,

Table 14.12 Concentrations of essential vitamins and minerals added to rabbit and non-human primate open formula diets

Supplement	Unit/kg	Rabbit (NIH-09)	Non-human primate
Methionine	mg	1100	25
Vitamins			
A (retinol)	IU	6600	8800
D$_3$ (cholecalciferol)	IU	2200	6000
E (*RRR*-α-Tocopherol)	IU	44	41
K (menadione)	mg	3.1	8.8
C (ascorbic acid)	mg	0.0	990[a]
Choline	mg	530	290
Niacin	mg	22	57
Pantothenic acid	mg	6.6	55
Pyridoxine	mg	5.0	8.8
Thiamine	mg	4.4	20
Riboflavin	mg	3.3	5.3
Folic acid	mg	2.6	2.6
Biotin	μg	0.13	110
B$_{12}$	μg	11	6.6
Minerals			
Magnesium	mg	176	440
Iron	mg	22	33
Manganese	mg	22	15.4
Zinc	mg	22	4.4
Copper	mg	7.15	2.2
Cobalt	mg	1.54	0.44
Iodine	mg	1.1	1.43
Potassium	mg	0.0	990

[a] Dusted or sprayed on the outside of pellets or biscuits.

Table 14.13 Selected nutrient concentrations of rabbit and monkey open formula diets

Nutrient (unit)	Rabbit[a] (NIH-09)	Non-human primate[b]
Crude protein (%)	16.2 (0.64)	17.6 (1.68)
Crude fat (%)	2.2 (0.29)[c]	6.5 (0.64)[d]
Crude fibre (%)	16.6 (1.46)	4.7 (0.06)
Calcium (%)	1.3 (0.19)	1.0 (0.02)
Phosphorus (%)	0.65 (0.05)	0.64 (0.09)
Vitamin A (IU/kg)	11 900[e]	16 000[f]
Thiamine (mg/kg)	13.7[f]	14.4[f]
Vitamin C (mg/kg)	NA	1070 (290)

[a] Mean (SD) for five lots made between April 1996 and April 1997.
[b] Mean (SD) for four lots made between April 1996 and April 1997.
[c] Determined by Soxhlet extraction.
[d] Determined by acid hydrolysis.
[e] Value for one lot.
[f] Average for two lots.
NA, Not available or not applicable.

Table 14.14 Nutrient concentrations of open formula rat and mouse diets for safety studies[a]

Nutrient	NIH-07	NTP-2000
Crude protein (%)[b]	23.04 (0.88)	14.1 (0.9)
Crude fat (%)[b]	5.30 (0.43)	8.2 (0.4)
Crude fibre (%)[b]	3.40 (0.39)	9.4 (0.6)
Carbohydrates (%)[c]	52	53
Vitamins[d]		
A (IU/kg)[b]	8170 (3160)	5780 (1780)
D (IU/kg)	4450 (1382)[e]	1000[f]
E	35.2 (8.6)	83.8 (17.5)
K[f]	3.0	1.0
Thiamine[b]	18.1 (3.3)	10.1 (2.2)
Riboflavin	7.8 (0.9)	6.0 (1.7)
Niacin	98.7 (23.2)	75.3 (3.1)
Pantothenic acid	32.9 (8.9)	26.2 (2.9)
Pyridoxine	9.3 (2.49)	11.6 (1.4)
Folic acid	2.6 (0.7)	1.77 (0.48)
Biotin	0.27 (0.046)	0.29 (0.02)
B_{12} (μg/kg)	41.6 (18.6)	48 (NA)
Choline	2955 (382)	3000 (264)
Minerals[d]		
Calcium[b]	12 100 (1300)	9500 (600)
Phosphorus[b]	9400 (600)	5800 (400)
Potassium	8860 (590)	6650 (300)
Sodium	3160 (310)	1920 (300)
Magnesium	1650 (100)	1930 (100)
Iron	348 (84)	154 (18)
Manganese	93.3 (5.6)	51 (5)
Copper	11.6 (2.5)	5.9 (0.5)
Zinc	59.4 (9.7)	49 (3.8)
Iodine	3.5 (1.14)	0.55 (0.25)
Selenium[b]	0.34 (0.11)	0.21 (0.12)

[a] From the National Toxicology Program database.
[b] Mean (SD) for 197 lots of NIH-07 and 31 lots of NTP-2000.
[c] Other than crude fibre, average value calculated by difference including the correction for moisture and ash.
[d] As mg/kg, mean (SD) for 12 lots of NIH-07 diet analysed during 1985–1996, and average for three lots of NTP-2000 diet analysed during 1995–1997, unless stated otherwise.
[e] Mean (SD) for four lots.
[f] Added concentration, not analysed.
NA, not available.

and it will kill a high proportion of vegetative forms of bacteria and most parasites and insects. The pelleting process generally decreases or eliminates most *Salmonella* and coliform organisms. However, bacterial and fungal spores, parasites cysts, heat-resistant ova/eggs or cysts of insects may not be eliminated. Pelletisation is not known to cause a significant decrease of the nutrients, especially the heat-labile vitamins A and thiamine. To sterilise

Table 14.15 Selected nutrient concentrations of some rat and mouse diets available for safety studies

Nutrient	(Unit)[a]	NIH-31[b]	Kocanda[c]	Purina 5002[d]	Biosure		Purina 5056[f]	Altromin	
					SB[e]	SM[e]		1320[g]	1340[g]
Crude protein	(%)	18.7 (0.5)	25.2	21.1 (0.31)	19.7	14.4	14.1	19.0	12.5
Crude fat	(%)	5.5 (0.2)	4.8	4.5 (0.02)	3.4	3.2	3.3	4.0	3.0
Crude fibre	(%)	3.6 (0.4)	4.1	4.4 (0.33)	2.3	6.4	5.8	6.0	20
Calcium	(%)	1.14 (0.07)	1.32	0.84 (0.08)	0.71	0.71	0.70	0.9	0.9
Phosphorus	(%)	0.93 (0.04)	1.01	0.67 (0.06)	0.74	0.69	0.60	0.7	0.7
Vitamin A	(IU/kg)	25 000 (5000)	24 700	19 000 (4600)	NA	NA	26 400	15 000	15 000
Thiamine	(mg/kg)	83 (6.5)	23.9	13.9 (4.3)	NA	NA	17	NA	NA
Vitamin E	(mg/kg)	NA	97.2	71 (2.3)	NA	NA	99.2	75	75

[a] Mean (SD).
[b] For 35 lots of autoclavable diet during a 6-year period, analysed before autoclaving.
[c] For one lot of autoclavable diet made by mill Kocanda of Czech Republic in 1997, analysed before autoclaving.
[d] For 11 lots made in 1995.
[e] Biosure (England) standard breeding (SB) and standard maintenance (SM) diets from Roe (1991); SD not available.
[f] Based on ingredient analysis information as published by Purina Mills, Inc., (USA) in 1992.
[g] Based on ingredient analysis as published by Altromin International (Germany).
NA, not available.

Table 14.16 Selected nutrient concentrations of some rabbit, dog and monkey diets for safety studies

Nutrient	(Unit)[a]	Rabbit		Dog		Primate	
		Purina 5322[b]	Altromin 2020[c]	Purina 5007[b]	Altromin 4010[c]	Purina 5048[b]	Altromin 6010[c]
Crude protein	(%)	17.4 (0.28)	17.5	27.0 (0.51)	26.0	26.9 (0.4)	25.0
Crude fat	(%)	3.2 (0.14)	4.0	5.8 (0.04)	6.0	5.9 (0.46)	5.5
Crude fibre	(%)	15.4 (0.6)	14.5	2.9 (0.19)	4.2	4.2 (0.26)	4.5
Calcium	(%)	1.07 (0.12)	0.95	1.74 (0.18)	1.50	1.02 (0.08)	0.95
Phosphorus	(%)	0.53 (0.04)	0.70	1.06 (0.10)	1.10	0.66 (0.05)	0.70
Vitamin A	(IU/kg)	19 500 (1800)	15 000	42 000 (3800)	15 000	53 000 (12 000)	20 000
Thiamine	(mg/kg)	5.0 (2.1)	NA	10.1 (1.9)	NA	12 (2.1)	NA
Vitamin E	(mg/kg)	35 (3.2)	75	39 (6.7)	75	56 (3.2)	100
Vitamin C	(mg/kg)	NA	NA	NA	NA	1600 (190)	NA

[a]Mean (SD).
[b]For 12 lots made in 1995, analysis date provided by Purina Mills, Inc. USA.
[c]Based on ingredient analysis information as published by Altromin International (Germany).
NA, not available or not applicable.

(destroy all forms of insect, parasite and microbial contamination), the diets must be autoclaved at 120–130°C for 20–30 minutes. Autoclaving will decrease the vitamin A content of diets by 30–50% depending upon the physical form of the vitamin. Loss due to autoclaving of stabilised or microencapsulated forms of vitamin A may be considerably lower than the non-stabilised form. Autoclaving may destroy up to 90% of the thiamine in the diet. However, autoclaving decreased the volatile nitrosamine NDMA concentration by ∼ 70% (G. Rao, unpublished data). If the diet is to be sterilised by autoclaving, the vitamin A content should be three to five times and thiamine 10–15 times the recommended concentration before autoclaving. Steam sterilisation will be appropriate for pelleted form of diets, but the meal or powdered diets may become 'cakey' after autoclaving. Steam sterilisation may increase the pellet hardness of rodent diets (Thigpen et al., 1993). Treatment of pelleted as well as meal forms of diets at or below 25°C by ionising energy (irradiation), from gamma rays or X-rays at 25–50 kGy, is known to destroy most, if not all bacterial, parasitic and insect contamination without a significant loss of the essential nutrients such as Vitamins A, E and thiamine (Ley, 1972, 1975). However, ionising energy may increase the peroxide concentration of the diets and this increase is expected to be associated with the fat content, especially polyunsaturated fat. Irradiation of NTP-2000 diet (Tables 14.10 and 14.14) containing ∼ 8.5% fat derived from corn oil and soybean oil at 25–50 KGy at room temperature increased the peroxide content of the diet from 2.8 to 4.0 Meq/kg, when analysed about three weeks after irradiation (G. Rao, unpublished data). However, for diets containing ≤ 10% fat, the increase in peroxide content due to ionising radiation may not be markedly different than the peroxide accumulation during storage of diets (Fullerton et al., 1982).

Quality control and documentation

Toxicology and carcinogenesis study protocols should specify the type of diet to be used with ingredients, formulation and nutrient and contaminant concentrations to the extent possible. Each batch or lot (a lot is a mix of a few to several batches milled at the same time) of diet used should be analysed for macronutrients (proximate constituents) to confirm the formulation and for selected labile essential micronutrients such as vitamins A, thiamine and possibly E to ascertain the presence of adequate concentrations. In addition, randomly selected batches or lots used during the course of a safety study should be analysed for all essential micronutrients including amino acids and fatty acids to confirm the adequacy of the diet for the strain and species on study. Each batch or lot of diet used for safety studies should also be analysed for contaminants expected to be present in the ingredients (Rao, 1986; NRC, 1995). Contaminant concentrations in a selected batch or lot of diet can be controlled by pre-screening the ingredients for contaminants expected to be present in that ingredient (Rao and Knapka, 1987; Rao, 1991). Ingredients, diet formulation and nutrient and contaminant concentrations as determined by analyses either by the manufacturer or by the user should be retained and included in the safety study report (Rao, 1986).

Storage of diets

Environmental conditions of the storage area may affect the stability of some nutrients and may influence the growth of biological contaminants in diets not sterilised by heat or ionising energy. Natural ingredient diets may be stored in a dry (relative humidity $50 \pm 10\%$) and cool ($\leq 25°C$) environment or in a room with controlled temperature and relative humidity that is similar to or lower than that of the safety study room. Under the above type of conditions, the nutrients of cereal-based diets are expected to be stable and adequate for more than 168 days (Fullerton *et al.*, 1982) and therefore may be used for 5–6 months after manufacture (NRC, 1996). Since natural ingredient, non-purified diets contain antioxidants, storage of cereal-based diets at 4°C may not be necessary. However, diets with high fat content (>10%) may have to be stored at 4°C to retard the rancidity due to peroxide formation. Cereal-based diets with added vitamin C that is not protected by microencapsulation or other processes may have to be used within 3 months of manufacture due to gradual loss of vitamin C activity (NRC, 1996). The refined ingredients of purified diets will be generally free of antioxidants present in non-purified natural ingredients; therefore, purified diets should be stored at 4°C to reduce the loss of vitamins A, E and thiamine and to decrease peroxide formation.

Summary

Diet is one of the most important variables in safety studies. The ingredient, nutrient composition and chemical and biological contaminant concentrations of the diets may influence the physiology and, therefore, the results of toxicology and carcinogenesis studies. Cereal-based natural ingredient diets are the most commonly used diets in safety studies. Excesses of some nutrients such as protein, simple carbohydrates and fat-soluble vitamins may influence the metabolism and toxicity of chemicals under investigation. Deficiency of essential nutrients, improper proportions of some nutrients such as calcium and phosphorus, vitamins A and E, and some trace minerals may enhance spontaneous lesions such as nephropathy and dystrophic calcification of tissues. These changes may complicate the interpretation of biochemical effects and tissue lesions in toxicology and carcinogenesis studies. Non-purified natural ingredients of cereal-based diets contribute various contaminants such as nitrosamines, mycotoxins, heavy metals and pesticides. These contaminants may influence the toxic and carcinogenic responses of test chemicals and agents of the safety studies. The contaminant concentrations of cereal-based diets could be controlled by pre-screening the required non-purified ingredients for selected contaminants. Due to the use of refined ingredients, nutrient and contaminant concentrations of purified diets could be controlled within a narrow range. However, purified diets will be expensive, substantially different from recommended human diets, and may cause substantial changes in physiology including changes in gut flora. Such changes in turn may cause alterations in micronutrient requirements and metabolism of chemicals under investigation. However, when the chemical under investigation is a nutrient or a contaminant of natural ingredient diets, and the contribution of this chemical to the diets cannot be limited or controlled within a narrow range, it may be appropriate to use purified diets for such studies. Insect, parasite and microbial contamination of diets for safety studies should be controlled by heat treatment or irradiation. Safety study protocols should specify the ingredient formulation, nutrient composition and contaminant limits of the selected diet. All or selected batches/lots of diets used in the safety studies should be analysed for nutrients and contaminants, and the analysis reports, along with the formulation, should be included in the safety study report.

References

Abdo KM, Wenk ML, Harry JG, Mahler J, Goehl TJ and Irwin RD (1998) Glycine modulates the toxicity of benzyl acetate in F344 rats. *Toxicologic Pathology*, **26**, 395–402.

American Institute of Nutrition (1977) Report of the AIN Ad Hoc Committee on standards for nutritional studies. Report of the Committee. *Journal of Nutrition*, **37**, 1340–1348.

Anderson LM, Priest LJ, Budinger JM (1979) Lung tumorigenesis in mice after chronic exposure to early life to a low dose of dimethylnitrosamine. *Journal of the National Cancer Institute*, **62**, 1553–1555.

Beri, JG (1979) Letter to the editor. *Journal of Nutrition*, **109**, 925–926.

Bidlack WR, Brown RC and Mohan C (1986) Nutritional parameters that alter hepatic drug metabolism, conjugation and toxicity. *Federation Proceedings, Federation of American Societies for Experimental Biology*, **45**, 142–148.

Blakely SR, Grundel E, Jenkins MY and Mitchell GV (1990) Alterations in β-carotene and vitamin E status in rats fed β-carotene and excess vitamin A. *Nutrition Research*, **10**, 1035–1044.

Boyd EM, Dobos I and Taylor F (1970) Benzylpenicillin toxicity of albino rats fed synthetic high starch versus high sugar diets. *Chemotherapy*, **15**, 1–11.

Bus JS and Gibson (1979) Lipid peroxidation and its role in toxicology. *Reviews in Biochemical Toxicology*, **1**, 125–149.

Butler LE and Dauterman WC (1988) The effect of dietary protein levels on xenobiotic biotransformations in F344 male rats. *Toxicology and Applied Pharmacology*, **95**, 301–310.

Campbell TC and Hayes JR (1974) Role of nutrition in the drug-metabolizing enzyme systems. *Pharmacological Reviews*, **26**, 171–197.

Conner WM and Newberne PM (1984) Drug–nutrient interactions and their implications for safety evaluations. *Fundamental and Applied Toxicology*, **4**, S341–S356.

Daft FS, McDaniel EG, Herman LG, Romine MK and Hegener JR (1963) Role of coprophagy in utilization of B vitamins synthesized by intestinal bacteria. *Federation*

Proceedings, Federation of American Societies for Experimental Biology, **22**, 129–133.

Day HG and Pigman W (1957) Carbohydrates in nutrition. In *The Carbohydrates*, Pigman W (ed), Academic Press, New York, pp. 779–806.

Dillehay DL, Webb SJ, Schmelz E-M and Merill AH Jr (1994) Dietary sphingomylein inhibits 1,2-dimethylhydrazine-induced colon cancer in CF1 mice. *Journal of Nutrition*, **124**, 615–620.

Everitt JI, Ross PW, Neptun DA and Mangum JB (1988) Effect of purified diet on dystrophic cardiac calcinosis in mice. *Laboratory Animal Science*, **38**, 426–429.

Feldman DB, McConnell EE and Knapka JJ (1982) Growth, kidney disease, and longevity of Syrian Hamsters (*Mesocricetus auratus*) fed varying levels of protein. *Laboratory Animal Science*, **32**, 613–618.

Fleming SE and Lee B (1983) Growth performance and intestinal transit time of rats fed purified and natural dietary fibers. *Journal of Nutrition*, **113**, 592–601.

Fullerton FR, Hunziker J and Bryant P (1981) Evaluation of a new rat feeder for use in chemical toxicology and nutrition studies. *Laboratory Animal Science*, **31**, 276–279.

Fullerton FR, Greenman DL and Kendall DC (1982) Effects of storage conditions on nutritional qualities of semipurified (AIN-76) and natural ingredient (NIH-07) diets. *Journal of Nutrition*, **112**, 567–573.

Fullerton FR, Greenman DL, McCarty CC and Bucci TJ (1991) Increased incidence of spontaneous and 2-acetylaminofluorene-induced liver and bladder tumors in B6C3F1 mice fed AIN-76A diet versus NIH-07 diet. *Fundamental and Applied Toxicology*, **16**, 51–60.

Fullerton FR, Greenman DL and Bucci TJ (1992) Effects of diet types on incidence of spontaneous and 2-acetylaminofluorene-induced liver and bladder tumors in BALB/c mice fed AIN-76A diet versus NIH-07 diet. *Fundamental and Applied Toxicology*, **18**, 193–199.

Greenman DL, Oller WL, Littlefield NA and Nelson CJ (1980) Commerical laboratory animal diets: toxicant and nutrient variability. *Journal of Toxicology and Environmental Health*, **6**, 235–246.

Haseman JK, Huff JE, Rao GN, Arnold JE, Boorman GA and McConnell EE (1985) Neoplasms observed in untreated and corn oil gavage control groups of F-344/N rats and (C57BL/6NXC3H/HeN) F1 mice. *Journal of the National Cancer Institute*, **75**, 975–984.

Hayes JR and Campbell TC (1974) Effect of protein deficiency on the inducibility of the hepatic microsomal drug-metabolizing enzyme system. III. Effect of 3-methylcholanthrene induction on activity and binding kinetics. *Biochemical Pharmacology*, **23**, 1721–1731.

Hietanen E (1980) Modification of hepatic drug metabolizing enzyme activities and their induction by dietary protein. *General Pharmacology*, **11**, 443–450.

Institute of Laboratory Animal Resources (1978) *Control of Diets in Laboratory Animal Experimentation*, National Academy of Sciences, Washington, DC.

Ip C (1987) Fat and essential fatty acid in mammary carcinogenesis. *The American Journal of Clinical Nutrition*, **45**, 218–224.

Jackson CD, Weis C, Miller BJ and James SJ (1997) Dietary nucleotides: effects on cell proliferation following partial hepatectomy in rats fed NIH-31, AIN-76A, or folate/methyl-deficient diets. *Journal of Nutrition*, **127**, 834s–837s.

Johnston PV and Fritsche KL (1989) Nutritional methodology in dietary fat and cancer research. In *Carcinogenesis and Dietary Fat*, Abraham S (ed), Kluwer Academic, Boston, pp. 9–25.

Klahr S, Buerkert J and Purkerson ML (1983) Role of dietary factors in progression of renal disease. *Kidney International*, **24**, 579–587.

Knapka JJ, Smith PK and Judge FJ (1974) Effect of open and closed formula rations on the performance of three strains of laboratory mice. *Laboratory Animal Science*, **24**, 480–487.

Kritchevsky D (1977) Modification by fiber of toxic dietary effects. *Federation Proceedings, Federation of American Societies for Experimental Biology*, **36**, 1692–1695.

Lambert JV, Lambert JP, Rao GN and Wenk ML (1991) An innovative feeder for powdered mouse diet. *American Association for Laboratory Animal Science Bulletin*, **30**, 16–20.

Ley FJ (1972) The use of irradiation for the treatment of various animal feed products. *Food Irradiation Information*, **1**, 8–22.

Ley FJ (1975) Radiation sterilization. An Industrial process. Proceedings of the Fifth International Congress of Radiation Research, Seattle Washington, 14–20 July, 1974. In *Radiation Research, Biomedical, Chemical and Physical Perspectives*, Nygaard OF, Adler HI and Sinclair WK (eds), Academic Press, New York, pp. 118–130.

Longnecker DS, Roebuck BD, Yager JD Jr, Lilja HS and Siegmund B (1981) Pancreatic carcinoma in azaserine-treated rats; induction, classification and dietary modulation of incidence. *Cancer*, **47**, 1561–1572.

Maciorowski KG, Turner ND, Lupton JR, Chapkin RS, Shermer CL, Ha SD and Ricke SC (1997) Diet and carcinogen alter the fecal microbial populations of rats. *Journal of Nutrition*, **127**, 449–457.

McLean AEM and McLean KK (1966) The effect of diet and 1,1,1-tricholoro-2,2 bis (β-chlorophenyl) ethane (DDT) on microsomal hydroxylating enzymes and on sensitivity of rats to carbon tetrachloride poisoning. *The Biochemical Journal*, **100**, 564–571.

Medinsky MA, Popp JA, Hamm TE and Dent JG (1982) Development of hepatic lesions in male Fischer-344 rats fed AIN-76A purified diet, *Toxicology and Applied Pharmacology*, **62**, 111–120.

Megens WJ, Vane FM, Tannenbaum SR, Green L and Skipper PL (1979) In vitro nitrosation of methapyrilene. *Journal of Pharmaceutical Science*, **68**, 827–832.

Merrill AH Jr, Schmelz E-M, Wang E, Dillehay DL, Rice LG, Meredith F and Riley RT (1997) Importance of sphingolipids and inhibitors of sphingolipid metabolism as components of animal diets. *Journal of Nutrition*, **127**, 830s–833s.

Mertz W and Roginski EE (1969) Effect of chromium (III) supplementation on growth and survival under stress in rats fed low protein diets. *Journal of Nutrition*, **97**, 531–536.

Miller DL (1990) A new feeder for powdered diets. *Proceedings of the Society of Experimental Biology and Medicine*, **176**, 81–84.

National Research Council, Committee on Animal Nutrition (1977) *Nutrient Requirements of Rabbits*, National Academy Press, Washington, DC.

National Research Council, Committee on Animal Nutrition (1978a) *Nutrient Requirements of Laboratory Animals*, 3rd revised edn, No 10. National Academy of Sciences, Washington, DC.

National Research Council, Committee on Animal Nutrition (1978b) *Nutrient Requirements of Nonhuman Primates*, National Academy Press, Washington, DC.

National Research Council, Committee on Animal Nutrition (1982) *United States-Canadian Tables of Feed Composition*, National Academy Press, Washington, DC.

National Research Council, Committee on Animal Nutrition (1985) *Nutrient Requirements of Laboratory Dogs*, National Academy Press, Washington, DC.

National Research Council, Committee on Animal Nutrition (1995) Nutrient requirements of the laboratory rat and mouse. In: *Nutrient Requirements of Laboratory Animals*, National Academy Press, Washington, DC, pp. 11–102.

National Research Council, Institute of Laboratory Animal Resources (1996) *Guide for the Care and Use of Laboratory Animals*, National Academy Press, Washington, DC, p. 39.

Nettesheim P and Williams ML (1976) The influence of vitamin A on the susceptibility of the rat lung to 3-methylcholanthrene. *International Journal of Cancer*, **17**, 351–357.

Newberne PM (1975) Influence of pharmacological experiments of chemicals and other factors in diets of laboratory animals. *Federation Proceedings, Federation of American Societies for Experimental Biology*, **34**, 209–218.

Newberne PM (1978) Nutritional disease. In *Pathology of Laboratory Animals*, vol. II, Bernischke K, Garner FM, Jones TC (eds), Springer-Verlag, New York, pp. 2153–2154.

Newberne PM and Conner MW (1974) Effect of selenium on acute response to aflatoxin B1. In *Trace Substances and Environmental Health*, vol. 8, Hamphill D (ed), Univ. of Missouri, Columbia, MO, pp. 323–328.

Newberne PM and Conner MW (1986) Nutrient influences on toxicity and carcinogenicity, *Federation Proceedings, Federation of American Societies for Experimental Biology*, **45**, 149–154.

Nguyen HT (1982) Nephrocalcinosis induced by AIN-76 semipurified diet in rats: a nutritional and ultrastructural study. *Laboratory Animal Science*, **32**, 415.

Omaye ST (1986) Effects of diet on toxicity testing. *Federation Proceedings, Federation of American Societies for Experimental Biology*, **45**, 133–135.

Rao GN (1986) Role of diet in carcinogenicity testing. In *Long-Term and Short-Term Assays for Carcinogens*, International Agency for Research on Cancer, Scientific Publication No. 83, pp. 42–45.

Rao GN (1988) Rodent diets for carcinogenesis studies. A commentary. *Journal of Nutrition*, **118**, 929–931.

Rao GN (1991) Significance of dietary contaminants in diet restriction studies. In *Biological Effects of Dietary Restriction*, Fishbein L (ed), Springer-Verlag, New York, pp. 16–24.

Rao GN (1995) Husbandry procedures other than dietary restriction for lowering body weight and tumor/disease rates in Fischer 344 rats. In *Dietary Restriction: Implications for the Design and Interpretation of Toxicity and Carcinogenicity Studies*, Neumann DA, Hart RW, Robertson RT (eds), ILSI Press, Washington, DC, pp. 51–62.

Rao GN (1996) New diet (NTP-2000) for rats in the National Toxicology Program toxicity and carcinogenicity studies. *Fundamental and Applied Toxicology*, **32**, 102–108.

Rao GN (1997) New nonpurified diet (NTP-2000) for rodents in National Toxicology Program's toxicology and carcinogenesis studies. *Journal of Nutrition*, **127**, 842s–846s.

Rao GN and Haseman JK (1993) Influence of corn oil and diet on body weight, survival, and tumor incidences in F344/N rats. *Nutrition and Cancer*, **19**, 21–30.

Rao GN and Knapka JJ (1987) Contaminant and nutrient concentrations of natural ingredient rat and mouse diet used in chemical toxicology studies. *Fundamental and Applied Toxicology*, **9**, 329–338.

Rao GN, Piegorsch WW and Haseman JK (1987) Influence of body weight on the incidence of spontaneous tumors in rats and mice of long-term studies. *The American Journal of Clinical Nutrition*, **45**, 252–260.

Rao GN, Haseman JK, Grumbein S, Crawford DD and Eustis SL (1990) Growth, body weight, survival, and tumor trends in F344/N rats during an eleven year period. *Toxicologic Pathology*, **18**, 61–70.

Rao GN, Edmondson J and Elwell MR (1993) Influence of dietary protein concentration on severity of nephropathy in Fischer-344 (F-344/N) rats. *Toxicologic Pathology*, **21**, 353–361.

Rao GN, Edmondson J, Hildebrandt PK and Bruner RH (1996) Influence of dietary protein, fat, and fiber on growth, blood chemistry and tumor incidences in Fischer 344 rats. *Nutrition and Cancer*, **25**, 269–279.

Rao GN, Ney E and Herbert RA (1997) Influence of diet on mammary cancer in transgenic mice bearing oncogene expressed in mammary tissue. *Breast Cancer Research and Treatment*, **45**, 149–158.

Reeves PG, Nielsen FH and Fahey GC Jr (1993) AIN-93 purified diets for laboratory rodents: Final report of the American Institute of Nutrition Ad Hoc writing committee on reformulation of the AIN-76A rodent diet. *Journal of Nutrition*, **123**, 1939–1951.

Roe FJC (1991) 1200-rat Biosure study: design and overview of results. In *Biological Effects of Dietary Restriction*, Fishbein L (ed), Springer-Verlag, New York, pp. 287–304.

Roebuck BD, Wilpone SA, Fifield DS and Yager JD Jr (1979) Letter to the editor. *Journal of Nutrition*, **109**, 924–926.

Rogers AE (1983) Influence of dietary content of lipids and lipotropic nutrients on chemical carcinogenesis in rats. *Cancer Research*, **43**, 24775–24843.

Rogers AE and Newberne PM (1971) Diet and aflatoxin B_1 toxicity in rats. *Toxicology and Applied Pharmacology*, **20**, 113–121.

Rogers AE, Henderson BJ and Newberne PM (1973) Induction by dimethylhydrazine of intestinal carcinoma in normal rats and rats fed high or low levels of vitamin A. *Cancer Research*, **33**, 1003–1009.

Rowland IR, Mallett AK and Wise A (1985) The effect of diet on the mammalian gut flora and its metabolic activities. *CRC Critical Reviews in Toxicology*, **16**, 31–103.

Saffiotti V, Montesano R, Sellkumar AR and Borg SA (1967) Experimental cancer of the lung: inhibition by vitamin A of the induction of tracheobronchial squamous metaplasia and squamous cell tumors. *Cancer*, **20**, 857–864.

Scott ML (1978) Vitamin E. In *Handbook of Lipid Research, Vol. 2, The Fat Soluble Vitamins*, DeLuca HF (ed), Plenum Press, New York pp. 133–210.

Shakman RA (1974) Nutritional influences on the toxicity of environmental pollutants. *Archives of Environmental Health*, **28**, 105–113.

Shively CA, White DM and Takara SM Jr (1986) Diet induced alterations in the theobromine disposition and toxicity in the rat. *Toxicology and Applied Pharmacology*, **84**, 593–598.

Sontag JM, Page NP and Saffiotti (1976) *Guidelines for Carcinogenesis Bioassay in Small Rodents* (National Cancer Institute Carcinogenesis Technical Report Series No. 1, DHHS Publication No. NIH 76–801), Dept of Health and Human Services, Washington, DC.

Stoewsend GS, Anderson JL and Lee ZY (1973) Nitrate induced methemoglobinemia in guinea pigs: influence of diets containing beets with varying amounts of nitrate and the effect of ascorbic acid and methionine. *Journal of Nutrition*, **103**, 419–424.

Strother A, Throckmorton JK and Herzer C (1971) The influence of high sugar consumption by mice on the duration of action of barbiturates, aniline and *p*-nitroanisole. *The Journal of Pharmacology and Experimental Therapeutics*, **179**, 490–498.

Sunde RA, Weiss SL, Thompson KM and Evenson JK (1992) Dietary selenium regulation of glutathione peroxidase mRNA – Implications for the selenium requirement. *The Federation of American Societies for Experimental Biology Journal*, **6** (part 1), A1365.

Thigpen JE, Locklear J, Romines C, Taylor KA, Yearby W and Stokes WS (1993) A standard procedure for measuring pellet hardness of rodent diets. *Laboratory Animal Science*, **43**, 488–491.

Van Fleet JF (1976) Induction of lesions of selenium-vitamin E deficiency in pigs fed silver. *American Journal of Veterinary Research*, **37**, 1415–1420.

Van Fleet JF, Greenwood LA and Rebon AH (1981) Effect of selenium-vitamin E on hematologic alterations of adriamycin toxicosis in young pigs. *American Journal of Veterinary Research*, **42**, 1153–1159.

Voss KA, Chamberlain WJ, Bacon CW, Herbert RA, Walters DB and Norred WP (1995) Subchronic feeding study of the mycotoxin fumonisin B1 in B6C2F1 mice and Fischer 344 rats. *Fundamental and Applied Toxicology*, **24**, 102–110.

Welsh CU, Goodrich-Smith M, Brown CK and Crowe N (1981) Enhancement by retinyl acetate of hormone-induced mammary tumorigenesis in female GR/A mice. *Journal of the National Cancer Institute*, **67**, 935–938.

Williams RT and Millburn P (1975) Detoxification mechanisms – The biochemistry of foreign compounds. In *Physiological and Pharmacological Biochemistry*, Blaschko HDF (ed), University Park Press, Baltimore, Biochemistry Series 1, Vol. 12.

Woodard JC (1971) Relationship between the ingredients of semipurified diets and nutritional nephrocalcinosis of rats. *The American Journal of Pathology*, **65**, 269–278.

Yoshida T, Oowada T, Ozaki A and Mizutani T (1993) Role of gastrointestinal microflora in the mineral absorption of young adult mice. *Bioscience Biotechnology and Biochemistry*, **57**, 1775–1776.

Zannoni VG, Finn EJ and Lynch M (1972) Ascorbic acid and drug metabolism. *Biochemical Pharmacology*, **21**, 1377–1392.

Index

Page entries followed by a suffix refer only to a figure (f) or table (t), not to text.